Radionuclide Concentrations in Food and the Environment

FOOD SCIENCE AND TECHNOLOGY

Radionuclide Concentrations in Food and the Environment

Edited by
Michael Pöschl
Leo M. L. Nollet

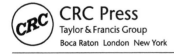

CRC Press
Taylor & Francis Group
Boca Raton London New York

CRC Press is an imprint of the
Taylor & Francis Group, an **informa** business

A TAYLOR & FRANCIS BOOK

CRC Press
Taylor & Francis Group
6000 Broken Sound Parkway NW, Suite 300
Boca Raton, FL 33487-2742

© 2007 by Taylor & Francis Group, LLC
CRC Press is an imprint of Taylor & Francis Group, an Informa business

First issued in paperback 2019

ISBN 13: 978-0-367-45349-7 (pbk)
ISBN 13: 978-0-8493-3594-5 (hbk)

Library of Congress Cataloging-in-Publication Data

Nollet, Leo M. L., 1948-
   Radionuclide concentrations in food and the environment / Leo M.L. Nollet and Michael Poschl.
      p. cm.
   Includes bibliographical references and index.
   ISBN 0-8493-3594-9 (9780849335945 : alk. paper)
   1. Radioactive pollution. 2. Radioactive contamination of food. I. Poschl, Michael. II. Title.

TD196.R3N65 2006
363.17'992--dc22   2006003723

Visit the Taylor & Francis Web site at
http://www.taylorandfrancis.com

and the CRC Press Web site at
http://www.crcpress.com

Preface

The environment that surrounds us contains small amounts of radioactive (unstable) elements or radionuclides (radioisotopes) that are derived from primordial and secondary cosmogenic sources. In addition to naturally occurring radioactive materials (NORMs), technologically enhanced naturally occurring radioactive materials (TENORMs) and man-made (artificially produced) radionuclides have been introduced into ecosystems due to the proliferation of different nuclear applications in industry, medicine, and research. Radionuclides in the air, soil, water, and rocks that make up Earth's geosphere and atmosphere can be transferred into the biosphere by many organisms and can also bioaccumulate in the food chain. This can result in an increase in population radiation doses, which requires an understanding of the environmental behaviors of different radionuclides and estimation of their human risks.

This new radioecologically concerned publication on *Radionuclide Concentrations in Foods and the Environment* addresses the key aspects of important and complex interdisciplinary issues concerning the relationship between natural and man-made sources of environmental radioactivity and the subsequent radionuclide concentrations in foods on an academic research level. It discusses the negative effects of environmental radioactivity on plants and animals, as well as the effects of radiocontaminated food on human health. It also offers perspectives for preventing the transfer of contaminants into foodstuffs and food raw materials.

In Chapter 1, fundamental data for understanding the substance of matter and its behavior patterns are presented. A history of the atom and radioactivity, and important information about basic radiological terms as the basic properties of radionuclides are also outlined.

A great deal of the book is devoted to the sources of radionuclides and the radionuclide content of the principal environmental components related to food production (soil and aquatic environments), as well as foodstuffs and food raw materials. Chapter 2 deals with the natural and anthropogenic (more accurately, primordial) sources of radionuclides found in the environment. It focuses on isotopic species that are important contributors to overall radionuclide abundances in various ecosystems.

Air radionuclides can be easily transported throughout the environment and become part of food, contributing to the total radiation exposure of biota, including human beings. The origins and characteristics of these radionuclides are analyzed in Chapter 3. Special attention is paid to man-made radionuclides released into the air from nuclear weapons testing and production, electricity generation in nuclear power plants, and nuclear accidents.

Water covers more than two thirds of the Earth's surface and is a necessary resource for human life: water is used for direct consumption, in the production of food, for many industrial activities, etc. Water is also a medium for the transport and interaction of radionuclides in different parts of the troposphere. Thus the radioactivity present in water can reach humans and ecosystems through many different mechanisms. These mechanisms are discussed in Chapter 4.

Chapter 5 discusses the behavior of radionuclides in soil, including the fractionation of radionuclides in soils, radionuclide migration along the soil profile, the role of microorganisms, and radionuclide bioavailability and transference into plants. Finally, some scientific and social applications of radionuclide concentration measurements in soils, such as dose assessment, earthquake prediction through radon measurements, and dating of a soil core, are discussed.

The transfer/transport of radionuclides through ecosystems is discussed in Chapter 6, with and emphasis on their transport from the environment into food raw materials and foodstuffs. Predictive modeling of these transfer processes is analyzed and clarified.

The physical and chemical aspects of ionizing radiation interactions and the biological consequences of radiation interactions (i.e., the effects of radioactivity on individual plants and animals), including information on the effects of radio-contaminated food on human health and further ecological consequences of radiation exposure are discussed in Chapter 7.

In order to assess the impact of food contamination exposure on humans, radioactivity monitoring programs for food were developed, including international safety and trade legislation, and public reassurance. Both the possible content of radionuclides in foods and the importance of monitoring food for levels of radioactivity are discussed in Chapter 8. Characteristics of the pathways of radionuclide transfer from the environment to food and specification of radionuclides of interest in important food groups are discussed. Examples of special investigations and routine programs are also presented.

Radiation detection and radioactivity analysis are the backbone of studies of environmental radioactivity as well as radionuclides in foods. These methods include techniques and principles that measure the disintegration rates of radionuclides and the types of radiation emanating from radioactive samples. Determining the energies of emanating particles or electromagnetic (EM) rays originating in radioactive decay (radiospectrometry) provides a qualitative measure of radionuclides. Determining the disintegration rates thus provides a quantitative measure of the amount of those radionuclides in the sample. Chapter 9 first focuses on the principles of radiation detection. Descriptions of the most used radiation detection and measurement systems and their main components follows. The precision and accuracy of radioactivity analysis of different environmental samples are determined by high-quality sample preparation, calibration of the detection system, quality control measures, and accurate radioactivity calculations. A good understanding of each of these aspects and practical experience are essential to performing accurate radioactivity analysis of foodstuffs and food raw materials.

A radiation protection program is, in effect, a management system that affords organizations the ability to anticipate, recognize, evaluate, and control sources of radiation that might be present in the workplace. The main aim of such activities is to prevent or minimize the harmful effects of radiation sources. Many radioactive sources are used by human beings: as encapsulated standards for the calibration of counting equipment or in dispersible forms for radiolabeling or internal standardization procedures; in the form of radiation-producing devices such as analytical x-ray machines, electron microscopes, or x-ray diffraction devices. Samples of food and environmental media contain myriad radionuclides in various concentrations stemming from natural sources or from environmental releases. With all of these different types of sources that might be present in any analytical lab, and the various pathways for potential exposure, the development of a vigilant radiation protection program to protect the health of individuals associated with laboratory activities is considered a necessity. Safety management in radioanalytical laboratories is analyzed in Chapter 10.

Ethnic, religious, social, political, and economic issues are causing complex conflicts in a number of critical regions of the world. One phenomenon of particular concern is the upsurge in global terrorist activity. A number of recent events show that terrorism is fast becoming a considerable threat to global security. While terrorist groups continue to use conventional weapons to conduct their operations, there is concern that some groups may be considering the use of radiological material. Relevant to this discussion are both nuclear (fissionable) and other radioactive materials, which, although disparate in terms of their potential to cause destruction, are of increasing concern to the worldwide community. Chapter 11 discusses and analyzes many issues: the nuclear and radiological terrorist threat, the categorization of nuclear and radiological materials, radiological scenarios, the illicit trafficking of radioactive materials, the role of scientific practitioners, radiation detection strategies (radionuclides and radiation detection systems of interest in border monitoring), masking of illicit materials, nuclear and radiological forensics, and a number of other subjects related to protection against the radiological terrorist threat.

The countermeasures limiting or preventing radiocontamination of plants and animals, which are the sources of plant- and animal-based foodstuffs, and which could also be the source of food contamination, are characterized in Chapter 12. International and national bodies have formulated maximum permissible contamination limits in response to the 1986 Chernobyl accident, and more recently in preparation for future radiological emergencies, either accidental or by malevolent intent. Individual countries have promulgated sets of regulatory limits, some based on international standards, some generated internally. To list control values for all countries would be impractical, therefore a limited selection of regulations and recommendations (relevant to radioactivity in food, the environment, and drinking water) from international agencies and some individual nations are presented. The radioactivity arising from naturally occurring radionuclides and man-made radioactive contamination are taken in the account in these regulations.

The increasing consumer demand for "fresh" and natural food products has led to the improvement of nonthermal technologies such as irradiation and freezing as food preservation processes (Chapter 13). Nonthermal technologies, such as irradiation, have the ability to inactivate microorganisms at ambient or near-ambient temperatures, thus avoiding the deleterious effects of heat on flavor, color, and nutrient value. Irradiation has become one of the most extensively investigated and controversial technologies in food processing. For this reason, "food irradiation" is discussed in this book. Experts have regularly evaluated studies on the safety and proprieties of irradiated foods and have concluded that the process and the resulting foods are safe. The World Health Organization (WHO) recently concluded on the basis of extensive scientific evidence that food irradiated to any dose appropriate to achieve the intended technological objective is both safe to consume and nutritionally adequate.

The editors do not claim that this book is exhaustive in its coverage of all aspects concerning the topic of radionuclides in foods. We are, however, very grateful to all the authors for their contributions, expertise, and unwavering commitment to this project. We also gratefully acknowledge the support of Patricia Roberson and Susan B. Lee (project coordinators, Taylor & Francis Group LLC) for their assistance in the preparation of this book.

The book was edited by two editors; however, the person who initiated the writing of this book is Leo M. L. Nollet, who made it possible for M. Pöschl to participate in the editing. To him, M. Pöschl wishes to express his sincere thanks, not only for being provided this opportunity, but also for the advice, recommendations, and experience he so willingly and unselfishly rendered.

Finally, and above all, we thank our wives, Vera and Clara, for their support, understanding, and patience during our months-long activities as editors of this book—it is little compensation for all the time we could not devote to them. We also dedicate this book to our sons and daughters.

Michael Pöschl and Leo M. L. Nollet

About the Editors

Michael Pöschl is associate professor of special animal husbandry in the Department of Radiobiology of Faculty of Agronomy at the Mendel University of Agriculture and Forestry (MUAF) in Brno, Czech Republic. His mean research interests are situated in the domain of radioecology, radio-spectrometry, and radio-contamination of foodstuffs. Dr. Pöschl is author or co-author of numerous scientific articles, abstracts, and presentations. He received the RNDr. (Degree of Doctor of Natural Sciences, Charles University in Prague, Czech Republic, 1976) and Ph.D. (1986) degrees in biology from the MUAF.

Leo M. L. Nollet is a professor of biochemistry, aquatic ecology, and ecotoxicology in the Department of Engineering Sciences, Hogeschool Gent, Ghent, Belgium. His main research interests are in the areas of food analysis, chromatography, and analysis of environmental parameters. He is the author or coauthor of numerous articles, abstracts, and presentations, and is the editor of *Handbook of Food Analysis*, 2nd ed. (three volumes), *Food Analysis by HPLC*, 2nd ed., and *Handbook of Water Analysis* (all titles, Marcel Dekker, Inc.). He received his M.S. (1973) and Ph.D. (1978) degrees in biology from the Katholieke Universiteit Leuven, Leuven, Belgium.

Contributors

Juan Pedro Bolívar
Dpto. Física Aplicada
Universidad de Huelva
Huelva, Spain

Maria Luísa Botelho
Nuclear and Technological Institute
Sacavém, Portugal

F. J. Bradley
New York, New York

Sandra Cabo Verde
Nuclear and Technological Institute
Sacavém, Portugal

Peter Carny
Abmerit
Trnava, Slovakia

M. A. Charlton
Department of Environmental Health
and Safety
University of Texas Health Science
Center at San Antonio
San Antonio, Texas

Mike Colella
Institute of Materials and Engineering
Science
Australian Nuclear Science and
Technology Organisation
Menai, Australia

Guillermo Manjón Collado
Departamento de Física Aplicada II
E.T.S. Arquitectura
Sevilla, Spain

Tony Dell
Radiochemistry Unit
Vet Lab Agency
New Haw, Addlestone, Surrey,
England

R. J. Emery
Department of Environmental Health
and Safety
University of Texas Health Science
Center at Houston
Houston, Texas

Pascal Froidevaux
Institut de Radiophysique Appliquée
Lausanne, Switzerland

Jeffrey S. Gaffney
Environmental Research Division
Argonne National Laboratory
Argonne, Illinois

Kathryn A. Higley
Department of Nuclear Engineering
and Radiation Health Physics
Oregon State University
Corvallis, Oregon

Ashraf Khater
Physics Department
College of Science
King Saud University
Riyadh, Saudi Arabia

Manuel García-León
Departamento de Física Atómica
Molecular y Nuclear
Universidad de Sevilla
Sevilla, Spain

Rafael García-Tenorio
Departamento de Física Aplicada II
Escuela Universitaria Superior de
  Arquitectura
Sevilla, Spain

G. Lima
Ecola Superior Agraria de Santarém
Santarém, Portugal

Nancy A. Marley
Environmental Research Division
Argonne National Laboratory
Argonne, Illinois

José Luis Mas
Departamento de Física Aplicada I
Universidad de Sevilla
Escuela Universitaria Politécnica
Sevilla, Spain

Paula Pinto
Ecola Superior Agraria de Santarém
Santarém, Portugal

Michael Pöschl
Mendel University of Agriculture and
  Forestry in Brno
Brno, Czech Republic

R. M. Pratt
New York, New York

Mark Reinhard
Institute of Materials and Engineering
  Science
Australian Nuclear Science and
  Technology Organisation
Menai, Australia

Antonieta Santana
Ecola Superior Agraria de Santarém
Santarém, Portugal

Stuart Thomson
Institute of Materials and Engineering
  Science
Australian Nuclear Science and
  Technology Organisation
Menai, Australia

Paul Tossell
Emergency Planning, Radiation, and
  Incidents Division
Food Standards Agency
London, England

Maria João Trigo
National Institute of Agrarian and
  Fishery Research
Quinta do Marquês
Oeiras, Portugal

Claudio Tuniz
Abdus Salam International Centre for
  Theoretical Physics
Trieste, Italy

C. M. Vandecasteele
Federal Agency for Nuclear Control
Brussels, Belgium

Table of Contents

1 What Are Radionuclides?

Michael Pöschl

CONTENTS

1.1 INTRODUCTION

A radionuclide (radioactive nuclide) is a nuclide with an unbalanced and unstable nucleus. A nuclide is an atom with a defined atomic number and a defined neutron number. The definition is immediately related to a number of other terms — atom, element, nuclide, isotope — and these are terms that we must define first (Section 1.3). In the following sections, the origin and nature of radionuclides (Section 1.4) and radioactive decay or radioactivity as the basic properties of radionuclides (Section 1.5) are described. The recent importance of radionuclides is discussed in Section 1.6, including their use and their health risks.

Since the history of radionuclides is immediately connected with our understanding of matter, and thus with the study of atoms and with the discovery of radioactivity, a brief discussion of the history of the atom and radioactivity is presented in Section 1.2.

1.2 HISTORY

1.2.1 The History of Atomic Theory

The history of atomic theory goes back about 2,500 years. Before the existence of the group of Greek thinkers seeking a rational explanation of the observable world through their "natural" philosophy, people believed in a world ruled by gods [1]. The Greek philosophers living between the 7th and 3rd centuries B.C., in particular Thales of Miletus, Anaximander, Anaximenes, Heraclitus of Ephesus, Xenophanes of Colophon, Parmedides, Empedocles of Agrigentum, Anaxagoras of Clazomenae, Plato, and Aristotle, promoted a number of "single" and "multiple" element (air, fire, Earth, water, or warm, dry, moist, cold) theories, by which they attempted to identify the universal and the essential, and explained natural processes and their substance. Pythagoreans had very specific attitudes about the world; for them the number was the primordial element, and these numbers were closely related to simple geometric objects. The idea of two basic elements, corpuscular and void, was fundamental for atomists of antiquity, whose proponents were Leucippus and Democritus. The idea of the indivisibility of matter (*atomos*) has been attributed to the latter, and also Epicurus, who claimed that to a certain extent the motion of atoms is random and at the same time deviation may happen. Democritus and Leucippus, Greek philosophers of the 5th century B.C., presented the first theory of atoms. They held that each atom had a different shape, like a pebble, that governed the atom's properties. Aristotle did not believe in atomism and introduced the idea of the primordial qualities of warm, cold, dry, moist.

Nearly 2,000 years later, in the 18th century, modern atomists represented by Lavoisier, Cavendish, Priestley, and later Dalton followed the Greek atomists. Dalton's work in the 19th century proved that matter was made up of atoms, but he knew nothing of their structure. This goes against the theory of infinite divisibility, which states that matter can always be divided into smaller parts.

The atomic theory became universally accepted by the end of the 19th century. Chemists were filling in the details of the periodic table and physicists were occupied with the kinetic theory of gases, Brownian motion, the determination of Avogadro's number, and the "counting" of atoms [1]. In 1897 the theory of "indivisible" atoms was put to rest with the discovery of the electron, the first of the subatomic particles, by J. J. Thomson [2]. This showed that atoms are, in fact, divisible. Ernest Rutherford's work helped to show that the positively charged nucleus did exist. Other elementary particles of matter were discovered much later.

All recent models of the atom have taken into account the existence of subatomic particles. Learning about the subatomic "world" is continuing. Among the most recent developments is the discovery of David J. Gross, H. David Politzer, and Frank Wilczek, that is, "the discovery of asymptotic freedom in the theory of the strong interaction," in the context of quantum chromodynamics. For this discovery they received the Nobel Prize in physics in 2004 [3].

J. J. Thomson's discovery of electrons was important not only because it was the beginning of studies of subatomic particles, but it was immediately associated with the discovery of radioactivity. Later it was discovered that β emission is actually a flow of electrons with high energy. The discovery of radioactivity, like electrons, was associated with electric discharges in gas and "cathode rays" in a cathode ray tube.

1.2.2 THE HISTORY OF RADIOACTIVITY

On November 8, 1895, Wilhelm Roentgen (Figure 1.1), a Prussian professor, director of the Wurzburg Physics Institute, covered with black paper an apparatus that he used to study electricity. He saw a surprising phenomenon: the screen placed nearby seemed to shine with a green light [4]. Moreover, his hand placed behind the screen showed the shadow of his hand bones. At the end of December he published a short article claiming fantastic news: the existence of an unknown and strange radiation that was quickly named "x-rays." For this discovery he received the first Nobel Prize in physics in 1901.

Subsequently Antoine Henri Becquerel (Figure 1.2), from the French Science Academy, decided to study the existence of a possible relation between those famous x-rays and the fluorescence phenomena. At that time he was studying the fluorescence of uranium salts. At first he assumed that after illumination with sunlight and showing fluorescence, the salts radiated X radiation. However, later, by coincidence, following many gray, cloudy days in Paris, he noted that the photographic plates were impressed with nonfluorescent uranium. The shadow of a copper cross that Becquerel had placed between the uranium and the covered plates was visible (Figure 1.3). The new radiation had not gone through it. Becquerel called them "U-rays," and in this way he actually discovered natural radioactivity.

This discovery and subsequent scientific work made the 20th century completely different from the previous ones. Marie Sklodowska joined this research and showed that, like uranium, thorium is also radioactive; with Pierre Curie in July 1898, she succeeded in isolating a new material, a million times more

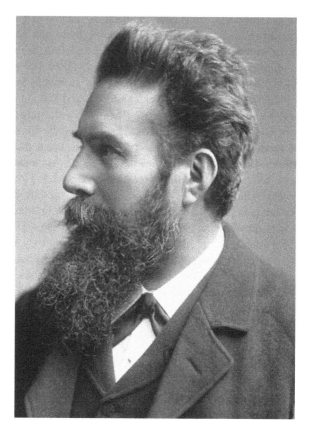

FIGURE 1.1 Wilhelm Conrad Roentgen. © The Nobel Foundation [14].

radioactive than uranium, that she called "polonium." Then, from many tons of pitchblende ore, Pierre and Marie (Figure 1.4) extracted by hand a few milligrams of another new material, 2.5 million times more radioactive than uranium: radium.

The next step in the history is made of long and patient studies, with many fundamental breakthroughs in understanding what matter is. Ernest Rutherford (Figure 1.5), James Chadwick, Marie Curie, and Paul Villard showed that emitted radiations are of three types: the helium nuclei (α radiation), electrons (β radiation), or very energetic photons (γ radiation).

The atomic nucleus was discovered around 1911, thanks to, among others, Ernest Rutherford, Hans Geiger, and Ernest Marsden. The knowledge about it improved rapidly: in 1932, James Chadwick discovered the neutron, while Irene and Frederic Joliot-Curie, having observed the neutron decay, did not recognize it as a new particle of the nucleus.

In 1934 Irene and Frederic Joliot-Curie (Figure 1.6) discovered artificial radioactivity, taking a great step toward the use and control of radioactivity. In 1938 some physicists realized the possibilities of nuclear energy (wrongly named atomic energy). In 1939, two German scientists, Otto Hahn and Fritz Strassmann,

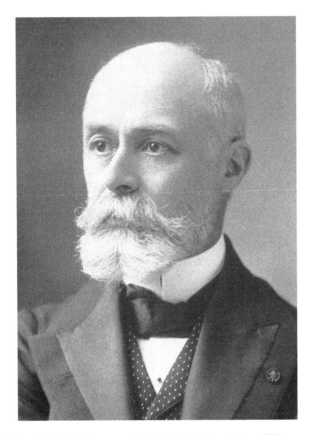

FIGURE 1.2 Antoine Henri Becquerel. © The Nobel Foundation [14].

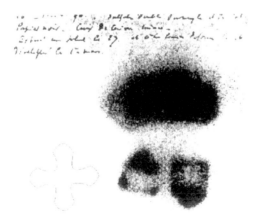

FIGURE 1.3 Photographic plate of Becquerel impressed with the radioactivity of uranium. (Photo courtesy of ACJC Curie and Joliot-Curie Fund.)

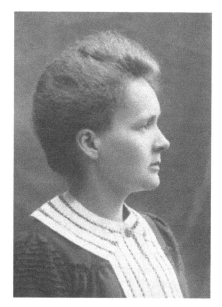 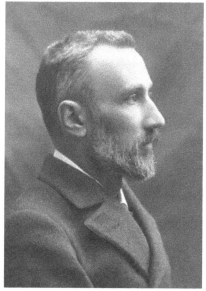

FIGURE 1.4 Marie Sklodowska-Curie and Pierre Curie. © The Nobel Foundation [14].

demonstrated that the uranium nucleus could be cut in two parts: this is fission of the nucleus. Some months later, Frederic Joliot-Curie and his colleagues Hans von Halban, an Austrian, and Lew Kowarski, a Russian, detected an emission of neutrons when a uranium nucleus was cut. The French team had advanced to the point of outlining an arrangement of uranium and a moderator that could sustain a chain reaction — a reactor.

This chapter in the history of radioactivity ends with the first nuclear bomb, which was detonated on July 16, 1945, in the desert of Alamogordo, New Mexico, near the town of Los Alamos. This complete transformation of the 20th century, with the horror of the two bombs of 1945 launched on human beings, was possible thanks to the discovery of radioactivity.

However, this did not bring the history of studies of the composition of matter, or the atom and radioactivity, to an end, evidence of which is the above-mentioned discovery in physics and the Nobel Prize for 2004. Further evidence is the standing exploitation of a number of methods useful for man using the phenomenon of radioactivity and seeking instruments for "safer" uses of nuclear energy.

1.3 ATOM, ELEMENT, NUCLIDE, AND ISOTOPE

The word "atom" is derived from the Greek *atomos*, "indivisible," from *a*-, "not," and *tomos*, "a cut." An atom is a microscopic structure found in all ordinary matter around us; it is the smallest part of a chemical element. Atoms exist in chemical reactions and are composed of three types of subatomic particles: electrons (with a negative charge), protons (with a positive charge), and neutrons

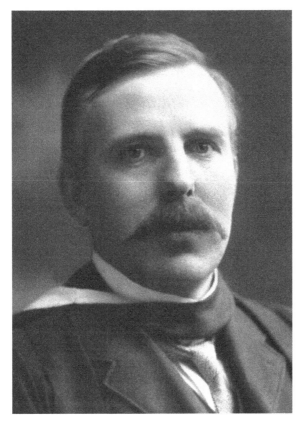

FIGURE 1.5 Ernest Rutherford. © The Nobel Foundation [14].

(with no charge). Protons and neutrons, in turn, are composed of more elementary particles known as quarks. Particle physics further distinguishes the so-called fundamental particles, which make up all the other particles found in nature and are not themselves made up of smaller particles.

Atoms are generally classified by their atomic number, which corresponds to the number of protons in the atom. The atomic number defines which element the atom is. All atoms with the same atomic number share a wide variety of physical properties and exhibit the same chemical behavior. The various kinds of atoms are listed in the periodic table in order of increasing atomic number. The mass number, atomic mass number, or nucleon number of an element is the total number of protons and neutrons in an atom of that element.

In general, an atom with atomic number Z and neutron number N is known as a nuclide. The total number of protons plus neutrons is known as the mass number A of a nuclide. Hence a nuclide can be specified as follows:

$$^A_Z X_N,$$

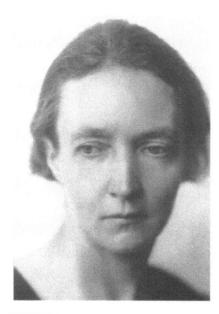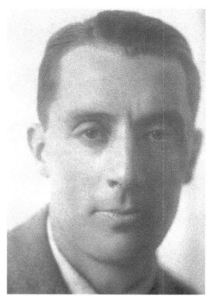

FIGURE 1.6 Irene and Jean Frederic Joliot-Curie. © The Nobel Foundation [14].

where Z is the atomic (proton) number, N is the neutron number, A is the (atomic) mass (or nucleon) number $(N + Z)$, and X is the chemical element symbol.

There are 116 [5] currently known chemical elements. Very recently, evidence for the existence of two new superheavy elements has been reported. Elements consist of atoms with a fixed number Z (the atomic number) of protons in the nucleus and an equal number of orbital electrons. In addition to protons, the nucleus contains a variable number of neutrons N. Atoms of the same element with different numbers of neutrons are known as isotopes of that element. Elements can have many isotopes, most of which are unstable.

The most widely accepted structure (model) of an atom is the wave model. It is based on the Bohr model, but takes into account recent developments and discoveries in quantum mechanics. Quantum mechanics was the focus of Niels Bohr, and his followers were Max Planck, Albert Einstein, Max Born, Werner Heisenberg, Erwin Schrödinger, Max Born, Paul Dirac, Wolfgang Pauli, and others. Some fundamental aspects of the theory are still actively studied.

1.4   RADIONUCLIDES

In any nuclide, the number of neutrons determines whether the nucleus is radioactive. For the nucleus to be stable, the number of neutrons should in most cases be a little higher than the number of protons. If the number of neutrons is out of balance, the nucleus has excess energy and sooner or later will discharge the energy by decay processes, that is, by emitting γ rays or subatomic particles. A nuclide with such an unbalanced nucleus is unstable and is called a radioactive nuclide, or radionuclide. Radionuclides are often referred to by chemists and biologists as radioactive isotopes or radioisotopes, and play an important part in the technologies that provide us with food, water, and good health. Radionuclides may occur naturally, but they can also be artificially produced.

A number of publications include lists of radionuclides and their characteristics [6,7] and these lists are also available on several Web sites [8–11].

Chapter 2 provides detailed data on the sources of radionuclides. In the following paragraphs only the general division is characterized.

1.4.1 NATURAL RADIONUCLIDES

Apart from stable chemical elements, very low concentrations of radioactive elements occur naturally in the environment. We can divide these natural radionuclides into three categories according to their origin and formation: primordial radionuclides, secondary radionuclides, and cosmogenic radionuclides [12].

1.4.1.1 Primordial Radionuclides

Primordial radionuclides are radionuclides that originated with other (stable) nuclei in the course of cosmic nucleogenesis by thermonuclear reactions in the core of a star, which then exploded as a supernova and enriched the nucleus cloud from which the sun and the solar system originated. They became part of the Earth at the time when the solar system was formed about 4 to 5 billion years ago. To the present day, only radionuclides with a very long half-life (i.e., more than about 10^8 years) were preserved.

The most widespread primordial radionuclide is ^{40}K; its average content in the crust of the Earth is about $3 \times 10^{-3}\%$. ^{40}K, with a half-life of $T_{1/2} = 1.277 \times 10^9$ years, disintegrates by β decay to ^{40}Ar (89%) and electron capture to ^{40}Ca (11%); both isotopes are stable.

Another natural primary radionuclide is ^{232}Th, which has a half-life of $T_{1/2} = 1.39 \times 10^{10}$ years and gradually disintegrates by α decay into a number of radionuclides of the so-called thorium decay chain (i.e., secondary radionuclides).

However, the most important natural radionuclides of primary origin in the Earth's crust are ^{238}U, with a half-life of $T_{1/2} = 4.468 \times 10^9$ years, and ^{235}U, with a half-life of $T_{1/2} = 7.038 \times 10^8$ years. Both of these isotopes of uranium are gradually transformed by α decay into a number of radionuclides of both uranium decay chains.

1.4.1.2 Secondary Radionuclides

The decay of primary radionuclides continuously gives rise to a number of secondary radionuclides. Natural radionuclides ^{232}Th, ^{238}U, and ^{235}U decay (by α and later also β decay) into nuclei, which are also radioactive, much like their other decay products (i.e., radioactive decay chains). In nature there are three radioactive decay chains: ^{232}Th, ^{238}U, and ^{235}U. To a certain extent these three natural decay chains are similar. They consist of isotopes of heavy elements mostly of α radioactivity (a smaller part is also β). Radon (the most stable isotope is ^{222}Rn) appears in the second half of the series; its decay products have a short half-life and disintegrate simultaneously by α and β decay. Radon is a radioactive noble gas, one of the heaviest gases. All three natural decay chains result in stable isotopes of lead.

1.4.1.3 Cosmogenic Radionuclides

Cosmogenic radionuclides are natural radionuclides that currently originate by nuclear reactions when high-energy cosmic radiation passes through the Earth's atmosphere. Examples include radiocarbon (^{14}C) and tritium (^{3}H).

1.4.2 ARTIFICIALLY PRODUCED RADIONUCLIDES

For the demands of present science and technology, industry, and health services, these few radionuclides of natural origin are far from sufficient. Therefore we must produce radionuclides artificially. Artificial radionuclides can be produced by nuclear reactors, by particle accelerators, or by radionuclide generators.

1.4.2.1 Radionuclides Produced by Nuclear Reactors

To produce a radioactive nucleus from a stable nucleus, it is necessary to change the number of protons or neutrons so as not to disturb the equilibrium configuration. This can be achieved by bombardment of the initial nucleus A with suitable particles — protons or neutrons (or α particles, deuterons, rarely also with heavy ions) — which enter the nucleus and cause the respective changes — nuclear reactions. The resulting nucleus B is formed (mostly in excited state B′), which is frequently radioactive.

The simplest bombardment of nuclei is with neutrons (n). Because the neutron has no electric charge, electric repulsive power does not function, and even a slow neutron will readily enter the nucleus. The use of neutrons generally results in nuclei with an abundance of neutrons and with β⁻ radioactivity. An intensive source of neutrons is the nuclear reactor, and so these β⁻ radionuclides are usually produced by bombardment of a suitable nuclear target in a special chamber of the reactor (Figure 1.7a). Some reactions in the production of radionuclides are ^{6}Li(n,)^{3}H, ^{14}N(n,p)^{14}C, ^{32}S(n,p)^{32}P, and ^{98}Mo(n,)^{99}Mo.

Nuclear reactors are also used in the separation of radionuclides from fission products of uranium. In the nuclear reactor, the nuclei of ^{235}U (or ^{238}U) split into two nuclei after the entrance of neutrons. In chemical terms they fall into the middle part of Mendeleyev periodic table and are mostly radioactive, for example,

$$^{235}U + n \rightarrow ^{236}U \rightarrow ^{131}J + ^{102}Y + 3n,$$
$$\rightarrow ^{137}Cs + ^{97}Y + 2n,$$
$$\rightarrow ^{133}Xe + ^{101}Sr + 2n,$$
$$\rightarrow ^{99}Mo + ^{135}Sn + 2n,$$
$$\rightarrow ^{155}Sm + ^{78}Zn + 3n,$$
$$...\text{and other radionuclides.}$$

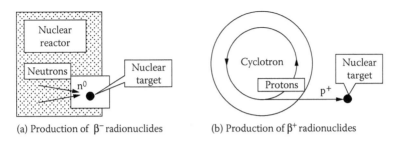

(a) Production of β⁻ radionuclides   (b) Production of β⁺ radionuclides

FIGURE 1.7 Production of radioisotopes by bombardment of nuclear targets in (a) a reactor or (b) a cyclotron.

The necessary radionuclides (e.g., ^{131}J, ^{99}Mo, ^{133}Xe, ^{137}Cs, ^{90}Sr, and others) are then isolated from these fission products by means of radiochemical separation methods. However, this is very difficult because the resulting radionuclide requires satisfactory purity.

1.4.2.2 Radionuclides Produced by Particle Accelerators

To produce positron (β⁺) radionuclides it is necessary to add protons (p) to the nucleus. For the proton p⁺ to enter the nucleus it must be accelerated to a high-energy state ranging from hundreds of kiloelectron volts (keV) to several mega-electron volts (MeV) to overcome by its own energy the repulsive coulomb power of the positively charged nucleus. The most frequently used accelerators of protons are cyclotrons. A cyclotron is a machine designed to accelerate clusters of charged particles by using a high-frequency alternating voltage and a perpendicular magnetic field to spiral the beam out. The proton cluster is then brought out of the circular path by the magnetic pole and falls onto a suitable target (Figure 1.7b).

With a view to nuclear reaction and transmutation, the nuclei can be bombarded with protons or other fast charged particles: deuterons (d) or heavier nuclei or ions. Nuclei with an abundance of protons are mostly β⁺ radioactive or they decay by electron capture; according to the mode of production, they are sometimes indicated as cyclotron radionuclides. Some reactions of radionuclide production are ^{18}O(p,n)^{18}F, ^{13}C(p,n)^{13}N, ^{11}B(p,n)^{11}C, ^{10}B(d,n)^{11}C, and ^{56}Fe(d,n)^{57}Co.

1.4.2.3 Radionuclides Produced by Generators

Radionuclide generators are used to obtain radionuclides with shorter half-lives from primary parent radionuclides with longer half-lives. Such a generator uses a moderately long-lived parent radionuclide that decays to produce a short-lived daughter radionuclide. The parent radionuclide is usually absorbed on support material, such as ion exchange resin, which is packed in a small, lead-shielded column. The short-lived radionuclide is then eluted from the support material with a solvent, when needed. Among the most important is the molybdenum-technetium generator for the preparation of ^{99m}Tc. Another example is the ^{81}Rb generator for the preparation of the radioactive krypton gas (^{81m}Kr).

1.5 RADIOACTIVITY

1.5.1 FUNDAMENTALS OF RADIOACTIVITY

Radioactivity is the fundamental property of unstable nuclei of radionuclides. Following the discovery of natural radioactivity by Becquerel in 1896, Frederic Soddy and Ernest Rutherford in 1902 defined radioactivity as a spontaneous disintegration of a radioactive element by the expulsion of particles with the result that new elements are formed. Today radioactivity is considered to be a phenomenon of spontaneous nuclear transformation of radionuclides (so-called radioactive decay), which is accompanied by the emission of particles (α, β^-, β^+), electron capture, proton emission, or the emission of fragments (i.e., the most common decay modes), and the emission of γ radiation. Radioactivity is also indicated as radioactive transmutation. Radioactivity can occur both naturally and through human intervention.

Empirically it was discovered that the nuclei of elements are stable, that is, they are not subject to radioactive decay, except under a particular neutron:proton ratio ($N{:}Z$). In stable, light nuclei ($Z \leq 20$), this ratio equals one, or is only a little larger than one (nuclei of $_1^1H$ and $_2^3He$ are exceptions). It increases to 1.52 in the heaviest stable nuclide $_{83}^{209}Bi$. If the composition of the nucleus deviates from the optimal range of the $N{:}Z$ ratio, that is, if the nucleus has too few or many neutrons for a certain proton number (e.g., in oxygen, the isotopes ^{14}O, ^{15}O, ^{19}O, ^{20}O), the nucleus becomes radioactive, that is, it decays spontaneously, most frequently to another nucleus. Symbolically the process can be described as follows:

$$_Z^A X \rightarrow (A_1, Z_1)Y + (A_2, Z_2) \text{ particle,}$$

where X is the "parent" nuclide and Y is the "daughter" nuclide.

In the decay, more than one light particle can be emitted and the process is usually accompanied by the emission of γ radiation.

In radioactive decay, energy is released (exoergic process) and the generated products always carry a certain kinetic energy. This is possible only if the primary nucleus has more rest energy (mass) than the sum of the rest energies (masses) of the products of the decay:

$$M(X) > M(Y) + M(\text{particle}).$$

This disparity is the basic condition of radioactivity. The energy equivalent to this difference in masses is the energy of radioactive decay. In radioactive decay, this release of energy occurs through emission (to a great extent) of one or more of the three types of radiation: α, β, and γ.

1.5.2 SIMPLE RADIOACTIVE DECAY, DECAY CONSTANT, HALF-LIFE, ACTIVITY

An unstable nucleus transforms into another nucleus spontaneously only with a certain probability (i.e., a consequence of the laws of quantum mechanics). It occurs according to the law of radioactive decay. Radioactive decay is a random process. The probability that an atom will decay during the time dt is given by λdt where λ is the constant of proportionality known as the decay constant. In a system where there are N_0 atoms present initially, the number of atoms decaying in time dt is given by

$$-dN = \lambda N dt.$$

In a limit of very small time intervals, the previous formula can be expressed as

$$-dN/dt = \lambda N,$$

and integration with respect to time gives the number of atoms present at any time, that is,

$$N_t = N_0 e^{-\lambda t}.$$

The law has a statistical character and can therefore be applied only for large groups of nuclides.

A clearer quantity used to characterize the radionuclide instead of the decay constant λ is half-life. The half-life $T_{1/2}$ is the time it takes for the number of atoms to decrease to half the initial value (i.e., $\frac{1}{2} = e^{-\lambda t}$). Thus the half-life is related to the decay constant through the equation

$$T = \ln 2/\lambda, \text{ that is, } T = 0.693/\lambda.$$

Half-lives vary greatly among different types of atoms, from less than a second to billions of years. For example, it will take about 4.5 billion years for half of the atoms in a mass of ^{238}U to spontaneously disintegrate, but only 24,000 years for half of the atoms in a mass of ^{239}Pu to spontaneously disintegrate. In contrast, ^{131}I, commonly used in medicine, has a half-life of only 8 days.

The quantity that characterizes the speed of radioactive decay is called activity (or emitter activity). The activity A is defined as the number of decays per unit time interval, or the loss in the number of as yet undecayed nuclei per unit time interval:

$$A_t = -dN_t/dt = \lambda N_t.$$

The unit of activity is the becquerel (Bq), one disintegration per second. The older unit of activity was the curie (1 Ci = 3.7×10^{10} Bq).

For practical purposes we define the so-called activity concentration as the proportion of the activity compared to the total mass of the radioactive substance (i.e., the sum of the masses of all radionuclides and stable nuclides contained in the substance).

1.5.3 RADIOACTIVE DECAY CHAIN

If the daughter nuclide in radioactive decay is also unstable, the decay continues further in a decay chain until a stable nuclide is reached. Each state or step will have its own unique characteristics of half-life and type of radiation emitted as the move is made to the next state. For example, the decay of ^{238}U, the primary source of natural radioactivity on Earth, is unusually complicated and proceeds as follows: ^{238}U (emits α) – ^{234}Th (emits β) – ^{234}Pa (emits β) – ^{234}U (emits α) – ^{230}Th (emits α) – ^{226}Ra (emits α) – ^{222}Rn (emits α) – ^{218}Po (emits α) – ^{214}Pb (emits β) – ^{214}Bi (emits β) – ^{214}Po (emits α) – ^{210}Pb (emits β) – ^{210}Bi (emits β) – ^{210}Po (emits α) – ^{206}Pb (which is stable).

1.5.4 TYPES OF RADIOACTIVE DECAY

We distinguish three groups of radioactive decay types:

- changing Z with constant A (β^- decay, β^+ decay, and electron capture),
- changing both A and Z (α decay, emission of nucleons, spontaneous fission, cluster emission),
- caused by de-excitation of the nucleus changing only the energy content of the nucleus (immediate and delayed γ emission and isomeric transition [IT]).

In general we can distinguish the pure decay modes — α decay, β^- decay, β^+ decay, electron capture (EC), spontaneous fission (SF), proton (p) decay, neutron (n) emission, and the so-called cluster emission (CM; a variety of rare decay processes) — and the mixed modes, that is, multiple pure decay modes or modes with various combinations of pure decay modes [13].

In the following sections, only processes arising from basic radioactive decays will be described in greater detail (i.e., α decay, β^- decay, β^+ decay, electron capture, γ emission, and isomeric transition).

1.5.4.1 Alpha Decay

Alpha decay is a type of radioactive decay characterized by α emission. Symbolically the process can be described as follows:

$$_{Z}^{A}X \longrightarrow {}_{Z-2}^{A-4}Y + {}_{2}^{4}He.$$

Alpha emission is a cluster of two neutrons and two protons (^{4}He^{2+}; i.e., a helium nucleus). α particles are slow moving (about 20,000 km/s, not of high energy) and easily stopped by a sheet of paper or a few centimeters of air. α particles are highly charged (+2) and thus are very harmful. The energy spectrum of α emission is discrete (linear). Nuclei of the following radionuclides decay with α emission: $^{241}_{95}\text{Am}$, $^{238}_{92}\text{U}$, $^{230}_{90}\text{Th}$, $^{227}_{89}\text{Ac}$, $^{227}_{88}\text{Ra}$, $^{212}_{84}\text{Po}$.

1.5.4.2 Beta Decay

Beta decay is a type of radioactive decay characterized by emission of β^- or β^+ particles (radiation). Symbolically the process can be described as follows:

$$^A_Z\text{X} \longrightarrow \,^A_{Z+1}\text{Y} + \,^0_{-1}\text{e} + \tilde{v}_e \text{ for } \beta^- \text{ (i.e., electron emission), or}$$

$$^A_Z\text{X} \longrightarrow \,^A_{Z-1}\text{Y} + \,^0_{+1}\text{e} + v_e \text{ for } \beta^+ \text{ (i.e., positron emission),}$$

where $\tilde{v}_e$ is an electron antineutrino and v_e is an electron neutrino.

A positron is an electron antiparticle that has the same rest mass, but opposite sign of electric charge. Neutrinos and antineutrinos are neutral particles with a zero or very small mass. The energy spectrum of β radiation is continuous. The principle of β decay is the decay of nucleons in the nucleus, that is, of neutrons into protons and vice versa according to the following:

$$^1_0\text{n} \longrightarrow \,^1_1\text{p} + \,^0_{-1}\text{e} + \tilde{v}_e, \text{ or}$$

$$^1_1\text{p} \longrightarrow \,^1_0\text{n} + \,^0_{+1}\text{e} + v_e.$$

The β particles emitted by the nucleus in β decay (β emission) are fast moving (about 280,000 km/s) and high-energy particles. β particles can travel father than α particles; a few meters of air or a sheet of aluminum is needed to stop them. Examples of β decay are

$$^3_1\text{H} \xrightarrow{\beta^- \text{decay}} \,^3_2\text{He} \text{ and } \,^{30}_{15}\text{P} \xrightarrow{\beta^+ \text{decay}} \,^{30}_{14}\text{Si}.$$

1.5.4.3 Electron Capture

In electron capture, an electron in an atom's inner shell is drawn into the nucleus where it combines with a proton, forming a neutron and a neutrino. The neutrino is then ejected from the atom's nucleus. Electron capture is also called K capture because the captured electron usually comes from the atom's K shell. The process is as follows:

$$^A_Z\text{X} + \,^0_{-1}\text{e} \longrightarrow \,^A_{Z-1}\text{Y} + v_e.$$

Although the nucleus transmutation must be induced by another particle (electron), the process may be spontaneous if the nucleus is part of the atom (i.e., has orbital electrons). It is customary to consider electron capture as a type of radioactive transition. In most cases the nucleus Y is excited, and so the electron capture appears either as a subsequent de-excitation of the photon, or characteristic x-ray radiation, or emission of the so-called Auger electrons.

1.5.4.4 Gamma Emission and Isomeric Transition

In addition to the above-mentioned radioactive changes where the type of the nucleus changes (change in Z and A numbers), there are also very often processes (mostly following radioactive changes) that result in changes in the composition of the atomic nucleus (e.g., α decay, β decay, electron capture) where only the energy state of the nucleus changes. This is the de-excitation of the nucleus (i.e., transition from the excited stage; all energy states but the basic) to the basic state, the lowest energy state. De-excitation occurs either by γ emission or isomeric transition.

Gamma radiation (γ emission) is a process of de-excitation of the atomic nucleus through the emission of a γ photon. The energy spectrum of γ radiation is discrete (linear). Since γ is one type of radioactive radiation, γ radiation is often considered a type of radioactive decay. However, in the case of γ emission, the composition of the atomic nucleus does not change (i.e., there is no change in the proton and neutron number). γ emission is not a particle, but a burst of very high energy as electromagnetic radiation of a very high frequency (wavelengths of 10^{-10} m). It is very hard radiation, very dangerous, and it can be blocked only by large amounts of lead or concrete.

Isomeric transition is a process of de-excitation of the atomic nucleus when the energy of the excited nucleus is transferred by means of direct electromagnetic interaction to an orbiting electron and the electron is ejected from the atom, the so-called Auger electron. Isomeric transition is a competitive process of γ radiation. The energy spectrum of conversion electrons is discrete (linear).

The above types of radiation do not have to occur as radioactive decay only, but may accompany random types of nuclear transmutations, including nuclear reactions, or even changes of elementary particles. In this general sense we usually talk about nuclear radiation.

The wavelength range of γ radiation overlaps with the range of X radiation (i.e., Roentgen radiation) (10^{-11} to 10^{-8} m) and "hard" x-rays overlap the range of long-wavelength (low energy) γ rays. Roentgen radiation (x-ray photons), however, is generated by energetic electron processes in the electron shell of the atom (e.g., in a Roentgen tube) or as bremsstrahlung radiation of electrons in the substance, while γ rays are produced by transitions within the atomic nuclei.

1.5.5 INTERACTIONS OF RADIATION WITH MATTER

The most important interactions of radiation with matter are interactions of α or β particles and γ photons with electrons of an atom. α and β particles are classed as ionizing particles. This is because they carry an electric charge that causes the atoms to separate into ions. Each separation creates an ion pair. γ rays are said to be indirectly ionizing, as described later in this section.

1.5.5.1 Interactions of α Particles

Alpha particles, with their charge of +2 and their mass of 4 amu, create intense ionization. In dry air, α particles generate about 50,000 ion pairs per centimeter of its path, giving up about 34 eV per pair produced. A 4 MeV α particle dissipates its energy in about 2.5 cm of travel. It slows, stops, and becomes a normal helium atom by adopting two electrons from its surroundings. Near the end of its path it transfers some energy to neighboring atoms by atomic excitation.

1.5.5.2 Interactions of β Particles

Beta particles, with their charge of –1 (or +1), a mass of 0.000548 amu, and very fast travel cause less intense ionization than α particles, typically 100 to 300 ion pairs per centimeter of path in dry air. Because of their small mass, β particles are deflected easily and do not travel in a straight line. In dry air, their total path length is typically 20 m or less. β particles are more penetrating than α particles. Generally 1 mm or so of a dense material is sufficient to stop them. Rapid slowing or quick changes in direction cause β particles to emit x-rays (so-called bremsstrahlung).

1.5.5.3 Gamma Ray Interactions with Atoms

Gamma rays do not interact with matter in the same way as α and β particles because they have no charge and no mass and do not lose energy steadily in small, scattered amounts. Instead, they give it away in larger chunks in direct interactions. Three reactions between γ rays and atoms are discussed in the following sections.

1.5.5.3.1 The Photoelectric Effect
The γ photon gives all of its energy to the orbiting electron and ceases to exist. The electron is ejected from the atom and behaves like a β particle. The ejected electron is called a photoelectron.

1.5.5.3.2 The Compton Effect
This γ ray interaction is most important for γ photons with energies between 0.1 and 10 MeV. The incident γ ray is "scattered" by hitting an electron. The electron receives some of the γ ray energy and is ejected from the atom. A Compton electron is usually much more energetic than a photoelectron. It causes ionization just as a β particle does.

1.5.5.3.3 Pair Production
This γ ray interaction always occurs near an atomic nucleus that recoils. The γ ray gives its energy to the creation of an electron-positron pair. The minimum γ photon

energy that can do this is 1.02 MeV (the energy equivalent of two electrons). The process most often happens for high-energy γ rays.

In addition to these basic interactions there are other interactions of individual products of radioactive decay, not only with atom electrons of matter, but also nuclei. The interaction of emitted particles or other products of radioactive decay with matter determines the effect of ionizing radiation on abiotic and living matter, and is the principle enabling the measurement of radiation.

1.6 RADIONUCLIDES TODAY

More than 1,500 radionuclides are known today. Some occur in nature, but most are produced artificially. However, only 10% are important and are applied in practice [12]. The main factor that decides the importance and application of radionuclides is their half-life. The majority of important radionuclides applicable in science, technology, and industry have a sufficiently long half-life — months, years, tens of years, and even more — allowing long-term application, especially in the form of so-called closed radio emitters. Thanks to their chemical and pharmacokinetic properties, short-lived radionuclides used in nuclear medicine can be applied in radionuclide diagnosis and therapy in the form of open radio emitters. These are called radiopharmaceuticals and are administered to the organism directly (in most cases intravenously or orally). This section will introduce some of these radioisotopes. The application of ionizing radiation from radionuclides is very versatile; however, radionuclides may be hazardous to people and the environment.

1.6.1 Radionuclides and Radioactivity: Uses

The applications of radionuclides and radioactivity have been constantly growing in number, especially in chemistry, biology, medicine, archaeology, sciences, the food industry, and others. The energy contained in nuclei is used to produce electricity. Radionuclides are used in two major ways: for their chemical properties and as a source of radiation.

In nuclear medicine, for example, radionuclides and radioactivity are used in diagnosis and research: radioactive tracers are used to determine the anatomy and functioning of specific organs; technetium-labeled (^{99m}Tc) radiopharmaceuticals have a wide range of applications in static and dynamic scintigraphy of the kidneys, liver, lungs, heart, brain, and other organs as well as in the diagnosis of tumors; radioiodine ^{125}I is used for *in vitro* radioimmunoassays (RIAs). More powerful sources (especially ^{60}Co) γ rays or β particles are used in radiotherapy, including brachytherapy, immunotherapy, ion beam therapy, and boron neutron capture therapy.

Industrially and in mining, radionuclides are used as radioisotope tracers, in radiography and gauging, and in radiation processing to examine welds, detect leaks, and study the rate of wear of metals, and for analysis of a wide range of minerals and fuels.

In agriculture and animal husbandry, radionuclides can be used to produce higher crop yields and disease- and weather-resistant varieties of crops, to study how fertilizers and insecticides work, and to improve the production and health of domestic animals. In food preservation, irradiation is used to stop the sprouting of root crops after harvesting and to kill parasites and pests in fruits and vegetables.

Environmentally radionuclides are used to trace and analyze pollutants, to study the movement of surface water, and to measure water runoff from rain and snow, as well as the flow rates of streams and rivers.

Some radionuclides (e.g., the uranium group) can be directly applied in human activities and, at the same time, they are much-feared products of nuclear power engineering. The most frequently used radionuclides and their characteristics are shown in Table 1.1.

1.6.2 Radionuclides and the Environment: Dangers

When ionizing radiation passes through matter, the component atoms may be ionized or excited. In the case of interaction with tissue, the ionization or excitation of molecules can pose a danger for livings cells and damage them.

A number of radionuclides occur in nature (see Section 1.4), either of cosmogenic or terrestrial origin. However, these sources of radioactive radiation in the environment are natural, and in normal concentrations they have no negative effect on plant and animal cells. The only exception is the radioactive gas radon, ^{222}Rn. This gas is the product of radioactive decay of ^{238}U released from rocks and soils, and in larger amounts it is hazardous to people.

If radionuclides, particularly those that are artificially produced or originating in nuclear power engineering, are released into the environment through accident, poor disposal, or other means (regrettably also by using or testing atomic weapons), they can pose a real danger of radioactive contamination.

Radioactive contamination is the uncontrolled distribution of radioactive material in a given environment. Such contamination is typically the result of a loss of control of radioactive materials during the production or use of radioisotopes. Radioactive contamination may also be an inevitable result of certain processes in nuclear fuel reprocessing.

Nuclear fallout is the distribution of radioactive contamination from a nuclear explosion. It commonly refers to the radioactive dust created when a nuclear weapon explodes, although it can also refer to nuclear accidents from reactors in nuclear power plants.

The hazards of radioactive contamination to people and the environment depend on the nature of the radioactive contaminant, the level of contamination, and the extent of the spread of contamination. The remaining chapters of this book discuss the hazards and radiation safety connected with radionuclides in foods and the environment.

Finally, the radioactivity of radionuclides is used in many different human activities. I hope that new possibilities for beneficial applications will be found.

TABLE 1.1
The Most Frequently Used Radionuclides and Their Selected Characteristics

Nuclide	Half-life ($T_{1/2}$)	Decay	Application
^{3}H	12.3 years	β^-	Biology, ecology
^{14}C	5730 years	β^-	Biology, ecology, archaeology, paleontology, chemistry
^{18}F	110 minutes	β^+, EC	Nuclear medicine
^{32}P	4.3 days	β^-	Biology, nuclear medicine
^{51}Cr	27.7 days	EC	Nuclear medicine
^{57}Co	271 days	EC	Source of γ
^{58}Co	70.8 days	β^+, EC	Biology, nuclear medicine
^{60}Co	5.271 years	β^-	Source of γ, medical (radiotherapy) and industrial applications
^{67}Ga	48 hours	EC	Nuclear medicine, γ imaging
^{68}Ga	68 minutes	β^+, EC	Nuclear medicine
^{81m}Kr	13 seconds	IT	Nuclear medicine, γ imaging
^{81}Rb	4.6 hours	EC	Generator of ^{81m}Kr, γ imaging
^{90}Y	64 hours	β^-	Nuclear medicine (brachytherapy, immunotherapy)
^{99}Mo	66 hours	β^-	Generator of ^{99m}Tc
^{99m}Tc	6 hours	IT	Nuclear medicine, γ imaging
^{111}In	2.8 days	EC	Nuclear medicine, γ imaging
^{123}I	13.2 hours	EC	Nuclear medicine, γ imaging
^{125}I	60 days	EC	Nuclear medicine (RIAs), brachytherapy
^{131}I	8.04 days	β^-	Nuclear medicine, γ imaging, immunotherapy
^{133}Xe	5.3 days	β^-	Nuclear medicine, γ imaging
^{137}Cs	30 years	β^-	Source of γ, radiotherapy, brachytherapy
^{192}Ir	74.2 days	β^-, EC	Source of γ, brachytherapy
^{201}Tl	73 hours	EC	Nuclear medicine
^{226}Ra	1602 years	α	Source of α
^{232}Th	1.41×10^{10} years	α	Nuclear fuel (prospective)
^{235}U	7.1×10^8 years	α	Nuclear fuel, fission material
^{238}U	4.51×10^9 years	α	Nuclear fuel
^{239}Pu	2.44×10^4 years	α	Fission material
^{241}Am	458 years	α	Source of α and γ
^{252}Cf	2.65 years	α, SF	Source of n

Note: EC, electron capture; IT, isomeric transition; SF, spontaneous fission.

This can be achieved only if scientists and other responsible people are able to make wise choices when applying scientific discoveries.

The existence of radionuclides in the environment from other than natural sources is also associated with nuclear explosions and nuclear accidents. It is necessary to avoid tests of nuclear weapons and their application (including weapons containing depleted uranium). We do not yet satisfactorily know how to destroy industrial radioactive wastes. They decay naturally with time, more or less rapidly, depending on their half-life. Consequently confinement and storage techniques require accelerated research. Also, a reduction in the volume and activity of radioactive wastes is a high-priority research goal. The study of the long-term behavior of waste packages is also a major line of research. The discovery of transmutation procedures, such as accelerator-driven transmutation technologies (ADTTs), and their potential application for the cleanup and destruction of high-level waste from nuclear power plants is an example.

REFERENCES

1. Pullman, B., *The Atom in the History of Human Thought*, Oxford University Press, New York, 2001.
2. Thomson, J.J., *The Corpuscular Theory of Matter*, Constable & Co., London, 1907.
3. Kungl. Vetenskapsakademien [The Royal Swedish Academy of Sciences], *Asymptotic Freedom and Quantum ChromoDynamics: The Key to the Understanding of the Strong Nuclear Forces*, advanced information on the Nobel Prize in physics, 2004.
4. *Centennial of the Discovery of Radioactivity*, http://web.ccr.jussieu.fr/radioactivite/english/indispensable.htm.
5. *Wikipedia 2004*, Free Software Foundation, Inc., http://en.wikipedia.org/.
6. Kuny, W. and Schnitlmeister, J., *Tabellen der Atomkerne*, Akademie Verlag, Berlin, 1959.
7. Magill, J., *Nuclides.net — An Integrated Environment for Computation on Radionuclides and Their Radiation*, Springer, Berlin, 2003.
8. Nuclear Data Evaluation Laboratory, Korea Atomic Energy Research Institute, http://atom.kaeri.re.kr/ton/nuc6.html.
9. National Nuclear Data Centre, Brookhaven National Laboratory, http://www.nndc.bnl.gov/index.jsp.
10. Nuclear Data Centre, International Atomic Energy Agency, http://iaeand.iaea.or.at/.
11. *Radiation Decay, version 3.6*, http://www.gu.edu.au/school/eng/mmt/RadDec.html.
12. Ullmann, V., *Nuclear Physics and Physics of Ionizing Radiation* [in Czech], Jaderna fyzika a fyzika ionizujiciho zareni, http://www.sweb.cz/AstroNuklFyzika/JadRadFyzika.htm.
13. Magill, J. and Galy, J., *Radioactivity, Radionuclides, Radiation*, Springer, Berlin, 2004, chap. 4.
14. *The Official Web Site of the Nobel Foundation*, http://nobelprize.org/physics/laureates/.

2 Radionuclide Sources

Jeffrey S. Gaffney and Nancy A. Marley

CONTENTS

2.1 INTRODUCTION

We live on a planet that was created by the initial forces of the "big bang" and continues to be affected by both natural events and human activities. The global environment that surrounds us contains small amounts of radioactive (unstable) elements or radionuclides (radioisotopes) that are derived from primordial, secondary, cosmogenic, and anthropogenic sources. Radionuclides in the air, soil, water, and rocks that make up the Earth's geosphere and atmosphere can be transferred into the biosphere by many organisms and bioaccumulated in the food chain. Indeed, the well-known uptake by living organisms of measurable amounts of naturally produced radionuclides, such as ^{14}C, is used as a means of differentiating living from "fossil" carbon. Most of the radioactivity to which we are exposed daily comes from background natural sources commonly occurring in our surrounding environment and the buildings in which we live.

Chapter 1 defines radionuclides and discusses the most common types of ionizing radiation, namely α particles (energetic helium nuclei), β particles (energetic electrons), and γ radiation (high-frequency, highly energetic electromagnetic radiation). This chapter deals with the natural and anthropogenic sources of radionuclides found in the environment. Addressing all of the more than 1,500 known radionuclides is beyond the scope of this chapter. We will focus on isotopic species that are important contributors to overall radionuclide abundances in various media, whose distributions in air, water, and soil are the topic of later chapters. More detailed information can be found in more extensive books on the sources of radionuclides, both natural and man-made [1].

Traditionally radionuclides have been separated into three categories or types: (1) primordial and secondary, (2) cosmogenic, and (3) anthropogenic. Primordial radionuclides, such as uranium, thorium, and certain isotopes of potassium, have very long lifetimes and were produced at or before the creation of planet Earth. Secondary radionuclides are derived through radioactive decay of the long-lived primordial parent nuclides. These decay products are commonly referred to as daughters. Along with the parent sources, the daughters constitute radiogenic decay families or "chains" that are an important source of natural radioactivity. Cosmogenic radionuclides are formed by the interaction of cosmic rays with Earth's atmosphere or lithosphere, while anthropogenic radionuclides are formed from human activities that create artificial radionuclides or enhance the levels of certain radionuclides already present on Earth. In this chapter we discuss the three types of radionuclide sources separately and highlight some of the more important examples.

2.2   PRIMORDIAL AND SECONDARY RADIONUCLIDES

The primordial radionuclides have radioactive decay half-lives that are approximately Earth's age or older (i.e., about 4 to 5 billion years). Primordial radionuclides (and the radioactive decay products they produce) are an important source of Earth's radioactivity. These radionuclides play an important role in the Earth's processes. Indeed, primordial radionuclides, in particular a potassium isotope of mass 40 (^{40}K), have been suggested as a key source of long-term heat in the Earth's core over the past 4.5 billion years [2]. The human population is exposed to radiation from primordial radionuclides directly, as a result of external exposure, or through incorporation of these radionuclides into the body through inhalation or ingestion. The primordial radionuclides present when the Earth was formed that have half-lives less than 10^8 years have since decayed to undetectable levels. Furthermore, the primordial radionuclides with half-lives greater than 10^{10} years do not make significant contributions directly to background radiation because their half-lives are long and their specific radioactivity levels are low. However, they do contribute significantly to natural background levels of radioactivity through their radioactive progeny or daughters, which often have much shorter half-lives and lead to a chain of radioactive isotope production.

The primordial radionuclides compose a significant portion of the natural radionuclides present on Earth because they are significantly long-lived and have half-lives long enough to have been present at the beginning of the Earth's formation. Table 2.1 lists some of the more important primordial radionuclides and their half-lives. Included are uranium and thorium isotopes having half-lives on the order of 1 to 10 billion years. ^{232}Th, one of the most abundant of the primordial radionuclides, has a half-life of 1.4×10^{10} years and is found at concentrations of 1.5 to 20 ppm in most crustal rocks [1]. ^{238}U, another abundant primordial radionuclide, is typically found at concentrations in the low parts per million in minerals and rocks. Both ^{232}Th and ^{238}U are concentrated in coals and peats, indicating that the bioaccumulation of these species has occurred over long

TABLE 2.1
Some Important Primordial Radionuclides

Radionuclide	Half-life (Years)	Estimated Abundance in Crust (ppm)
^{40}K	1.38×10^9	2–3
^{87}Rb	4.8×10^{10}	3–9
^{138}La	1.1×10^{11}	1×10^2 to 2×10^2
^{147}Sm	1.1×10^{11}	0.5–1
^{187}Re	4.0×10^{10}	3–5×10^4
^{232}Th	1.4×10^{10}	1–20
^{235}U	7.0×10^8	0.3×10^2 to 3×10^2
^{238}U	4.5×10^9	0.5–5

periods of time. The humin and humic materials that are known to produce coals and peat are strong chelating agents for these and other radionuclides [3]. Indeed, the first discoveries of radioactivity and the isolation of important radionuclides by the Curies and other pioneers in this area came in work with pitchblende and peat known to be enriched in radionuclides through the interaction of organic materials with rocks and minerals containing radioactive isotopes and elements.

Uranium was identified as an element by the German chemist Martin Klaproth, who isolated it from samples of pitchblende in 1789. It was not until 1841 that uranium was isolated in metallic form by the French chemist Eugene-Melchior Peligot. Most of the early interest in this element grew from its ability to add color to ceramics and paints. In 1896 the applied physicist Antoine Henri Becquerel reported that all uranium salts are radioactive. This work led to his sharing the 1906 Nobel Prize in physics with Pierre and Marie Curie for the discovery of spontaneous radioactivity [4]. The three naturally occurring isotopes of uranium are ^{234}U, ^{235}U, and ^{238}U. ^{238}U, by far the most abundant of the three, has a half-life of 4.47×10^9 years. Thus about half of its original primordial level at Earth's formation remains. In comparison, ^{235}U is fairly depleted from its original levels, having passed through more than six half-lives since Earth's origin. These two isotopes are both primordial, but ^{234}U, having a much shorter half-life, would have essentially disappeared from the planet after more than 18,000 half-life periods since its formation. However, ^{234}U is a good example of a secondary radionuclide, as it is produced in small quantities by the radioactive decay of the parent ^{238}U (see Figure 2.1). As we discuss later, ^{235}U and other isotopes that are fissionable by neutrons have played an important role in anthropogenic radionuclide production.

The uranium isotopes are all radioactive, and their decay produces a number of secondary radioactive elements that continue to decay until they reach stable nuclei. This decay chain of radionuclides is commonly referred to as the uranium decay series. Similarly thorium, another primordial isotope with a long half-life, also has a decay series that leads to the formation of numerous naturally occurring

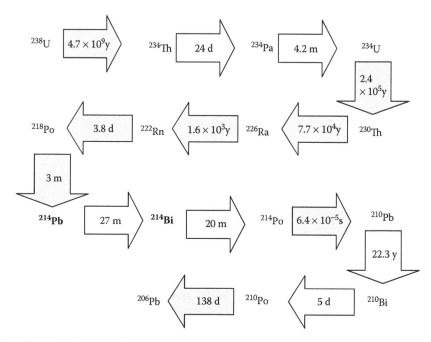

FIGURE 2.1 Uranium 238 decay, showing the main paths for the production of various radionuclides. Clear arrows indicate β decay and gray arrows are α processes. Half-lives for the decay processes are indicated inside the arrows. The major γ emitters are in bold letters. For complete radioactive decay processes, refer to *Table of Isotopes* and updates [5–7].

secondary radionuclides. Thus the key primordial radionuclides of uranium and thorium decay to many other radioactive isotopes that occur in the environment at different levels of abundance, depending on their own decay rates and those of their parents. Figure 2.1 and Figure 2.2 show the decay schemes for primordial ^{238}U and ^{232}Th, respectively. Figure 2.3 shows the decay processes for ^{235}U. Only the major pathways are shown in these figures, with the significant γ emitters highlighted in bold type. More detailed information on the isotopic decay processes, including minor pathways, can be obtained from the *Table of Isotopes* [5–7].

Other primordial isotopic species on the Earth's surface include ^{40}K, which has a half-life of 1.28×10^9 years. Potassium is quite an abundant element, composing more than 2% of the Earth's crustal mass. Of that amount, about 1.0×10^{-4} (0.01%) is ^{40}K atoms. ^{40}K can decay by γ emission (11% of the decay pathway) to give ^{40}Ar, and this is the basis for the potassium/argon methods used to age date very old rocks, meteorites, etc. ^{40}K can also emit a β particle and lead to the formation of ^{40}Ca (89% of the decay processes). Because of its ubiquity and biological uptake, ^{40}K is the most significant natural source of radioactivity ingested by humans.

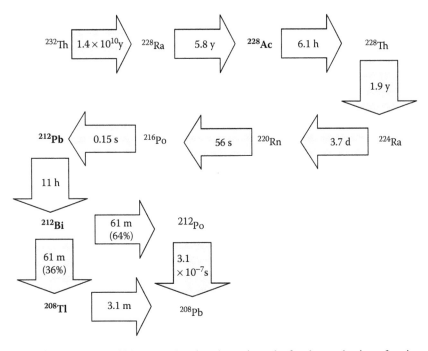

FIGURE 2.2 Thorium 232 decay, showing the main paths for the production of various radionuclides. Clear arrows indicate β decay and gray arrows are α processes. Half-lives for the decay processes are indicated inside the arrows. The major γ emitters are in bold letters. For complete radioactive decay processes, refer to *Table of Isotopes* and updates [5–7].

A very important and widespread secondary radionuclide is ^{222}Rn. This noble gas, with a half-life of 3.8 days, is produced from the longer-lived ^{226}Ra (half-life 1,600 years) formed by the decay of ^{238}U (see Figure 2.1). As a gas, ^{222}Rn can diffuse through the crustal material into the atmosphere, where it can be transported over continental regions. Its decay products attach themselves to fine atmospheric aerosols in the respirable size range. The dominant secondary radionuclide in this chain is ^{210}Pb, which has a half-life of 22.3 years. The fine aerosol ^{210}Pb and its daughters ^{210}Bi (half-life 5 days) and ^{210}Po (half-life 138 days) have been used to estimate the residence times of submicron aerosols in the environment [8–10]. ^{222}Ra and its progeny have been of particular concern as environmental hazards, particularly in homes and buildings where air infiltration rates can be low. Significant ^{222}Rn from ground-source uranium parents (see Figure 2.1) can concentrate in the lower levels of buildings (cellars, basements, etc.) and lead to potential inhalation risks in indoor environments [11].

^{210}Pb is another very ubiquitous secondary radionuclide that is formed from ^{238}U decay via ^{222}Rn (see Figure 2.1). Because it attaches itself to fine aerosols

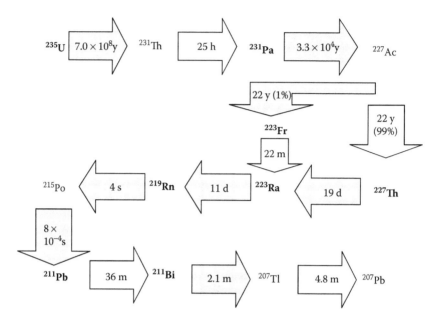

FIGURE 2.3 Uranium 235 decay, showing the main paths for the production of various radionuclides. Clear arrows indicate β decay and gray arrows are α processes. Half-lives for the decay processes are indicated inside the arrows. The major γ emitters are in bold letters. For complete radioactive decay processes, refer to *Table of Isotopes* and updates [5–7].

in the lower to mid troposphere once it is produced from the gaseous ^{222}Rn, ^{210}Pb can spread over significant distances. Indeed, a significant amount of ^{210}Pb is usually present in the upper sections of soil cores because of the atmospheric deposition of ^{210}Pb (half-life 22.3 years). Concentrations of ^{210}Pb usually decrease as a function of distance downward in soil cores, gradually diminishing from the surface to a fairly constant level within about 1 m of the surface. The background level of ^{210}Pb in subsurface soils is due to ^{222}Rn decay as the gas diffuses from soil and rock matrices. This background level of ^{210}Pb is considered to be supported by the local soil environment. The "excess" ^{210}Pb found in the soil closer to the surface is due to ^{222}Rn gas that is dispersed through the lower atmosphere and decays to produce ^{210}Pb, which becomes attached to fine aerosol particles and is deposited on soil surfaces by wet and dry deposition. The presence of this "excess" ^{210}Pb in surface soils due to atmospheric deposition has been useful for estimating soil sedimentation rates and erosion rates in many environments [12–17].

While many of the primordial and cosmogenic radionuclides are concentrated in Earth's lithosphere, significant amounts of ^{14}C, ^{238}U, and other radionuclides are found in the oceans as well. These accumulations are due to the equilibration of ^{14}CO$_2$ with ocean waters and the dissolution of minerals into fresh and ocean waters from rocks and soil erosion. Many primordial and secondary radionuclides are also found in fresh surface waters and groundwaters at low concentrations.

These are typically chemically bound or chelated by dissolved organic substances, principally humic and fulvic acids, that can limit the bioavailability of these materials in the natural environment [3].

2.3 COSMOGENIC RADIONUCLIDES

Cosmogenic radionuclides are formed by interactions of highly energetic cosmic particles with Earth's atmosphere and surface that lead to the formation of radioactive isotopes [18]. Some important cosmogenically produced radionuclides and their lifetimes are shown in Table 2.2.

Galactic cosmic rays that are capable of nuclear interactions lead to the direct formation of radionuclides and also generate secondary particles, particularly neutrons, that can result in the production of important radionuclides including ^{3}H, ^{7}Be, ^{10}Be, ^{14}C, and ^{22}Na. Most of these interactions occur in Earth's atmosphere, particularly in the stratosphere and upper troposphere. However, some minor production of radioisotopes also occurs at the Earth's surface (e.g., ^{10}Be, ^{26}Al, and ^{21}Ne) and their presence is an important indicator of cosmic ray activity. The differences in production rates in the atmosphere and surface are primarily due to the strong attenuation of many cosmic particles and secondary particles by Earth's atmosphere, with the result that more high-energy particle interactions occur in the upper atmosphere than at the surface, where the flux is smaller.

Production rates of many cosmogenic radionuclides depend on incoming cosmic particle intensities, which can be affected by Earth's magnetic field or can vary due to solar activity (e.g., sunspots or solar flares). The variations in the cosmic radiation fluxes lead to some temporal and spatial variability in the production of these radionuclides. Thus relatively short-term variations (on the order of days) and seasonal variations can result from solar events and changes in cosmic ray intensities. In addition, variability in latitudinal production arises because Earth's magnetic field can focus incoming cosmic rays, leading to more significant production at higher latitudes. The northern lights (the aurora borealis)

TABLE 2.2
Some Important Cosmogenically Produced
Radionuclides and Their Half-Lives

Radionuclide	Half-Life	Major Source
^{3}H	12.3 years	Atmospheric N, O
^{7}Be	53.3 days	Atmospheric N, O
^{10}Be	1.5×10^6 years	Atmosphere N, O, surface O
^{14}C	5.73×10^3 years	Atmospheric N
^{26}Al	7.1×10^5 years	Surface Si, meteorites
^{36}Cl	3.1×10^5 years	Surface Ca, K

are evidence of the increased production of radionuclides and the atmospheric effects of cosmic rays on the atmosphere at higher latitudes.

Cosmic radiation consists primarily of highly energetic particles, including α particles and neutrons. Their effects in the upper atmosphere lead to nuclear interactions with nitrogen and oxygen atoms and molecules resulting in the production of ^{14}C and ^{7}Be and other radionuclides, directly or via secondary neutron interactions. These same types of nuclear reactions can occur during aboveground nuclear tests that release energetic particles into the atmosphere. These reactions produce secondary particles (neutrons, protons, etc.) that can generate the same radionuclides as normal cosmic radiation exposures. Thus, during the 1950s, significant amounts of "bomb carbon" (^{14}C produced from aboveground nuclear tests) were produced, along with other radionuclides that will be discussed later in this chapter, by the same processes that occur naturally.

^{14}C is one of the more important natural radionuclides, being produced in the atmosphere by cosmic particle bombardment of nitrogen atoms. Once formed, the atomic ^{14}C is rapidly oxidized to carbon dioxide in the upper atmosphere. The ^{14}C-labeled carbon dioxide, quite a stable molecule, is mixed from the upper atmosphere down into the troposphere, where it is taken up by plants during photosynthesis. As herbivores and omnivores ingest plants for food, the ^{14}C is carried throughout the food chain, ultimately labeling all living things on the surface of the planet. With a half-life of 5.73×10^3 years, the abundance of ^{14}C has been used to differentiate recent carbon present in samples from "fossil" carbon derived from petroleum that is hundreds of millions of years old and is quite "dead" with regard to ^{14}C content [19]. ^{14}C is also the basis for carbon dating of organic artifacts in archeology.

Cosmic particle-driven neutron spallation reactions near the Earth's surface can lead to the formation of some important radionuclides that have been used for geochronology, such as ^{10}Be, ^{26}Al, and ^{36}Cl. Estimation of the production rates of cosmogenic nuclides requires an understanding of the cross sections for the nuclear reactions, along with estimates of cosmic ray fluxes that vary with geomagnetic latitude and altitude. Modeling that incorporates experimentally derived cross sections for gases and minerals has been used to estimate radionuclide production rates [20,21]. These production rates are then compared with direct measurements to evaluate the estimated results and also to probe past cosmic ray activity by examining the variance and concentrations of surface radionuclides of various lifetimes. Since the first measurements of ^{14}C by Willard Libby and coworkers [22], these cosmogenic isotopes have been used for geochronology, becoming important tools for the "dating" of events in geochemistry and geomorphology.

An extraterrestrial source for some of the heavier cosmogenic nuclides such as ^{26}Al is meteoric material that strikes the atmosphere or Earth's surface. Cross sections for atmospheric production of this radioisotope are small, because ^{26}Al is largely produced from argon, which composes only 1% of the atmosphere by volume. In contrast, the production of ^{26}Al can be quite high on the mineral surfaces of meteors because of the higher cosmic ray exposures in space. This difference has led to the use of ^{26}Al to evaluate meteoritic material deposition on the Earth's surface and to measure ice surface ages in the Antarctic [23,24].

There are indeed many trace-level cosmogenically produced radionuclides besides the ones we have discussed here, including ^{18}F, ^{22}Na, ^{24}Na, ^{31}Si, ^{32}Si, ^{32}P, ^{33}P, ^{35}S, ^{37}Ar, ^{38}Cl, ^{38}Mg, ^{38}S, ^{39}Ar, ^{39}Cl, and ^{80}Kr, as well as stable radionuclides like ^{3}He [1]. Many of the cosmogenic radioisotopes with longer half-lives are difficult to measure with conventional radiochemical counting methods. Because they have low radioactivity levels, they are measured directly by using accelerator mass spectrometry methods that have enhanced sensitivity and speed. Cosmogenic radioisotopes have been used to estimate surface ages of the Earth because their general production rates have remained fairly constant over time. Examination of the surface concentrations of the longer-lived radionuclides clearly indicates that Earth's surface has been exposed to cosmic radiation for millions of years, at a minimum. These data have been used as an effective argument against the concept of a much shorter time for Earth's creation that has been put forth by some creationist philosophies.

2.4 ANTHROPOGENIC SOURCES

Most of the radionuclides present on Earth are from primordial or cosmogenic sources, as noted above. During the early 1930s, a series of events that would change history and the world we live in began in the physics and chemistry communities. Following Enrico Fermi's lead in exploring the interactions of heavy nuclei with neutrons, Otto Hahn and Fritz Strassman attempted to make heavier elements (transuranics) by bombarding uranium with neutrons. They were able to identify the production of ^{141}Ba, which was correctly explained by Lise Meitner and Otto Frisch [25] as a fission product of ^{235}U. Soon, Niels Bohr and others recognized that the release of very large amounts of energy from nuclear fission might be useful for both peaceful and military applications. Letters from Bohr to Einstein and from Einstein to President Franklin Roosevelt ultimately led to the initiation of the Manhattan Project in the U.S. in June 1942 [26].

As part of the Manhattan Project, a group led by Enrico Fermi began to build a uranium-based reactor that they hoped would demonstrate the potential for a controlled chain reaction starting with ^{235}U. On December 2, 1942, the first self-sustained chain reaction, using enriched uranium oxide moderated by graphite rods, was achieved at the University of Chicago's Stagg Field stadium. This initial experiment demonstrating controlled nuclear fission led to the development of atomic weapons and nuclear industries in medicine and energy [26]. It also was the dawn of development of many radionuclides produced by humans for widely ranging uses including nuclear reactors, nuclear medicine, and nuclear weapons.

Nuclear fission is the process by which neutrons produce chain reactions in a nuclear reactor. When a fissionable nucleus is hit by a thermal or slow neutron, the nucleus can interact with the neutron and divide (fission) into two smaller nuclei, releasing neutrons and energy that initiate the splitting of more fissionable atoms, leading to a chain reaction. ^{235}U is the most abundant naturally available isotope that can undergo fission. Gaseous diffusion and other methods are used to enrich and separate the small amount of ^{235}U (0.72% natural abundance) from the predominantly ^{238}U found in nature. For most nuclear reactors, such as the light-water reactors, the enrichment required for a sustained nuclear reaction is approximately 10-fold. The more significant enrichment of ^{235}U required for atomic weapons is a difficult and expensive task.

In a nuclear reactor, the chain reaction with ^{235}U releases energy and neutrons and produces a number of side products, including isotopes of plutonium from neutron capture by ^{238}U in the fuel rods. ^{239}Pu produced through exposure of ^{238}U to neutrons is also fissionable. Both ^{235}U and ^{239}Pu have been used in nuclear reactors and in atomic weapons. Indeed, the first atomic weapons used in World War II, "Little Boy" and "Fat Man," were bombs that used ^{235}U and ^{239}Pu, respectively. Other fissionable materials, including ^{233}U and ^{232}Th, could conceivably be used in nuclear fuel cycles, although currently ^{235}U and ^{239}Pu are the main fuels used. ^{239}Pu is produced from ^{238}U by neutron irradiation, usually in $^{235}U/^{238}U$ "breeder" reactors.

Fission reactions lead to the formation of many isotopes (both stable and radioactive) from a wide variety of elements, as many fragment combinations are possible and do occur. For ^{235}U, the addition of one neutron would lead to two fission nuclei of 118 mass units if the process gave two equally sized nuclei. However, the fission reaction leads mostly to fragments of unequal sizes. For the case of ^{235}U, the major fission products are ^{137}Cs and ^{90}Sr. During aboveground testing of atomic bombs, a significant amount of anthropogenic radionuclides was released into the stratosphere and upper troposphere. This material became attached to particulate matter in the atmosphere and was deposited worldwide as "radioactive fallout."

Early on, bombardment of ^{238}U with neutrons was considered the only source of ^{238}Pu, ^{239}Pu, ^{240}Pu, and ^{241}Pu because plutonium was not a known natural radionuclide until its discovery in 1940 by Glenn Seaborg and colleagues. The 15 known isotopes of plutonium are mostly short-lived. The most important of these, as noted above, is ^{239}Pu, which is fissionable and has a long half-life (2.4×10^4 years). Not until the early 1970s did discovery of the remains of a natural fission reactor system in the Oklo district of Gabon, Africa, provide evidence that plutonium production could occur naturally [27–29]. The Oklo area is very high in uranium. Analysis of mines there yielded anomalous isotopic data indicating that neutron chain reaction events might have occurred under natural water mediation of the deposits. Furthermore, very low levels of ^{239}Pu produced more recently by normal neutron capture in uranium cores were measured in samples from the site [27,29]. Although these results demonstrate that natural production of ^{239}Pu is possible, it is safe to say that most of the plutonium currently present on Earth came from anthropogenic sources.

Many of the anthropogenic radionuclides produced from nuclear power or nuclear bomb tests have reasonably short half-lives with the exception of ^{239}Pu. Some other anthropogenic radionuclides include ^{131}I, which has a half-life of

TABLE 2.3
Some Anthropogenically Produced Radionuclides
and Their Half-Lives

Radionuclide	Half-life (Years)	Major Source
^{3}H	12.3	Atmospheric weapons tests, reactors
^{14}C	5.73×10^3	Atmospheric weapons tests
^{90}Sr	2.9×10^1	Reactors, weapons tests
^{99}Tc	2.1×10^5	^{99}Mo decay, nuclear medicine
^{129}I	1.6×10^7	Reactors, weapons tests
^{137}Cs	3.0×10^1	Reactors, weapons tests

8 days and is used in the treatment of thyroid cancer. Space limitations allow us to mention only some of the more important members of this large group. Since the cessation of aboveground testing, a number of the shorter-lived radioisotopes have already decreased and eventually will be lost; these include ^{90}Sr and ^{137}Cs, which have half-lives of approximately 30 years. In addition, a number of radio-isotopes, including ^{3}H, ^{11}C, ^{13}N, ^{14}C, ^{15}O, ^{99}Tc, ^{123}I, ^{125}I, and ^{131}I, are produced by the use of special equipment (nuclear reactors, cyclotrons, etc.) developed in the high-energy physics community and used routinely in nuclear medicine [30]. Some of the more important anthropogenic radionuclides are listed in Table 2.3, along with their half-lives.

2.5 CONCLUDING REMARKS

It should be noted that the sources of radioactivity to which the average person is exposed during a lifetime are dominated by the natural sources (i.e., the primordial and secondary radionuclides and the cosmogenic radionuclides). Anthropogenic material accounts for a small fraction of naturally occurring radioactivity. As estimated by the National Council on Radiation Protection and Measurement [31], exposure to radiation from artificial sources is only about 18% of the total human exposure in the U.S., and most of that exposure is from medical x-rays, nuclear medicine, etc. Exposures due to nuclear energy and fallout are responsible for less than 1% of the background exposure (see Figure 2.4). Many fallout materials have fairly short half-lives, and their levels are decreasing rapidly. Aboveground testing largely stopped when the U.S., the USSR, and the U.K. signed a nuclear test ban treaty on August 5, 1963. France and the Republic of China continued to test nuclear weapons aboveground and in the oceans until 1996, but these tests were few in comparison with the aboveground tests of the U.S. and USSR. Although it has not been approved by the U.S., a comprehensive test ban treaty drawn up by 37 nations in 1996 is likely to prevent the kind of aboveground nuclear testing that led to the dispersal of significant amounts of radionuclides globally, barring a nuclear war.

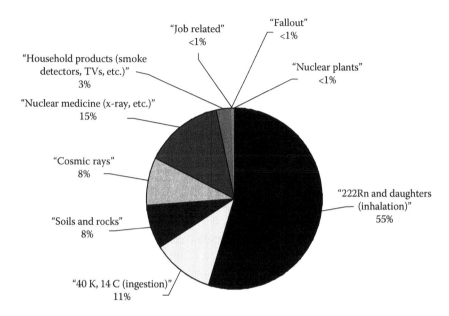

FIGURE 2.4 Relative radiation exposure estimates for the U.S. population, based on estimates from Curtis et al. [29].

Most of the radionuclides to which we are currently exposed in our foods and the environment come primarily from the naturally occurring primordial, secondary, and cosmogenic sources. Only during catastrophic events such as the 1986 Chernobyl reactor disaster or the testing of an atomic device aboveground are releases of anthropogenic radionuclides significant on a regional or global scale. Other sources of radionuclide release are tied to the nuclear energy industry in the transport of fuel rods and the reprocessing and disposal of spent fuel rods. In many instances spent uranium fuel rods are allowed to sit in interim cooling sites (ponds or air-cooled containers) so that the short-lived radionuclides produced during fission and neutron release can decay before the rods are reprocessed with the extraction of ^{239}Pu and unburned ^{235}U. Alternatively, the longer-lived radionuclide waste is placed in a geologic repository like the Yucca Mountain site. Other sources of radioactivity include medical radioactive sources used for nuclear medicine, typically operated in hospitals in major cities. These are localized sources and are not considered in this chapter. As they are of potential concern as sources of radioactivity, they are strongly regulated by various federal government agencies, as well as by the International Atomic Energy Agency.

ACKNOWLEDGMENTS

The submitted manuscript has been created by the University of Chicago as operator of Argonne National Laboratory under contract no. W-31-109-ENG-38 with the U.S. Department of Energy. The U.S. government retains for itself, and others acting on its behalf, a paid-up, nonexclusive, irrevocable worldwide license in said article to reproduce, prepare derivative works, distribute copies to the public, and perform publicly and display publicly, by or on behalf of the government. The authors' work is supported by the U.S. Department of Energy, Office of Science, Office of Biological and Environmental Research under contract no. W-31-109-ENG-38.

REFERENCES

1. Eisenbud, M. and Gesell, T., *Environmental Radioactivity from Natural, Industrial and Military Sources*, 4th ed., Academic Press, New York, 1997.
2. Murthy, V.R., Van Westernen, W., and Fei, Y., Experimental evidence that potassium is a substantial radioactive heat source in planetary cores, *Nature*, 423, 163–165, 2003.
3. Gaffney, J.S., Marley, N.A., and Clark, S.B., eds., *Humic/Fulvic Acids and Organic Colloidal Materials in the Environment*, ACS Symposium Series 651, American Chemical Society, Washington, DC, 1996.
4. Becquerel, A.H., Biography, in *Nobel Lectures. Physics 1901–1921*, Elsevier, Amsterdam, 1967.
5. Firestone, R.B., Shirley, V.S., Baglin, C.M., Chu, S.Y.F., and Zipkin, J., eds., *Table of Isotopes*, 8th ed., John Wiley & Sons, New York, 1996.
6. Firestone, R.B., Chu, S.Y.F., and Baglin, C.M., *Update to the 8th Edition of Table of the Isotopes*, John Wiley & Sons, New York, 1998.
7. Firestone, R.B., Chu, S.Y.F., and Baglin, C.M., *Update to the 8th Edition of Table of the Isotopes*. John Wiley & Sons, New York, 1999.
8. Gaffney, J.S., Marley, N.A., and Cunningham, M.M., Natural radionuclides in fine aerosols in the Pittsburgh area. *Atmos. Environ.*, 38, 3191–3200, 2004.
9. Marley, N.A., Gaffney, J.S., Orlandini, K.A., Drayton, P.J., and Cunningham, M.M., An improved method for the separation of ^{210}Bi and ^{210}Po from ^{210}Pb using solid phase extraction disk membranes: environmental applications, *Radiochim. Acta*, 85, 71–78, 1999.
10. Marley, N.A., Gaffney, J.S., Cunningham, M.M., Orlandini, K.A., Paode, R., and Drayton, P.J., Measurement of ^{210}Pb, ^{210}Po, and ^{210}Bi in size fractionated atmospheric aerosols: an estimate of fine aerosol residence times, *Aerosol Sci. Technol.*, 32, 569–583, 2000.
11. U.S. EPA, *A Citizen's Guide to Radon: The Guide to Protecting Yourself and Your Family from Radon*, EPA 402-K-02-006, Indoor Environments Division (6609J), U.S. Environmental Protection Agency, Washington, DC, revised May 2004.
12. Walsh, J.J., Premuzic, E.T., Gaffney, J.S., Rowe, G.T., Harbottle, G., Balsam, W.L., and Betzer, P.R., Organic storage of CO_2 within the last century on the continental slope off the mid-Atlantic bight, *Deep Sea Res.*, 32, 853–885, 1985.
13. Matisoff, G., Bonniwell, E.C., and Whiting, P.J., Soil erosion and sediment sources in an Ohio watershed using beryllium-7, cesium-137, and lead-210. *J. Environ. Qual.*, 31, 54–61, 2002.
14. Walling, E.E. and Woodward, J.C., Use of radiometric fingerprints to derive information on suspended sediment sources, in *Erosion and Sediment Transport Monitoring Programmes in River Basins*, publication 210, International Association of Hydrological Sciences, Wallingford, UK, 1992, pp. 153–164.

15. Olley, J.M., Murray, A.S., Mackenzie, D.H., and Edwards, K., Identifying sediment sources in a gullied catchment using natural and anthropogenic radioactivity, *Water Resour. Res.*, 29, 1037–1043, 1993.

16. Walling, D.E., Owens, P.N., and Leeks, G.J.L., Fingerprinting suspended sediment sources in the catchment of the River Ouse, Yorkshire, UK, *Hydrol. Processes*, 13, 955–975, 1999.

17. Owens, P.N., Walling, D.E., and Leeks, G.J.L., Use of floodplain sediment cores to investigate recent historical changes in overbank sedimentation rates and sediment sources in the catchment of the River Ouse, Yorkshire, UK, *Catena*, 36, 21–47, 1999.

18. Bierman, P.R., Using in situ produced cosmogenic isotopes to estimate rates of landscape evolution: a review from the geomorphic perspective, *J. Geophys. Res.*, 99, 13885–13896, 1994.

19. Tanner, R.L. and Gaffney, J.S., Carbon isotopes as tracers of biogenic and fossil-fuel derived carbon transport in the atmosphere, in *Fossil Fuels Utilization: Environmental Concerns*, R. Markuszewski and B.D. Blaustein, eds., ACS Symposium Series 319, American Chemical Society, Washington, DC, 1986, pp. 267–276.

20. Masarik, J. and Reedy, R.C., Terrestrial cosmogenic-nuclide production systematics calculated from numerical simulations, *Earth Planet. Sci. Lett.*, 136, 381–395, 1995.

21. Lal, D., Cosmic ray labeling of erosion surfaces: in-situ nuclide production rates and erosion models, *Earth Planet. Sci. Lett.*, 104, 424–439, 1991.

22. Arnold, J.R. and Libby, W.F., Age determinations by radiocarbon content: checks with samples of known age, *Science*, 110, 678–680, 1949.

23. Evans, J.C. Rancitelli, L.A., and Reeves, J.H., ^{26}Al content of Antarctic meteorites: implications for terrestrial ages and bombardment history, *Proceedings of the 10th Lunar and Planetary Science Conference*, Lunar and Planetary Institute, Houston, 1061–1072, 1979.

24. Evans, J.C. and Reeves, J.H., ^{26}Al survey of Antarctic meteorites, *Earth Planet. Sci. Lett.*, 82, 223–230, 1987.

25. Meitner, L. and Frisch, O.R., Disintegration of uranium by neutrons: a new type of nuclear reaction, *Nature*, 143, 239–240, 1939.

26. U.S. DOE, *The First Reactor: 40th Anniversary Commemorative Edition*, DOE/NE-0046, Office of the Assistant Secretary for Nuclear Energy, U.S. Department of Energy, Washington, DC, 1982.

27. Cowan, G.A., A natural fission reactor, *Sci. Am.*, 235, 36, 1976.

28. Myers, W.A. and Lindner, M., Precise determination of the natural abundance of ^{237}Np and ^{239}Pu in Katanga pitchblende, *J. Inorg. Nucl. Chem.*, 33, 3233–3238, 1971.

29. Curtis, D., Fabryka-Martin, J., Dixon, P., and Cramer, J., Nature's uncommon elements: plutonium and technetium, *Geochem. Cosmochim. Acta*, 63, 275–285, 1999.

30. Rayudu, G.V., Production of radionuclides for medicine, *Semin. Nucl. Med.*, 20, 100–110, 1990.

31. NCRP, *Ionizing Radiation Exposure of the Population of the United States*, report 93, ISBN 0-913392-91-X, National Council on Radiation Protection and Measurements, Bethesda, MD, 1987.

3 Radioactivity in the Air

Peter Carny

CONTENTS

3.1 COSMIC RAYS

Cosmic radiation contributes to a great extent to the total radiation exposure of human beings. This radiation has its origins in outer space; one component (protons with energies ~100 MeV) is generated by the Sun, all other components are primarily from our galaxy, and the origin of some high-energy protons (with energies ~10^{19} eV) is probably extragalactic.

Cosmic rays enter our atmosphere as protons, α particles, heavier nuclei, and electrons. These cosmic particles have an energy from 10^8 eV to greater than 10^{20} eV. After their interaction with atoms and molecules in the atmosphere, a lot of secondary charged and uncharged particles are generated: protons, neutrons, pions, nuclei with lower Z values, and further nucleonic cascades, electrons, muons, and photons. Exposure from cosmic rays at ground level is primarily from muons, electrons, photons, and neutrons. This exposure is realized as external exposure. The intensity of cosmic rays and the dose absorbed depends on the layer of the atmosphere above the ground; in other words, it quite strongly depends on the

TABLE 3.1
Typical Volume Activities of the Most Important
Cosmogenic Radionuclides in the Air, Typical
Annual Effective Dose Caused By These Nuclides

Nuclide	^3H	^{14}C
Average volume activity in air (Bq/m³)	1.4×10^{-3}	56.3×10^{-3}
Annual effective dose (µSv/year)	0.01	12

altitude and on geographic latitude. The thicker the layer of atmosphere, the lower the absorbed dose. At sea level, the typical annual effective dose due to cosmic rays is about 350 µSv/year (from this, 80 µSv/year is typically due to neutrons). According to the United Nations Scientific Committee on the Effects of Atomic Radiation (UNSCEAR) [1], the world average (altitude and latitude averaged) annual effective dose due to cosmic rays is about 460 µSv/year (from this 120 µSv/year is due to neutrons). People living at altitudes of 2 to 3 km above the sea level could obtain an annual effective dose from cosmic rays of up to 2000 µSv/year.

3.2 COSMOGENIC RADIONUCLIDES

Radioactivity in air due to cosmic radiation is a source of external irradiation of human beings as well as internal irradiation. Internal irradiation is caused by cosmogenic radionuclides present in the air. Cosmogenic radionuclides are products of cosmic ray interactions in the atmosphere. As a result of these interactions, many lower Z nuclei are created. The most important cosmogenic nuclei are ^3H and ^{14}C. Their importance is shown by their role in human body metabolism. They are contributors to the internal irradiation of human beings via inhalation and ingestion. Typical average volumes in air and average annual effective doses from these cosmogenic radionuclides are given in Table 3.1 (according to UNSCEAR [1]).

The global inventory of ^3H is about 1275×10^{15} Bq and the annual production rate is 72×10^{15} Bq/year. The global inventory of ^{14}C is about 13×10^{18} Bq and the annual production rate is 1.5×10^{15} Bq/year. Both these cosmogenic nuclides (^3H and ^{14}C) are released to the environment as man-made nuclides from nuclear installations and have been released during nuclear weapons tests.

3.3 TERRESTRIAL RADIATION

3.3.1 TERRESTRIAL RADIATION: RADON AND DECAY PRODUCTS IN THE AIR AND OTHER RADIONUCLIDES THAT CAN BE INHALED

Radionuclides that have a terrestrial origin (primordial radionuclides) are present at various levels in every kind of matter in nature. This means they are naturally present, even in the human body.

TABLE 3.2
Typical Volume Activities of Radionuclides From the Uranium and Thorium Series in Air (Bq/m³), with the Exception of ^{222}Rn and ^{220}Rn

Nuclide	^{238}U	^{230}Th	^{226}Ra	^{210}Pb	^{210}Po	^{232}Th	^{228}Ra	^{228}Th	^{235}U
Average volume activity	1×10^{-6}	0.5×10^{-6}	1×10^{-6}	500×10^{-6}	50×10^{-6}	0.5×10^{-6}	1×10^{-6}	1×10^{-6}	0.05×10^{-6}

Terrestrial radiation is formed mainly by radionuclides from the ^{238}U and ^{232}Th series and from ^{40}K. These radionuclides irradiate our body with γ radiation (externally and internally) and β and α radiation (mainly internally). External irradiation is caused by radioactivity present in the soil and in any other material surrounding our bodies, including the air. Internal irradiation is caused by radionuclides that are inhaled or ingested. In this chapter we discuss radioactivity in the air; therefore, the most important exposure pathway is inhalation.

Irradiation and effective doses caused by inhalation of terrestrial nuclides from the air result from the presence of dust particles containing radionuclides from the ^{238}U and ^{232}Th series. Typical amounts of ^{238}U and ^{232}Th in the air are about 1 μBq/m³. If the dust particles in air are formed by organic matter, then their uranium and thorium content is significantly lower. On the other hand, if dust particles are formed by fly ash (from the burning of coal), then the uranium and thorium content may be much higher. Typical volumes of uranium and thorium series radionuclides in air (according to UNSCEAR [1]) are shown in Table 3.2. The average annual effective dose from inhalation of uranium and thorium series radionuclides in air (without contributions of radon [^{222}Rn] and thoron [^{220}Rn]) is typically about 5 to 10 μSv/year.

The most important and dominant contributors to inhalation dose are decay products of radon. Radon and its decay products in the air are the main natural sources of irradiation in human beings.

Inhalation of radon (and its decay products) and thoron (so-called thoron) from the air causes their deposition on the lining of the lungs. These deposited radionuclides irradiate the lungs and other tissues, especially by α particles, as well as β and γ radiation.

What is the mechanism by which radon and thoron enter the atmosphere? Both nuclides are the gaseous products of the decay of radium isotopes ^{226}Ra and ^{224}Ra, which belong to the uranium and thorium series and are present in any terrestrial materials (in solid matrix). Some radon atoms are released from the solid matrix and escape from the mineral grain into the pore space. These radon atoms are then transported by diffusion and advection, and are either decayed or released to the atmosphere. As a result, the volume activity of radon and its daughter products in the air is observed. The process of radon emanation (escape from the solid matrix) and transportation is influenced by many factors such as moisture, geological factors, and climate or meteorological conditions. Radon and its decay products are released not only from the soil or from the mineral grains, but can also be released from various building materials. Radon can penetrate from the ground around the foundations of buildings. Under some special conditions radon can be "withdrawn" from the ground to the atmosphere of buildings at higher entry rates. These phenomena can cause indoor radon activity to be higher than outdoor radon activity. The volume activity of radon in the air is therefore classified as "outdoor" activity and "indoor" activity.

The typical outdoor volume activity of radon and thoron in the air is 10 Bq/m³. There are many places in the world with lower volume activities (from 1 Bq/m³) and with higher average activities (more than 100 Bq/m³) of radon and thoron in the air. Lower activities are typical for coastal regions and small islands. Higher activities are typical for sites with higher radon emanation and release to the atmosphere. The typical outdoor volume activity of radon results in a typical annual effective dose of about 100 μSv/year. Significant variations in radon volume activity in the air are usually observed in a given place during the day (solar radiation causes heating and transport of radon to higher layers of the atmosphere, thus expected air volume activity near the ground will be lower; at night and in the early morning, temperature inversions cause radon atoms to be closer to the ground, thus expected air volume activity near the ground will be higher), as a result of precipitation (rain can wash radon and its decay products from the higher air layers, causing an increase in radon levels near the ground), or as a result of winds.

The typical indoor volume activity of radon is about 10 to 100 Bq/m³ and thoron is about 2 to 20 Bq/m³. The typical indoor volume activity of radon produces a typical annual effective dose of about 1000 μSv/year (1 mSv/year) (Table 3.3). The indoor volume activity of radon varies significantly depending on geological conditions and the building materials used. Numerous surveys in many countries have been performed to determine the radon activity in dwellings. For example, the mean radon volume activity in dwellings in the Czech Republic

TABLE 3.3
Typical Volume Activities of ²²²Rn and ²²⁰Rn in the Air (Outdoor and Indoor) and Typical Annual Effective Doses (Outdoor and Indoor)

Nuclide	²²²Rn	²²⁰Rn
Average volume activity in outdoor air (Bq/m³)	10	10
Average volume activity in indoor air (Bq/m³)	10–100	2–20
Annual effective dose (μSv/year), outdoor	100	~10
Annual effective dose (μSv/year), indoor	1000	~90

Note: Values are based on data from UNSCEAR [1].

TABLE 3.4
Typical Content of Radionuclides in Building Materials in Slovakia (According to Cabanekova [4]) and Typical Mass Activity (in Bq/kg)

	^{40}K	^{226}Ra	^{232}Th
Bricks	600 (varies from 100 to 1000)	60 (varies from 30 to 300)	70 (varies from 100 to 600)
Concrete	300 (varies from 100 to 600)	50 (varies from 10 to 100)	30 (varies from 5 to 70)

is about 140 Bq/m^3, but buildings with values as high as 20,000 Bq/m^3 have been found. The mean radon volume activity in dwellings in Slovakia is about 90 Bq/m^3 and the highest values found have been about 4000 Bq/m^3 (see Table 3.4). On the other hand, the mean radon volume activity in dwellings in Egypt is about 9 Bq/m^3 and maximal values found have been about 20 Bq/m^3.

As was stated above, building materials (and the radioactivity of the uranium and thorium series in them) can affect indoor radon activities. Therefore in many countries there is legislation that defines the maximal permitted activity in building materials. For example, in Slovakia, the maximal permitted mass activity of ^{226}Ra in building materials is 120 Bq/kg.

3.3.2 TERRESTRIAL RADIONUCLIDES IN THE AIR DUE TO INDUSTRIAL ACTIVITIES (OTHER THAN NUCLEAR ENERGY)

Natural (terrestrial) radionuclides can be and are released to the atmosphere as a result of the industrial processing of various raw materials. Mineral processing and the combustion of fossil fuels are the most important processes that contribute to the emission of uranium and thorium series radionuclides to the environment, increasing their air volume activities and causing exposure of human beings.

The main radionuclide released from industrial activities is radon. Radon is released in the process of burning natural gas, as well as in the phosphates and cement industry and gas and oil extraction. Iron and steel production processes and cement and phosphorus production result in the release of ^{210}Pb.

Radionuclides released to the atmosphere can be transmitted over large distances (especially if they are released as a result of a thermal process) or can be released in the form of dust or fly ash in the vicinity of the industrial plant. Radionuclides released to the atmosphere from industrial activities other than nuclear energy contribute mainly to the internal exposure of human beings via inhalation and ingestion. For example, in the case of coal-burning power plants, the annual effective dose from natural radionuclides present in emissions is assumed to be maximally 10 to 50 μSv/year. According to UNSCEAR [1], the overall average annual effective dose due to emissions from industrial activities

TABLE 3.5
Typical Annual Releases of ^{222}Rn from Various Industrial Plants

Industrial Plant	Release of ^{222}Rn (Bq/year)
Coal-fired power plant	34×10^9
Gas-fired power plant	230×10^9
Oil extraction	540×10^9
Iron production	180×10^9

TABLE 3.6
Typical Air Volume Activities of Natural Radionuclides in the Environment

Nuclide	Average Volume Activity (Bq/m³)
^{3}H	1.4×10^{-3}
^{14}C	56.3×10^{-3}
^{238}U	1×10^{-6}
^{230}Th	0.5×10^{-6}
^{226}Ra	1×10^{-6}
^{210}Pb	500×10^{-6}
^{210}Po	50×10^{-6}
^{232}Th	0.5×10^{-6}
^{228}Ra	1×10^{-6}
^{228}Th	1×10^{-6}
^{235}U	0.05×10^{-6}
^{222}Rn outdoor	10
^{222}Rn indoor	10–100
^{220}Rn outdoor	10
^{220}Rn indoor	2–20

(other than nuclear) ranges between 0.001 and 20 μSv/year. The highest values for members of critical groups could be about 1000 μSv/year. Examples of typical releases of radon to the atmosphere from various industrial plants are shown in Table 3.5 (values are from UNSCEAR [1]).

3.3.3 SUMMARY: AIRBORNE ACTIVITY DUE TO NATURAL RADIATION SOURCES

Table 3.6 shows typical air volume activities (in Bq/m³) of natural radionuclides in the environment.

3.4 MAN-MADE RADIONUCLIDES IN THE AIR

3.4.1 MAN-MADE RADIONUCLIDES IN THE AIR DUE TO NUCLEAR WEAPONS TESTS AND PRODUCTION

Nuclear weapons tests in the atmosphere were performed between 1945 and 1980 by the U.S., the Soviet Union, the U.K., France, and China. During these tests (especially when performed in the atmosphere), many radioactive materials were released directly into the environment without any restrictions. As a result, the world's population was exposed to these materials via exposure from the ground deposition, inhalation of airborne nuclides, and ingestion. According to UNSCEAR [1], the average annual effective dose resulting from atmospheric nuclear tests was highest in 1963, about 110 μSv/year. At the end of the 20th century it was less then 6 μSv/year.

Many radionuclides were deposited as local or intermediate fallout and created deposits on the ground; however, large amounts of volatile radionuclides like ^{90}Sr, ^{137}Cs, and ^{131}I were dispersed in the world's atmosphere (Table 3.7). In the 1960s, the highest average airborne volume activities of ^{90}Sr in the air near the ground were about 10^{-3} Bq/m^3, while in the 1980s they were only about 10^{-7} to 10^{-6} Bq/m^3.

The effective dose from the inhalation (total effective dose due to inhalation resulting from all tests) of radionuclides produced in atmospheric tests was about 150 μSv. The annual effective dose due to inhalation was highest in 1963, about 36 μSv. The most important contributors to this exposure pathway were ^{144}Ce, ^{106}Ru, ^{95}Zr, and ^{90}Sr. After the atmospheric tests ceased, airborne activity of these radionuclides decreased rapidly and inhalation as an exposure pathway due to nuclear tests became practically negligible (Table 3.8).

There are still two other contributors to exposure that are widely dispersed in the atmosphere (and especially in the biosphere), namely ^3H and ^{14}C. However, their contribution to the inhalation dose is negligible and they contribute to effective dose via ingestion only. The estimated global release of ^{14}C in atmospheric tests was about 213×10^{15} Bq. The global inventory of ^{14}C as a cosmogenic

---

TABLE 3.7
Average Annual Airborne Volume Activity for the Northern Hemisphere of ^{90}Sr Due to Releases From Atmospheric Tests (According to UNSCEAR [1])

Year	Average Annual Volume Activity in Air (Bq/m^3)
1957	0.23×10^{-3}
1963	2.17×10^{-3}
1970	0.12×10^{-3}
1983	0.001×10^{-3}

TABLE 3.8
**Average Effective Dose Due to Inhalation (Total
Effective Dose Due to Inhalation Resulting From All
Tests) Caused By the Most Important Radionuclide
Contributors Produced in Atmospheric Tests**

Nuclide	Effective Dose Due to Inhalation (Total From All Atmospheric Tests) (μSv)
^{131}I	2.6
^{95}Zr	2.9
^{144}Ce	53
^{106}Ru	35
^{90}Sr	9.2
^{137}Cs	0.3
Pu, Am	38

nuclide is about 13×10^{18} Bq and the annual production rate due to cosmic radiation is 1.5×10^{15} Bq/year. From this it can be seen that atmospheric tests quite significantly influenced the natural state.

3.4.2 MAN-MADE RADIONUCLIDES IN THE AIR DUE TO ELECTRICITY GENERATION IN NUCLEAR POWER PLANTS: FUEL PRODUCTION AND OPERATION OF NUCLEAR POWER PLANTS

Global radionuclides released from the nuclear fuel cycle are nuclides that are fairly long-lived and are dispersed in the atmosphere and biosphere and irradiate the world population as a whole. These nuclides are ^3H (half-life 12.26 years), ^{14}C (half-life 5,730 years), ^{85}Kr (half-life 10.7 years), and ^{129}I (half-life 1.6×10^7 years). Again it should be emphasized that ^3H and ^{14}C are cosmogenic nuclides; this means they are also present naturally in the environment.

The total activity of global radionuclides released from the nuclear fuel cycle (nuclear power plants and reprocessing plants, release activity from the entire nuclear power industry at the end of 1997, according to UNSCEAR [1]), together with the average annual effective doses to individuals due to releases of global radionuclides (world average) are shown in Table 3.9.

Common releases caused by normal long-term operation of nuclear power plants consist of not only global radionuclides, but many other radionuclides. As an example, Table 3.10 and Table 3.11 list common atmospheric discharges from a nuclear power plant (VVER-440 MW type).

The activity of aerosols in normal effluents from power reactors is a function of the state of the fuel. If there is a problem with the tightness of the fuel in the reactor, contamination of the primary circuit is increased and consequently effluents of aerosols can be higher.

TABLE 3.9
Activity of Global Radionuclides Released to the Atmosphere From the Nuclear Fuel Cycle Through the End of 1997, According to UNSCEAR [1], and World Average Annual Effective Dose Due to These Releases

Global Nuclide	Activity in Effluents, Sum From the Whole Nuclear Fuel Cycle (Bq)	Annual Effective Dose (World Average)
^{3}H	~300 × 10^{15}	~0.005 µSv/year
^{14}C	~3 × 10^{15}	Maximally 1 µSv/year
^{85}Kr	~3.3 × 10^{18}	~0.1 µSv/year

TABLE 3.10
Common Activity of Noble Gasses Measured in Atmospheric Discharges From a Nuclear Power Plant VVER-440 (According to Tecl [8])

Nuclide	Half-Life	Typical Activity in Atmospheric Discharges From a Nuclear Power Plant VVER-440
^{41}Ar	110 minutes	500–700 Bq/m^3
^{133}Xe	5.2 days	70–80 Bq/m^3
^{85}Kr	10.7 years	20–30 Bq/m^3

TABLE 3.11
Atmospheric Effluents of Aerosols: Typical Values in Discharges From a Nuclear Power Plant VVER-440 (According to Rulik et al. [5])

Nuclide	Common Discharge Activity Per Quarter (VVER-440)
^{137}Cs	1E+4 to 1E+5 Bq
^{242}Cm	1E+3 to 1E+5 Bq
^{238}Pu	1E+3 to 1E+4 Bq

The reported annual effective dose in individuals living in the vicinity (up to 50 to 100 km from the site) of a nuclear power reactor is between 1 and 500 µSv/year. According to UNSCEAR [1], the typical annual effective dose to individuals resulting from nuclear reactor effluents to the atmosphere is between 0.04 µSv/year and 10 µSv/year (per reactor; this means that the dose is realized in human beings living up to approximately 50 km from the reactor).

3.4.3 MAN-MADE RADIOACTIVITY IN THE AIR IN CASE OF NUCLEAR ACCIDENT

The operation of nuclear power plants is one human activity that, if a serious accident occurs, can lead to very significant radioactive pollution of the environment and can cause increased irradiation of the population, especially in the vicinity of the plant (up to 100 to 300 km from the site of release). The possible impacts of a serious accident are the main reason why the nuclear industry is under very strict and sophisticated controls. These controls cover the nuclear power plant (the physical and chemical principles of the processes and the barriers preventing radionuclides from the reactor core from being released to the environment; one such barrier is modern containment, in which the reactor and all other systems that might be in contact with radioactivity from the core are covered and protected), training of the operators, safety procedures, etc. These controls have greatly improved because of the serious nuclear accidents that have taken place in the last 30 years.

Two such accidents were Three Mile Island, in the U.S., and Chernobyl, in Ukraine (former USSR). The Three Mile Island accident occurred in 1979. The initial cause of the accident was the loss of primary coolant. Consequently partial core damage occurred (half of the reactor core melted). As a result, an increase in radioactivity in the air due to the release of radionuclides to the atmosphere was observed. Effective doses to the inhabitants in the vicinity of the plant were relatively low, about 10 μSv per individual. This dose was realized in about 2 million people living in the vicinity of the plant.

The most catastrophic and severe nuclear accident happened in 1986 at the Chernobyl nuclear power plant. There was almost total damage of the core, with very high releases of radioactive substances from the reactor core to the atmosphere and the environment. Radioactive products were also emitted from the fires and explosions in the reactor. Released radionuclides were dispersed over long distances and pollution was measured all over Europe. The Chernobyl accident was the most severe accident that could be imaged in the context of the peaceful use of nuclear power.

For a better understanding of what could be expected in case of such a severe nuclear accident (as an example), the radiological conditions of a Chernobyl-type release are shown in Table 3.12, based on computer model calculations. The source term (the total release of radionuclides to the atmosphere) applied in the model calculations was the same as that estimated for the Chernobyl accident. The meteorological conditions applied were prepared (artificial) ones. The point of release assumed in the model calculations is identical with the former Chernobyl nuclear power plant site in Ukraine. It should be stated here that all three remaining reactors of the Chernobyl nuclear power plant have been shut down and decommissioned. The model calculations were performed using the *este* code — the computer code that is used by emergency response workers and crisis staff in case of a nuclear accident [2]. The results (the maps of radiological impacts calculated by *este*) are shown in Figure 3.1 and Figure 3.2. The estimated total release of radionuclides (the source term) in case of a Chernobyl-type accident is shown in Table 3.12.

TABLE 3.12

Estimated Total Release of Radionuclides (the Source Term) From the Core of a Chernobyl-Type Reactor in the Case of a Severe Accident with Total Melting of the Core (Core Damage) and Bypass of or Damage to the Reactor Building (According to Carny [6])

Nuclide	Estimated Core Inventory of the RBMK 1000 Reactor. T is the time from the end of the chain reaction (Bq).		Core Inventory of the Chernobyl Nuclear Power Plant at the Time of the Accident, According to OECD [7] (Bq)	Total Release to the Environment. The most severe source term for the RBMK 1000 reactor: total melting of the core (core damage) and bypass of or damage to the reactor building.		Total Release to the Environment During the Chernobyl Accident, Estimation According to OECD [7]
	T = 1.5 Hours	T = 24 Hours		(Bq)	Percent of the Core	Percent of the Core
85mKr	7.6E+17	2.2E+16		2.2E+16	100.00	
85Kr	2.1E+16	2.1E+16	(2.5–3.3)E+16	2.1E+16	100.00	100
87Kr	1.0E+18	3.6E+12		3.6E+12	100.00	
88Kr	2.0E+18	7.2E+15		7.2E+15	100.00	
86Rb	9.6E+14	9.3E+14		2.2E+14	23.99	
88Rb	1.9E+18	8.1E+15		1.9E+15	23.99	
89Sr	3.5E+18	3.4E+18	(2.3–4.0)E+18	1.6E+17	4.80	4.0–6
90Sr	1.4E+17	1.4E+17	(1.7–2.3)E+17	6.6E+15	4.80	4.0–6
91Sr	3.8E+18	7.0E+17		3.4E+16	4.80	
90Y	1.4E+17	1.4E+17		3.1E+14	0.22	
91mY	1.3E+18	4.5E+17		9.8E+14	0.22	
91Y	4.4E+18	4.4E+18		9.7E+15	0.22	
95Zr	5.6E+18	5.5E+18	(5.1–5.8)E+18	1.2E+16	0.22	3.5
97Zr	5.3E+18	2.1E+18		4.5E+15	0.22	

(continued)

TABLE 3.12 (continued)
Estimated Total Release of Radionuclides (the Source Term) From the Core of a Chernobyl-Type Reactor in the Case of a Severe Accident with Total Melting of the Core (Core Damage) and Bypass of or Damage to the Reactor Building (According to Carny [6])

Nuclide	Estimated Core Inventory of the RBMK 1000 Reactor. T is the time from the end of the chain reaction (Bq).		Core Inventory of the Chernobyl Nuclear Power Plant at the Time of the Accident, According to OECD [7] (Bq)	Total Release to the Environment. The most severe source term for the RBMK 1000 reactor: total melting of the core (core damage) and bypass of or damage to the reactor building.		Total Release to the Environment During the Chernobyl Accident, Estimation According to OECD [7]
	T = 1.5 Hours	T = 24 Hours	OECD [7] (Bq)	(Bq)	Percent of the Core	Percent of the Core
^{95}Nb	5.6E+18	5.6E+18		1.2E+16	0.22	
^{97}Nb	2.4E+18	2.2E+18		4.9E+15	0.22	
^{99}Mo	5.9E+18	4.6E+18	(4.8–7.3)E+18	9.2E+15	0.20	>3.5
^{99m}Tc	5.2E+18	4.4E+18		8.7E+15	0.20	
^{103}Ru	4.1E+18	4.0E+18	(3.8–5.0)E+18	8.0E+15	0.20	>3.5
^{105}Ru	2.3E+18	6.3E+16		1.3E+14	0.20	
^{106}Ru	9.3E+17	9.2E+17	(0.8–2.1)E+18	1.8E+15	0.20	>3.5
^{103m}Rh	2.1E+18	4.0E+18		8.0E+15	0.20	
^{105}Rh	1.8E+18	1.4E+18		2.7E+15	0.20	
^{127}Sb	2.2E+17	1.9E+17		2.3E+16	11.99	
^{129}Sb	1.0E+18	2.6E+16		3.1E+15	11.99	
^{127}Te	2.2E+17	1.8E+17		2.1E+16	11.99	
^{129m}Te	2.0E+17	1.9E+17		2.3E+16	11.99	
^{129}Te	1.1E+18	3.0E+16		3.5E+15	11.99	

^{131m}Te	4.7E+17	2.8E+17		3.3E+16	11.99	
^{132}Te	4.4E+18	3.6E+18	(2.7–4.4)E+18	4.3E+17	11.99	25–60
^{131}I	3.1E+18	2.9E+18	(2.4–3.1)E+18	7.0E+17	23.99	50–60
^{132}I	4.4E+18	3.7E+18		8.9E+17	23.99	
^{133}I	6.1E+18	2.8E+18		6.8E+17	23.99	
^{134}I	3.2E+18	4.0E+10		9.5E+09	23.99	
^{135}I	5.0E+18	4.5E+17		1.1E+17	23.99	
^{133m}Xe	2.2E+17	1.6E+17		1.6E+17	100.00	
^{133}Xe	6.3E+18	6.0E+18	(6.2–7.8)E+18	6.0E+18	100.00	100
^{135}Xe	1.6E+18	1.4E+18		1.4E+18	100.00	
^{138}Xe	3.3E+17	1.4E−12		1.4E−12	100.00	
^{134}Cs	2.8E+17	2.8E+17	(1.1–2.0)E+17	6.7E+16	23.99	33–43
^{136}Cs	1.1E+17	1.1E+17		2.5E+16	23.99	
^{137}Cs	1.7E+17	1.7E+17	(2.2–2.9)E+17	4.2E+16	23.99	33–43
^{138}Cs	1.1E+18	1.7E+05		4.0E+04	23.99	
^{140}Ba	5.9E+18	5.6E+18	(5.4–6.1)E+18	2.7E+17	4.80	4.0–6.0
^{140}La	5.9E+18	5.9E+18		1.3E+16	0.22	
^{143}Pr	4.8E+18	4.6E+18		1.0E+16	0.22	
^{147}Nd	2.2E+18	2.1E+18		4.6E+15	0.22	
^{141}Ce	5.5E+18	5.4E+18	(5.1–5.6)E+18	1.1E+16	0.21	3.5
^{143}Ce	4.7E+18	2.9E+18		6.0E+15	0.21	
^{144}Ce	3.1E+18	3.1E+18	(3.2–3.9)E+18	6.5E+15	0.21	3.5
^{239}Np	5.8E+19	4.4E+19	(2.7–6.7)E+19	9.2E+16	0.21	3.5
^{238}Pu	2.1E+15	2.1E+15	(0.7–1.6)E+15	4.4E+12	0.21	3.5
^{239}Pu	7.8E+14	7.8E+14	(8.0–9.6)E+14	1.6E+12	0.21	3.5
^{240}Pu	7.8E+14	7.8E+14	(1.2–1.6)E+15	1.6E+12	0.21	3.5
^{241}Pu	1.3E+17	1.3E+17	(1.7–1.9)E+17	2.6E+14	0.21	3.5

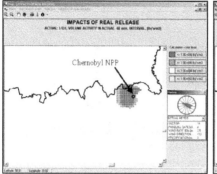
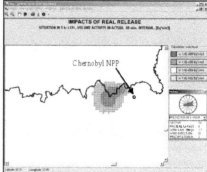

Actual situation, cloud due to 4 h release.   Projected cloud in 3 h.

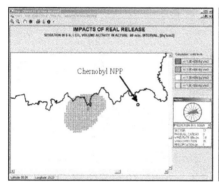
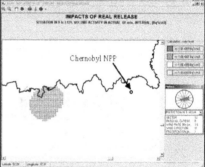

Projected cloud in 6 h.   Projected cloud in 9 h.

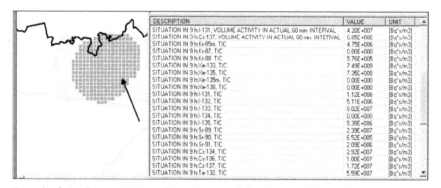

Example of air volume activities and time integrals of air volume activities at chosen point.

FIGURE 3.1 Example of the maps of ^{131}I air volume activity in the vicinity of the point of release as a function of time from the beginning of release. The point of release is the site of the Chernobyl nuclear power plant. The source term applied is the estimated source term for the Chernobyl accident. Meteorological conditions are modeled without relation to the real conditions during the accident at Chernobyl. Modeled by the computer code *este*. Actual situation, cloud 4 hours after release. Projected cloud in 3 hours. Projected cloud in 6 hours. Projected cloud in 9 hours. Example of air volume activities and time integrals of air volume activities at chosen point.

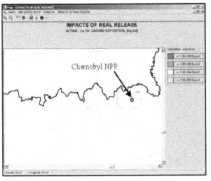

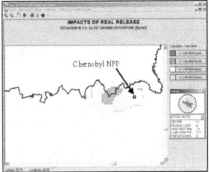

Actual situation, deposition due to 4 h release.   Projected deposition in 3 h.

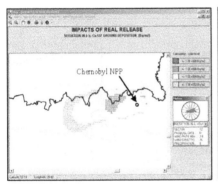

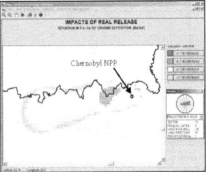

Projected deposition in 6 h.   Projected deposition in 9 h.

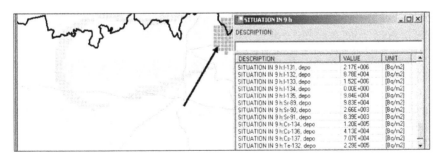

Example of expected ground deposition at chosen point in 9 h.

FIGURE 3.2 Example of the maps of ^{137}Cs ground deposition in the vicinity of the point of release as a function of the time from the beginning of release. The point of release is the site of the Chernobyl nuclear power plant. The source term applied is the estimated source term for the Chernobyl accident. Meteorological conditions are modeled without relation to the real conditions during the accident at Chernobyl. Modeled by the computer code *este*. Actual situation, deposition 4 hours after release. Projected deposition in 3 hours. Projected deposition in 6 hours. Projected deposition in 9 hours. Example of expected ground deposition at the chosen point in 9 hours.

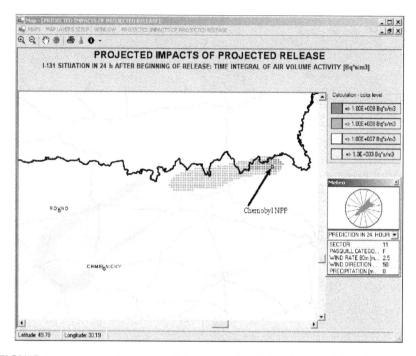

FIGURE 3.3 Example of the map of time integrals of air volume activity of ^{131}I in the vicinity of the point of release. Predicted situation 24 hours from the beginning of the release. The point of the release is the site of the Chernobyl nuclear power plant. The source term applied is the estimated source term for the Chernobyl accident. Meteorological conditions are modeled without relation to the real conditions during the accident at Chernobyl. The sites of other Ukrainian nuclear power plants — Rovno and Chmelnitsky — can be seen on the map. Modeled by the computer code *este*.

Examples of maps of radiological impacts due to a very serious nuclear accident are shown in Figure 3.3 and Figure 3.4. All the maps and results have been calculated using *este* [2]. From the figures, the expected range of air volume activities of ^{131}I can be seen. The radiotoxicity of ^{131}I occurs because iodine is inhaled with the air or ingested with food and causes irradiation of internal organs, especially irradiation of the thyroid gland. During longer periods after the accidental release, other nuclides (due to their longer half-life and expected larger amounts in the release) are expected to take the role of the most radiotoxic one, namely ^{134}Cs and ^{137}Cs. Therefore, ground deposition of ^{137}Cs is shown.

Finally, Figure 3.5 and Figure 3.6 show maps of avertable doses. Avertable doses (doses to human beings that could potentially be saved) serve as a criteria for interventions in case of a nuclear (radiological) accident (e.g., for the evacuation of inhabitants, for sheltering, for administration of iodine prophylaxis, etc.). Values of airborne activity that demand protective measures (urgent or precautionary measures) are shown in Table 3.13 [3].

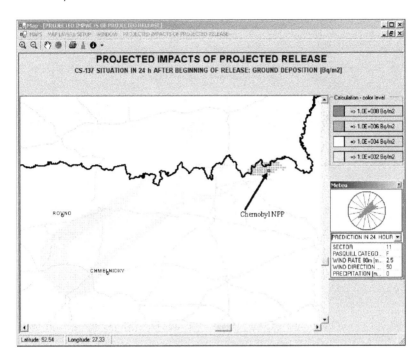

FIGURE 3.4 Example of the map of ground deposition of ¹³⁷Cs in the vicinity of the point of release. Predicted situation 24 hours from the beginning of the release. The point of the release is the site of the Chernobyl nuclear power plant. The source term applied is the estimated source term for the Chernobyl accident. Meteorological conditions are modeled without relation to the real conditions during the accident at Chernobyl. The sites of other Ukrainian nuclear power plants — Rovno and Chmelnitsky — can be seen on the map. Modeled by the computer code *este*.

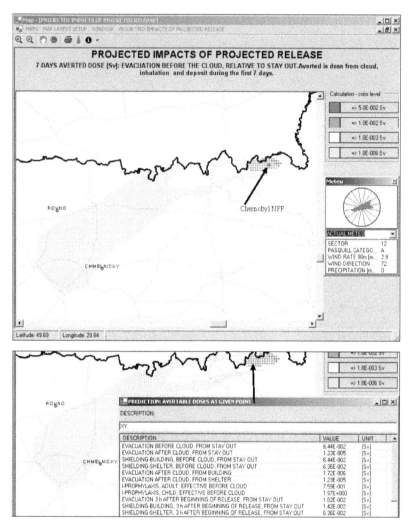

FIGURE 3.5 Example of the map of avertable dose: the dose averted by evacuation of inhabitants before the cloud enters a given region on the map. The intervention level for evacuation is usually the effective dose averted (= 50 mSv). (The value of the intervention level can vary country by country.) This means that evacuation of inhabitants is optimized if the effective dose averted by evacuation is 50 mSv or more. In some circumstances evacuation can be imposed according to other criteria. Predicted avertable doses, situation 24 hours from the beginning of the release. The point of the release is the site of the Chernobyl nuclear power plant. The source term applied is the estimated source term for the Chernobyl accident. Meteorological conditions are modeled without relation to the real conditions during the accident at Chernobyl. Modeled by the computer code *este*.

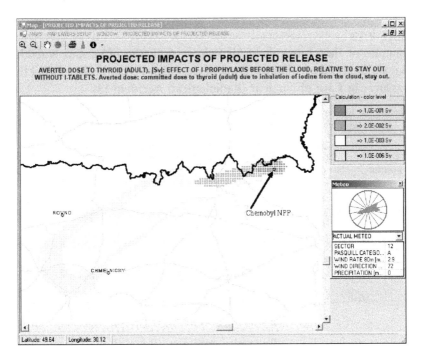

FIGURE 3.6 Example of the map of avertable dose to thyroid: the dose to thyroid averted by iodine prophylaxis implementation (iodine tablets are swallowed by inhabitants before the cloud enters a given region on the map). The intervention level for iodine prophylaxis implementation is usually the dose to thyroid averted (= 100 mGy). (The value of the intervention level can vary country by country. In some countries, special lower values of intervention levels for children are defined and used.) This means that implementation of iodine prophylaxis to inhabitants is optimized if the dose to thyroid averted by iodine tablet ingestion is 100 mGy or more. Predicted avertable doses to thyroid, situation 24 hours from the beginning of the release. The point of the release is the site of the Chernobyl nuclear power plant. The source term applied is the estimated source term for the Chernobyl accident. Meteorological conditions are modeled without relation to the real conditions during the accident at Chernobyl. Modeled by the computer code *este*.

TABLE 3.13
Examples of Time Integrals of Air Volume Activities of Various Nuclides That Should Lead to Administration of Urgent or Precautionary Protective Measures in Case of Nuclear (Radiological) Accident [3]

Operational Intervention Level (Bq/h/m³)		Intervention: Urgent Protective Measures, Precautionary Protective Measures, or Measures in the Field of Agriculture	Nuclide
Dry Deposition	Wet Deposition (5 mm/h)		
8E+05	3E+04	Sheltering	^{137}Cs
	9E+05	Wear (provisional) filter masks	
8E+06	3E+05	Evacuation	
	5E+02	Protection of workers exchanging filters in buildings	
	4E+03	Exchange filters in trucks	
4E+06	2E+04	Avoid staying outdoors, change clothing after staying outdoors	
	4E+02	Immediate harvest of agriculture products	
		Cover plants with foils	
		Close greenhouses	
		Close stables, sheds	
		Put livestock in stables	
		Stop inflow into cisterns	
	7E+04	Iodine prophylaxis for children and pregnant women	^{131}I
7E+05	6E+04	Sheltering	
	1E+06	Wearing (provisional) filter masks	
	7E+05	Iodine prophylaxis for adults	
7E+06	6E+05	Evacuation	
	1E+04	Protection of workers exchanging filters in buildings	
	1E+05	Exchange filters in trucks	
1E+06	3E+04	Avoid staying outdoors, change clothing after staying outdoors	
	2E+02	Immediate harvest of agriculture products	
		Cover plants with foils	
		Close greenhouses	
		Close stables, sheds	
		Put livestock in stables	
		Stop inflow into cisterns	

REFERENCES

1. United Nations Scientific Committee on the Effects of Atomic Radiation, UNSCEAR 2000 Report to the General Assembly, with scientific annexes, UNSCEAR, Vienna, Austria, 2000.
2. Carny, P., New functions of the *este system* — new possibilities for emergency response, paper presented at the conference "The 27th Days of Radiation Protection," Liptovsky Jan, Slovakia, 2005, Conference Proceedings ISBN 80-88806-53-4.
3. Carny, P., Procedures of the State Office for Nuclear Safety of the Czech Republic to the Catalogue of countermeasures in case of event with no insignificant radiological impacts, technical report ABment, Trnava, Slovakia, 2003.
4. Cabanekova, H., Building materials as the source of radiation load of Slovak population, paper presented at the conference "The 27th Days of Radiation Protection," Liptovsky Jan, Slovakia, 2005, 2005, Conference Proceedings ISBN 80-88806-53-4.
5. Rulik, P., Pfeiferova, V., Staubr, R., Tecl, J., Holgye, Z., and Schlesingerova, E., Independent monitoring of the aerosols effluents from NPP provided by SURO, paper presented at the conference "The 27th Days of Radiation Protection," Liptovsky Jan, Slovakia, 2005, Conference Proceedings ISBN 80-88806-53-4.
6. Carny, P., Database of basic source terms of European NPPs for emergency response purposes, technical report ABmerit, Trnava, Slovakia, 2003.
7. Devell, L., Guntay, S., and Powers, D.A., The Chernobyl accident source term. Development of a consensus view, NEA/CSNI/R(95)/24, OECD/NEA, Issy-les-Moulineaux, France, 1995.
8. Tecl, J., Results of independent monitoring of releases of noble gasses from nuclear facilities collected by the SURO Prague, paper presented at the conference "The 27th Days of Radiation Protection," Liptovsky Jan, Slovakia, 2005, Conference Proceedings ISBN 80-88806-53-4.

4 Radionuclide Concentrations in Water

José Luis Mas, Manuel García-León,
Rafael García-Tenorio, and Juan Pedro Bolívar

CONTENTS

4.1 INTRODUCTION

Different kinds of water cover more than two thirds of the Earth's surface. This resource is extremely important for human life: water is used for direct consumption, it is used in the production of food, it is used for many industrial activities, etc. Thus radioactivity present in water can reach humans and the environment through many different mechanisms.

Water is a medium for the transport and interaction of radionuclides with and within different compartments of the troposphere: soils, sediments, crustal rocks, biota, and even air are continuously exchanging their radioactive contents with water. The nature of the compartment determines the nature of the dominant interaction mechanisms. The properties of the compartments depend, of course, on the nature of the ecosystem where the compartment is located. Therefore, a systematic categorization can be established according to the possible scenarios where water is considered an important medium for the exchange, supply, or storing of radioactivity.

In this chapter, four different compartments are considered. In Section 4.2, rivers and lakes, which act as a water supply source to the sea, are described in detail. An overview of radioactivity in the oceans is presented in Section 4.3. Rainwater is discussed in Section 4.4. Underground reservoirs are intensively used for different human activities; these are discussed in Section 4.5. Finally, drinking water is analyzed in Section 4.6.

4.2 RADIONUCLIDES IN RIVERS AND LAKES: LEVELS AND BEHAVIOR

The natural compartment analyzed in this section could first be characterized by the fact that it does not contain any intrinsic radionuclides in its composition. The presence of natural and artificial radionuclides at different levels in surface waters is clearly correlated with the existence of some coupling between the different compartments. In fact, surface waters are coupled to subsurface aquifers, to soils, and to the atmosphere, allowing incorporation of several radionuclides following different routes. Indeed, some radionuclides previously dissolved in deep underground aquifers may reach surface waters, other radionuclides may be directly incorporated in surface waters by deposition from the atmosphere, and a large fraction of the radionuclides in aquatic systems have their origins in the underlying soils, from where they can be transported to surface waters through runoff or leaching into the groundwater. The first and last routes are the most important ones explaining the presence of natural radionuclides in rivers and lakes, while the second and third routes, together with direct discharges from nuclear facilities, are the main ways artificial radionuclides are deposited in aquatic ecosystems.

Once radionuclides are incorporated in a body of water, their dispersion and behavior is hard to predict in a general or straightforward way. Each stream, river, lake, etc., has its own mixing characteristics that vary from place to place and time to time [1], the rate of mixing being dependent on the depth of the water, the type of bottom, the shoreline configuration, wind, etc., and on the different chemical, physicochemical, and biological processes. Modeling of the hydrologic behavior of a water body requires site-specific parameters that limit its general applicability in water dispersion studies. Furthermore, the fate of a radionuclide can be complicated by its physicochemical behavior. If the radionuclide is present in the water body as a suspended solid, it can be deposited to the bottom or can pass to solution via desorption. On the other hand, if the radionuclide is incorporated in the solution phase, it can be adsorbed on suspended organic and inorganic solids, and then settle to the bottom. This physicochemical behavior is obviously element dependent; in addition, it depends on other factors such as pH, redox conditions, the total amount of solids, etc., as is shown later in this chapter [1].

All these facts make it quite difficult to predict, especially in rivers, the behavior and dispersion of radionuclides. However, if sufficient information can be obtained about their physical characteristics, it is possible to estimate with some degree of certainty the dispersion of some specific radionuclides. More advances have been made in the prediction of radionuclide behavior in lakes. Models for predicting the migration of radionuclides through the biotic and abiotic components of lacustrine environments have been clearly identified and are widely accepted by the scientific community [2].

For some radionuclides, such as ^{137}Cs and ^{90}Sr, a quantitative evaluation of the most important transfer parameters through lacustrine ecosystems has been performed. To do that, experimental studies following the most significant nuclear accidents (Chernobyl, Kysthym) were developed. Today, it is possible to obtain levels of uncertainty of a factor of two to three when models for these nuclides are applied as generic tools for predicting their behavior in the abiotic components of the lacustrine environment. These uncertainties can be decreased if a detailed study of site-specific values of the model's parameters is performed. Nevertheless, for several important radionuclides, the parameters are not yet available with enough uncertainty, and further assessments are necessary, mainly in relation to the evaluation of model uncertainties [2].

In surface water bodies such as rivers and lakes, an understanding of the role of bottom sediments is essential to understanding the behavior and fluxes of radionuclides incorporated from the coupled ecosystems (atmosphere, soils, groundwater, etc.). On a long time scale, the bottom sediments can be considered, at least temporally, as sinks for a fraction of the material in the different chemical and biological aquatic cycles. Radionuclides adsorbed onto organic or inorganic material in the water or forming part of the crystalline structure of suspended inorganic material can be incorporated into the sediments. Once a radionuclide has been incorporated to the sediment phase, its future depends on a great number of complex factors. In fact, radionuclides can either be permanently linked to a sediment component or can be liberated and take part in different biogeochemical reactions. Consequently the ability to predict the future behavior of a radionuclide initially incorporated in the sediment is one of the key factors in evaluating its effect on the environment. For this reason, it is insufficient to determine its total content in the sediment in order to understand its behavior. It is necessary, in addition, to obtain information about the path or mechanism followed by the radionuclide in its linking to the sediment.

In order to do this, it is necessary to distinguish between the residual and nonresidual fractions in the sediment. This separation is very important in relation to the possible liberation of radionuclides (both natural and artificial) incorporated in the sediment. The radionuclides forming part of the residual phase can be considered immobile (i.e., not reactive in the environment), while the radionuclides associated with the nonresidual fraction can be considered potentially mobile. Consequently this mobile phase can be considered as reactive in the different chemical and biological processes that occur in the water–sediment interface.

Among the different natural radionuclides that can be found in nature, there are the radionuclides belonging to the uranium and thorium series and ^{40}K, the isotopes that may be present at higher levels in water. Both uranium and thorium are initially in the valence state +4 in igneous rocks and primary minerals, but uranium, in contrast to thorium, can experience oxidation in the valence states of +5 and +6. In oxidized environments, uranium will be in the state +6, forming the quite soluble uranyl ion (UO_2^{2+}), which plays an essential role in the transport of uranium in the environment. For this reason, uranium can be found in dissolution in most surface water systems. In contrast, thorium is quite insoluble in the majority of natural waters, being present or transported in the suspended matter of water bodies. Even in the case when thorium is generated as a daughter of uranium in dissolution, it is quickly hydrolyzed and adsorbed to the surfaces of the particulate matter fraction.

Few studies have been conducted on riverine uranium. A global survey of uranium concentrations in dissolution from 43 rivers ranging in flow from less than 1 km³/year to 6930 km³/year was published by Palmer and Edmond [3], estimating the average concentration of uranium in river water at 2.3 mBq/l. Recently this database was extended to include smaller watersheds (an additional 29 rivers with flow rates ranging from less than 1 km³/year to 100 km³/year); the result when the two datasets are combined does not change the previously indicated average concentration of dissolved uranium in rivers [4]. Nevertheless, the authors of these studies pointed out (1) the difficulty in obtaining representative samples from rivers, which show large fluctuations in runoff and dissolved load, and (2) the scatter of the uranium concentrations in the different rivers that can vary considerably in relation to the worldwide average value. Values 10 times higher than the average have been determined, for example, in the upper parts of the Ganges River, while concentrations two to three times higher have been determined in the Guadalquivir (Spain) and Seine (France) rivers. Values one order of magnitude lower than the average worldwide uranium concentration have been found in the Amazon River system.

The higher or lower values of uranium in dissolution in rivers and lakes can be associated with the characteristics and relative influence of the different sources terms of this element. The bedrock type of the aquifers feeding their waters into the analyzed river as well as the soil types in the river basins and their drainage area are important factors in the levels of uranium in dissolution in the waters incorporated into the river. As explained by Schmidt [4], the high values of uranium in dissolution in the Seine River are associated with the main characteristics of its drainage basin, which is rather homogeneous with sedimentary rocks, mainly carbonate rocks, such as limestone. This explanation follows the suggestion of Broecker [5], indicating that uranium variations in river water may be due to variations in the carbonate concentrations in dissolution, because the uranium in carbonate form is quite stable and soluble. It is also well known that high levels of uranium can be found in water from granitic aquifers, while lower values are found in water from sandy ones.

A high positive correlation has been observed between the level of uranium in dissolution in river water and the concentration of NO_3 [6] and the total amounts of solids in dissolution [7]. In several rivers, an inverse correlation between the uranium in dissolution and silicon/total anions has been found. This indicates that the dominant control on uranium in dissolution is probably the chemical weathering of nonsilicate minerals [8].

At this point it is necessary to remark about what is meant by uranium in dissolution: this term is applied to the uranium activity (or mass) that is associated with the fraction passing filters with a pore size of 0.45 μm. It has been observed in several rivers, and associated to the filtered fraction, that a large proportion (30 to 90%) of the uranium is carried by colloids, a fact that is compatible with a possible uranium complexation with humic acids [9].

In addition to natural uranium inputs, the presence of uranium with an anthropogenic origin should be considered. It has been suggested [10] that some high values in specific rivers may be due to the extensive use of phosphate fertilizers in agriculture, which have uranium contents up to 1 Bq/g. In contrast, Mangini and Dominik [6] conclude that the uranium from phosphate fertilizers is mainly adsorbed to the surface layers of the sediment. However, phosphate fertilizers may also affect the uranium in dissolution via a more indirect route, because high phosphate levels can lead to eutrophication and to an increase in the biological breakdown of organic matter, which may result in enhanced uranium in dissolution.

A number of investigations have been performed in the mouths of the rivers, studying the influence of dissolved uranium in the complex interactions between fresh- and saltwater. In estuarine zones, where a pronounced gradient of salinity can be observed, the iron and manganese dissolved in river water can precipitate as oxihydroxides, provoking the coprecipitation of uranium and its incorporation in the sediment together with the organic matter in dissolution [11]. Nevertheless, this process is not general. A good number of studies show the conservative behavior of uranium in estuaries, with a positive correlation between uranium concentrations and water salinity. This correlation is due to the higher levels of uranium in seawater in relation to freshwater. This conservative behavior has been observed, for example, in the estuary of the Seine River [4], and can be correlated with the proportion of uranium present in the water in colloidal form. Studies performed by Porcelli et al. [9], in a river discharging in the Baltic Sea, suggest that while solute uranium behaves conservatively during estuarine mixing, colloid-bound uranium is lost due to rapid flocculation of colloidal material. Thus the association of uranium with colloids may play an important role in determining uranium estuarine behavior.

Regarding the characteristics of the main source terms and the routes followed by the natural radionuclides for their incorporation in water bodies, it can be seen in rivers and lakes that there is a clear fractionation or disequilibrium between radionuclides belonging to the same natural series. The water passes through the solid grain either in the bedrock of the aquifers or in the soils from the drainage area. The rate of this weathering is not the same for the different radionuclides, some elements being more soluble than their parents or daughters under different redox and pH conditions. The result is a liquid phase enriched in radionuclides of one natural series and depleted in others. Later, the soluble radionuclides can even decay into daughters with less solubility than their progenitors. It is possible to observe other fractionation processes through precipitation and adsorption onto the surface of the particulate matter of some radionuclides.

The processes indicated below can explain, for example, the high level of disequilibrium observed in river and lake daughters between ^{234}U and its daughter ^{230}Th. $^{230}Th/^{234}U$ activity ratios are clearly lower than those observed in the studied water bodies because (1) the uranium under oxidized conditions is clearly more soluble than thorium, and for that reason the groundwater and the leached soil waters are enriched in ^{234}U in relation to ^{230}Th; and (2) even when the ^{230}Th is formed inside the surface water body due to the decay of its progenitor, ^{238}U, it tends to incorporate to the solid phase by precipitation or adsorption. These processes also explain the very low levels of ^{210}Pb and ^{210}Po in dissolution in river and lake waters due to their low solubility and tendency to be associated with particulate matter.

In the river and lake waters, a clear disequilibrium has also been observed between two radionuclides that belong to the same natural series and are isotopes of the same element (^{238}U and ^{234}U). Studies have been carried out in a number of rivers distributed all over the world and with quite a broad range of flow rates. A general consensus has been reached indicating that $^{234}U/^{238}U$ activity ratios are in the range of 1.20 to 1.30 [12]. This fractionation cannot be explained simply by a combination of dissolution/precipitation processes in the previously explained way, because both radionuclides are isotopes of the same chemical element. It is necessary to explain the observed disequilibrium on the basis of other type of processes.

The preferential presence of ^{234}U in relation to ^{238}U in dissolution can be explained by a process called the Szilard-Chalmers effect. This process is based on the increased vulnerability of the daughter nuclide to the dissolution process. In solid grains, and due to the decay of ^{238}U by emitting an α particle, the crystalline structure is destroyed in the route followed by the recoil daughter. The daughter can end up hosted in an inhospitable place in the crystalline structure and can present, as a result of the nuclear transformation, an unstable electronic configuration. As a consequence, this nuclide can be more vulnerable to dissolution than the neighboring atoms, including other members of the same series with long half-lives or even other isotopes of the same chemical species. This process is especially significant in the activity isotope ratios $^{234}U/^{238}U$ and $^{228}Th/^{232}Th$.

Relatively few studies exist about ^{226}Ra investigations in riverine systems. Several authors concluded their investigations by indicating that the concentrations of ^{226}Ra in dissolution in freshwater ecosystems are generally low (although higher than the thorium concentrations) because of the tendency of this radionuclide to be associated by adsorption to the surface of the suspended particulate matter in water. But they also found, in general, a noticeable increase in the concentrations of this radionuclide in dissolution in estuarine environments. This increase is clearly correlated with the increase in the gradient of salinity due to the mixture of fresh- and saltwater. In this case, and because of the low concentrations of ^{226}Ra in the marine environment, the ^{226}Ra concentration in estuaries cannot be associated with inputs from the oceans, as in the case of uranium. In the case of radium, the explanation is related to a change in its chemical behavior, with a noticeable increase in the desorption of this radionuclide initially bound to particle surfaces as the particles transported by the rivers enter the high ionic strength estuarine water. The increments in the concentrations of competing ions in the processes of adsorption to the surface particles induce a clear decrease in the radium adsorption coefficients, as was proved by Li et al. [13]. These authors concluded that the release of radium from river-borne particles is the main mechanism that explains the increments of radium in dissolution in estuarine environments.

In addition to the modern inputs of uranium and other natural radionuclides related to increased agriculture, some specific rivers around the world have not been free of anthropogenic inputs of natural radionuclides due to releases produced by nuclear and nonnuclear industries or activities. Indeed, the contamination is clearly evident in uranium and its daughters in some rivers due to uranium mining activities in the drainage area. But even so, anthropogenic inputs of uranium associated with other mineral mining activities have been observed, such as the ones related with pyrite extraction. In this last case, the mining of heavy metal sulfates and the use of river water for mineral washing induces the production of sulfuric acid, the consequent acidification of the water, and an increase in uranium dissolved from the river bed. Also, saline water from underground coal mines contains natural radioisotopes, mainly ^{226}Ra from the uranium decay series and ^{228}Ra from the thorium series, and this water is sometimes released into surrounding rivers.

Furthermore, several industrial activities exist that, in their production processes, form by-products and wastes that are radionuclide enriched (technologically enhanced naturally occurring radioactive material [TENORM]). Such industries release, or have released in the past, a fraction of these radionuclides to freshwater or estuarine aquatic systems. This is the case, for example, in the production of phosphoric acid for phosphate fertilizers, which use as a primary mineral sedimentary phosphate rocks and release, or have released, into riverine or estuarine environments large amounts of phosphogypsum, which contains ^{226}Ra (up to 1 Bq/g) and ^{210}Pb (up to 1 Bq/g) [14]. This is also the case in the production of titanium bioxide pigments. These wastes produce a clear radioactive impact in relatively local zones of the aquatic systems that receive the releases. These zones have been used as natural laboratories to obtain information about the behavior of several natural radionuclides [14].

At the beginning of the 21st century, the levels of artificial radionuclides in rivers and lakes are fairly low, with the exception of limited rivers affected by the releases of some nuclear facilities. The main historical source of artificial radionuclides on a global scale, the fallout from nuclear weapons tests, affected water bodies worldwide mainly in the middle of the 20th century. The great majority of these artificial radionuclides that were incorporated in surface waters have either been transported to the oceans or have been accumulated and fixed in the sediment. This is even true for some European rivers contaminated by the Chernobyl accident; only small amounts of radionuclides are present today. Aarkrog [15] estimated that historically about 9% of the ^{90}Sr inventory on land would be removed by runoff and incorporated in surface waters, while this percentage is about 2% for ^{137}Cs and even lower for plutonium isotopes. The amount of radionuclides that can be mobilized through runoff depends on the tendency of the chemical species considered to be fixed or associated to particulate matter. For example, the quite soluble behavior of ^{90}Sr and the more reactive character of plutonium isotopes are well known.

Today, the concentrations of artificial radionuclides in dissolution are generally below the detection limit in most rivers and lakes. This is the case observed in some artic lakes, where the concentrations of ^{241}Am and ^{137}Cs were less than 1 µBq/l and less than 0.3 mBq/l, respectively, while the $^{239+240}$Pu concentrations in filtered water ranged between 3 and 6 µBq/l [16]. This clearly indicates that these radionuclides are effectively scavenged from the water column. The same effect was observed in the four largest rivers in Slovenia, where the concentration of ^{137}Cs could only be found in traces up to a maximum of 0.5 mBq/l. As an aside, in these Slovenian rivers, it is possible to find higher concentrations of ^{131}I released from nuclear medicine centers than ^{137}Cs. Levels of ^{131}I in the studied Slovenian rivers range from 10 to 21 mBq/l.

Authorized releases from nuclear power plants introduce into surface waters only small amounts of ^{3}H, with a negligible radiological impact, as well as very small amounts (so small they are difficult to be detected) of other artificial radionuclides. Water concentrations of ^{3}H of several tens of becquerels per liter can be found in some rivers where authorized releases from nuclear power plants occur. Due to the conservative behavior of this nuclide in water, ^{3}H routinely released by nuclear power plants has been used as a radiotracer to determine the longitudinal dispersion coefficient and velocity of the river water [17].

Higher concentrations of artificial radionuclides can be found in water bodies affected by releases from other nuclear facilities, such as reprocessing plants and reactors for plutonium production. This is the case in the Rhone River (France), which was affected by releases from the Marcoule fuel reprocessing plant. This plant was shut down some years ago and is now being dismantled. Nevertheless, this has not reduced, until now, the discharge activities of plutonium isotopes, as washing effluents continue to be produced and released [18]. The authors reported that the annual amount of $^{239+240}$Pu carried toward the Mediterranean Sea by the Rhone River is about 1 GBq/year. They state that the $^{239+240}$Pu, ^{241}Am, and ^{137}Cs concentrations in the Rhone River due to Marcoule releases are about 0.025, 0.041, and 2 mBq/l, respectively. These values are clearly higher than those found in rivers not affected by local sources of artificial radioactivity.

The radioactivity released by nuclear reprocessing plants and reactors may be incorporated in water bodies, eventually reaching the sediments. The magnitude of this effect is variable and depends on (1) the composition of the particulate matter (its capacity for sorption and ion exchange), which can vary from place to place in the same river, (2) the salinity of the overlying water, and (3) the radionuclide considered. In studies carried out in the Clinch River (Tennessee; below the Oak Ridge nuclear facility), it was estimated that from the total amount of radioactive material released during a 20-year period, the sediments contained 21% of the ^{137}Cs and only about 0.2% of the ^{90}Sr, reflecting the behavior of both radionuclides in freshwater aquatic systems [1].

One of the freshwater systems most contaminated historically by artificial radionuclides is the Techa River, in the former Soviet Union. The main source of contamination on this river is the Mayak Nuclear Complex, which began operations in 1948. It includes reactors for plutonium production, radiochemical facilities for plutonium separation, and reprocessing plants.

A historical overview of contamination of the Techa River can be found in Kryshev et al. [19]. They indicate that in the period 1949 to 1952, about 10^{17} Bq of liquid radioactive waste were discharged into this river system. Radionuclide transport was reduced through the construction of a system of bypasses and industrial reservoirs for the storage of low-activity liquid wastes. They also indicate that at the present time, the main source of radionuclide intake in the Techa River is the transport of ^{90}Sr through the bypasses. About 6×10^{11} Bq/year of ^{90}Sr, on average, entered the Techa River through the bypasses in the period 1981 to 1995. Finally, they report that the highest radionuclide concentrations in the river were observed in the period 1950 to 1951, at a distance of 78 km from the discharge site: there the amount of ^{90}Sr in the water was 27,000 Bq/l and that of ^{137}Cs was 7500 Bq/l. Thereafter a decrease in radionuclide concentrations in the water was observed (by a factor of approximately 1000). In the period 1991 to 1994, the annual average amount of ^{90}Sr ranged from 6 to 20 Bq/l, while the annual average amount of ^{137}Cs ranged from 0.06 to 0.23 Bq/l. The concentration of $^{239+240}$Pu in the water during this time ranged from 0.004 to 0.019 Bq/l.

The contamination of freshwater bodies due to the release of artificial radio-nuclides produced by nuclear facilities has affected very limited or local zones.

But this fact should not cause us to underestimate its importance both in the environment and in humans. In fact, in most cases these contaminated water bodies play an essential role in the development and life of the people who use these waters, as in the case of the Techa River, where the water is used extensively in agriculture and as a drinking water supply [19].

4.3 RADIONUCLIDES IN THE SEA AND OCEAN

4.3.1 SYSTEM OVERVIEW

Ocean waters are continuously interacting with different substrates, which act either as sources or sinks for radionuclides. A summary of the interaction mechanisms of radionuclides is shown in Figure 4.1.

The three major mechanisms for radionuclide incorporation in the ocean system are (1) atmospheric input, (2) riverine input, and (3) radionuclide input associated with the interaction of ocean water and the crustal oceanic basalts. These input mechanisms are in competition with radionuclide removal processes. First, the radionuclides can be removed from the water column to the sediment thorough adsorption onto sinking particles, so-called particles scavenging. Second, they can be incorporated in biota thorough direct uptake mechanisms, thereafter

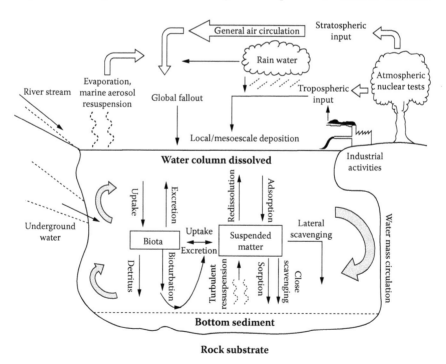

FIGURE 4.1 A simplified schematic diagram of radionuclide exchange paths within a sea compartment model.

being incorporated in the sediment as biological detritus. Uptake by biota is dependent, however, on present and past radioactive levels, and the rates of decay, dispersion, uptake, and biological elimination. Third, the radionuclides can also be redissolved or chemically desorbed from particles while traveling through an oxic environment, being transferred again to the water column. All these mechanisms are present simultaneously and affect radionuclides with different intensities according to their respective geochemical behaviors. Finally, the radioactive decay must be kept in mind; this mechanism acts as a source for the corresponding daughter product and a sink for the corresponding parent.

The distribution of radionuclides between the different compartments considered here (seawater, biota, and sediment) are usually characterized in terms of two parameters, the concentration factor (CF) and the partition (or distribution) coefficient (K_D). These are defined for biota and sediment, respectively, as

$$CF = \frac{\dfrac{Activity\ of\ nuclide\ in\ biota}{Mass\ of\ biota}}{\dfrac{Activity\ of\ nuclide\ in\ seawater}{Mass\ of\ seawater}}$$

and

$$K_D = \frac{\dfrac{Activity\ of\ nuclide\ in\ sediment}{Mass\ of\ sediment}}{\dfrac{Activity\ of\ nuclide\ in\ seawater}{Mass\ of\ seawater}}$$

usually in liters per kilogram. There is, however, some concern regarding the definition and application of these coefficients. First, they only offer a global overview of the redistribution process. Second, K_D values can be very different depending on the geochemical nature of the analyzed sediment fraction (reduced, oxidized, refractory, etc.), and the same can be said for CF, as the different organs can show very different behaviors regarding the concentration capacity for certain elements. Actually, kinetic transfer coefficients are being used in order to do numerical simulations of radioisotopes speciation in the environment [20,21], and CF values are now being established for individual organs instead of whole-body values. However, since these concepts are widely used, they will be used in what follows in order to identify potentially troublesome species. Furthermore, there is a large amount of literature for calculating CF and K_D values for different radionuclides; only field collected data will be reported here, because laboratory experiments show a general trend for overestimating these values.

It is accepted by the scientific community that ocean composition is almost constant and homogeneous as a consequence of dilution mechanisms. However, different water mixing processes can cause the redistribution of radionuclides within the water column. This fact is associated with water dynamics, which is governed by ocean currents and wind effects. Because of this mechanical mixing, vertical gradients of salinity and temperature are almost uniform. According to this, the concentration profiles of many natural radionuclides should also be uniform. This is not true, however, due to the previously referred to intake/loss balance mechanisms, which depend on local environment conditions and the characteristics of the radionuclide's geochemical behavior.

Although the behavior of artificial radionuclides in the different compartments of the ocean is restricted to the same mechanisms as natural radionuclides, the major difference between them is related to the source term: the range, frequency, and intensity of the input of artificial radionuclides to the oceans follow very different systematics. Some artificial radionuclides can also be generated in natural ways (e.g., tritium, ^{14}C, ^{129}I); however, they are discussed in the artificial isotopes section because these make a larger contribution to the world's inventory.

4.3.2 Sources and Sinks of Natural Radionuclides in the Ocean

Among the primordial available radionuclides in the ocean, only ^{40}K and ^{87}Rb are significant from the point of view of exposure to man [22]. Potassium represents approximately 1.1% of dissolved salts in seawater (approximately 392 ppm), while the cosmogenic radionuclide ^{40}K is 0.0118%. It remains dissolved in the seawater column under a wide range of Eh-pH conditions, although it can be incorporated as a nutrient by biota. Its activity concentration in seawater correlates with salinity; as a result, there is not a well-defined average value. The typical range of activity concentration is 11 to 12 Bq/l [1], although different values have been found in different places around the world [23,24]. Because of its very long half-life and natural origin, low concentrations of ^{40}K are usually considered to be natural background levels for both seawater and biota (and the human body itself). It should be noted that Alam et al. [24] reported low CF values for ^{40}K in two different species of mussels, which are considered to be natural bioaccumulators (2 to 7 l/kg for the soft body and 6 to 12 l/kg for the shell).

^{87}Rb, which is 27.8% abundant in natural rubidium, has been reported at levels of 104 mBq/l in ocean water, and within a range of 0.3 to 3.0 mBq/g in marine fish and invertebrates [1]. This would produce a corresponding CF in the range of 2.9 to 29 L/kg. Thus the highest range is about three times less than the radionuclide concentration in the human body itself.

A major source of natural radionuclides in seawater should be the decay of their corresponding parents (^{238}U, ^{232}Th, and ^{235}U). However, seawater represents a rich environment with many possible mechanisms for producing secular equilibrium. These series (and that of ^{232}Th) include a wide variety of isotopes from 10 different elements. A complete and systematic description of these series from different points of view (especially the geochemical one) can be found in the books of Ivanovich and Harmon [25] and Bourdon et al. [26]; these books are strongly recommended for those interested in a comprehensive study of these natural series in different environmental compartments. Here, only a summarized overview of their levels and behavior in the oceanic system is included.

Under oxic conditions, dissolved uranium in seawater remains stable as a carbonate ion $UO_2(CO_3)^3$. The determination of uranium concentrations in Atlantic and Pacific seawater was carried out by Chen et al. [27]. Their results reflected concentrations in the range of 3.16 to 3.28 ng/g, (i.e., about 40 mBq/l) in Atlantic seawater samples, while about 1% higher concentrations were found at Pacific collection sites. Several deviations were reported in the past, resulting in estimates in the range of 1 to 5 ng/ml. However, these differences could be associated with analytical artifacts. The development of relatively recent high-precision techniques such as secondary focusing inductively coupled plasma mass spectrometry (SF-ICP-MS) and new advances in the thermal ionization mass spectrometry (TIMS) technique closed this discussion: recent work shows local values quite similar to that of Chen et al. [28,29]. A recent data update using the TIMS technique on samples collected at Indian, Pacific, and Atlantic Ocean sites and in the Mediterranean Sea produced results quite similar to those from Chen et al., without systematic differences between the oceans [30]. Indeed, the values for the Mediterranean Sea seem to be compatible with those found in open oceans, in agreement with the general correlation with salinity. A clear correlation with the salinity profile has also been found for deep uranium concentration profiles. These detected deviations seem to be associated with changes in redox conditions, which could be linked to natural fluctuations in the organic carbonate composition of seawater.

The isotope ratios collected in seawater are quite homogeneous in the water column (~1.140) for $^{234}U/^{238}U$ in terms of activity ratio; this value deviates slightly from previous assays as a result of an update in their corresponding isotopic half-lives [8]. The origin of the isotope ratio deviation from the secular equilibrium condition is based on the different weathering conditions at the seawater sources (i.e., preferential leaching for ^{234}U). The homogeneity of both the concentration and isotope ratio shows the very long residence time of uranium in seawater, which is greater than the water mixing time (~10^3 years versus 4×10^5 years residence time). This fact ensures homogeneous mixing. On the other hand, ^{235}U remains in seawater and sediments at the natural ratio (7.3×10^{-1}% or 0.73% of natural uranium), as ^{235}U and ^{238}U are weathered at the same rate as ocean sources of uranium. Thus no isotope fractionation mechanisms are involved for these decay series parents and any deviation from the natural value must be associated with anthropogenic pollution episodes.

Uranium is not considered a nutrient for biota. CF values for mussels have been reported in the range of 75 to 100 l/kg, showing a positive correlation with the size of the animal [24]. Indeed, at very contaminated sites, the time variations in the uranium concentration in marine organisms such as mussels and winkles show good agreement with the history of discharges. The experimental values of CF are in agreement with those recommended by the International Atomic Energy Agency (IAEA). The same can be said for K_D values.

[232]Th is the parent of another natural decay series, and there are several long-lived thorium isotopes within the uranium series. Thorium is much less stable than uranium in seawater, as it becomes rapidly adsorbed onto sinking particles; the residence time for thorium in seawater has been estimated to be in the range of 0.7 years [31]. A study of [232]Th concentrations in seawater was performed by Huh et al. [32]. These more recent data show values in a range of approximately 0.02 to 1.7 µBq/l. Higher concentrations have been reported in surface waters, a fact that could be indicating either thorium intake as atmospheric dust, or thorium riverine intake, as this effect seems especially important close to coastal regions. In fact, thorium concentrations in sediments increase toward estuarine and coastal areas [33].

An important thorium isotope fractionation occurs in the open ocean, as the remaining thorium isotopes have additional in situ sources in the ocean. These are decay products from [234]U ([230]Th), [235]U ([231]Th), and [228]Ac ([228]Th). A dataset obtained after analysis of Japanese waters indicated that the concentration of [230]Th increases with collection depth both for particulate thorium and dissolved thorium [34]. Furthermore, a systematic trend was found for the activity concentration (a, in Bq/m^3) of the different thorium isotopes: $a(^{232}Th) < a(^{230}Th) < a(^{228}Th)$. The [230]Th depth profiles are in accordance with its longer half-life (7.5 × 10^4 years), the almost homogeneous concentration of parent uranium in seawater, and the high scavenging rate of thorium [35].

Concentration factor values as high as 600 to 700 l/kg have been reported for mussels collected in Bangladesh [24]. Because of the normally low thorium content of seawater, its isotopes are not usually of special concern from a radiologic point of view. For example, McDonald et al. [31] published an exhaustive report on radionuclide concentrations in different coastal compartments along the British coast, reporting [232]Th concentrations usually less than 1 Bq/kg, with similar or slightly smaller ranges than those for [230]Th. This is an extremely interesting issue, as several of the sampled locations were highly polluted by [238]U series radionuclides. Field results from Martin et al. [36] seem to confirm the low biological affinity for thorium isotopes.

Because of their very distinct characteristics, disequilibria between thorium and uranium (and protactinium) isotopes can be used in oceanic sciences. Thus the [234]U/[238]U ratio has been used for dating manganese nodules and fossil corals [30,37,38]. The dynamics of particle inputs near the seafloor were studied using the excess of [234]Th in basin sediments, which is associated with the inflow of suspended particles. However, diffusion of the dissolved nuclide to deep sea sediments complicates interpretation of the results. A very interesting tool in paleoceanographic studies is the [231]Pa/[230]Th ratio. It is being successfully applied in the estimation of scavenging rates in pelagic sediments. Thus even syndepositional redistribution of the sediment can be taken into account and calculations for biological productivity within a date range of 200,000 to 300,000 years can be performed. The basis of this tool (or "proxy") is as follows: These radionuclides are both α emitters arising from the [235]U and [238]U series, respectively. It is well known that both radionuclides show a high reactivity with particles. Such affinity for particles is especially strong in the case of thorium; this is the reason why its residence time in seawater is shorter than that of [231]Pa. These particles are related to bioproductivity and their incorporation in sediments can be traced to an excess [231]Pa/[230]Th ratio.

Seawater is depleted in radium isotopes regarding uranium as a consequence of thorium removal from the water column. The presence of [230]Th in sediment particles and its corresponding α decay are thought to be one of the sources for the increasing [226]Ra activity with depth, a fact well established in the literature. Radium atoms are diffused from bottom sediments following [230]Th decay. Nozaki et al. [35] reported very homogeneous values for [226]Ra activities in surface waters all over the world, with average values in the range of 1.1 to 1.4 mBq/l. The vertical gradients of [226]Ra do not follow the same trends in the Atlantic and Pacific Oceans because of the different effects of biogenic activity on its removal/desorption. Higher values can be easily found in coastal zones. Examples of local variations are those reported for the Red Sea and Bay of Bengal, which are associated with the upwelling effect and intake from the Ganga-Brahmaputra Delta, respectively. These concentrations are more than 10 times higher than the theoretical decay-only contribution. This fact supports the existence of additional sources of radium in the ocean. The influence of the radium content in groundwater has already been established at about 10% of the overall ocean radium inventory [39]. The lack of agreement between this amount and riverine and groundwater inputs supports the importance of diffusion from bottom sediments as the dominant source of radium isotopes in the ocean.

Although radium remains stable when dissolved in seawater, its substitution by calcium isotopes in microorganisms increases its mobility: first, it is depleted in biota-rich environments; then, it is enriched in bottom sediments as foraminifera skeletons become part of the detrital component; finally, it is released by excess [230]Th. The CF values reported for mussels were of the same order of magnitude as those associated with uranium [24], and additional recent reports do not show very high radium isotope concentrations in marine biota and food samples [40,41]. The other relevant radium isotope, [228]Ra, has a half-life (5.75 years) much shorter than seawater mixing time, and its distribution is characterized by the high activities that can be reached in the shallow water column over shelf areas [42]. Surface concentrations throughout the world can vary over more than two orders of magnitude (0.08 to 4 mBq/l), depending on local factors such as input from coastal sediments, bottom depth (i.e., sediment to surface distance), etc. [35].

[228]Ra profiles in surface seawater samples have allowed researchers to calculate eddy diffusivity coefficients of coastal sites [5]. To do this, a single model that considers decay, diffusion, and eventually advection is used. This model is summarized in the following diffusion equation [43]:

$$\frac{dA}{dt} = K \frac{\partial^2 A}{\partial x^2} - \varpi \frac{\partial A}{\partial x} - \lambda A \qquad (4.1)$$

where A is the nuclide concentration, K is the eddy diffusivity coefficient, x is the distance from the shoreline, ω is the advection velocity, and λ is the corresponding decay constant. It is possible, neglecting the advection near the shoreline (located at position x_0), to get a steady-state solution given by

$$\ln A (x) = \ln A (x_0) - \sqrt{\frac{\lambda}{K}} (x - x_0). \qquad (4.2)$$

Measurements of short-lived radium nuclides at different distances provide activity data, allowing a linear fit that provides a reasonable approach to find K. This short half-life precludes its application as a large-scale oceanic tracer, in contrast to ^{226}Ra.

^{226}Ra should be in near-secular equilibrium with its short half-life daughter ^{222}Rn. Depth profiles for ^{222}Rn and ^{226}Ra concentrations were recorded during the Geochemical Ocean Section Study (GEOSECS) program. They reflected two natural sites for deviations: (1) the sediment-water interface, where ^{222}Rn diffuses from bottom sediments and there is a greater radon concentration due to its less reactive nature; and (2) the sea-air interface, where there is a depletion of radon because of its diffusion to the atmosphere [44]. These phenomena allowed the application of a single model similar to that previously described for calculating eddy diffusion coefficients in vertical mixing.

^{210}Pb and ^{210}Po have been extensively used in environmental and dating studies because of the large differences in both their half-lives and chemical properties. Those geochemical differences are translated to their respective ocean half-lives of 4 years (polonium) and 50 years (lead) in deep water. The ^{210}Pb levels in ocean waters vary over a wide range depending on the location. In surface waters, its most important source is the local decay of ^{226}Ra and the atmospheric transport of ^{222}Rn from continental and coastal areas. Nearshore waters reflect both a low ^{210}Pb concentration and a low ^{210}Pb/^{226}Ra activity ratio. Besides the proximity of continental areas in these regions (and local strong sources for atmospheric ^{222}Rn), there is usually high productivity that enhances reactive lead removal to sinking particles. On the other hand, such removal processes are reduced in the open ocean; the sinking processes for lead are also reduced and therefore the ^{210}Pb/^{226}Ra activity ratio increases. A ^{210}Pb world map of surface open ocean waters can be found in Ivanovich and Harmon [25]. Activity concentrations for ^{210}Pb in these waters range from 0.13 mBq/kg to 0.42 mBq/kg. This activity ratio increases in bottom waters, where production through radium decay can be 2 to 20 times higher than the atmospheric contribution. This fact is reflected in the nature of suspended lead, which appears to be associated with colloidal suspended matter in the open ocean and as solid particles near the shorelines.

In accordance with the previously mentioned partitioning behavior, sediments usually appear to be more enriched in ^{210}Pb than biota. Thus the IAEA [45] recommendations for K_D and CF values are K_D: 5000–100000 l/kg and CF: 100–1000 l/kg, respectively (for mussels, winkles, and seaweed). Experimental field values from McDonald et al. [46] revealed K_D values in accordance with such recommendations, although CF factors were higher than the upper limit by a factor of six to seven at selected polluted places on the British coast.

This additional supply (or excess, $^{210}Pb_{ex}$) produced by atmospheric ^{222}Rn decay is incorporated and retained in the sediments. As it decays following the radioactive law, a sediment depth profile concentration can provide a time scale within a range of about 120 years. This approach also allows for the estimation of changes in the sedimentation rate. This time frame also covers the industrial era, providing support for man-made impacts on the environment. Unfortunately sediments are not a closed system. Different mechanisms such as sediment mixing (bioturbation, storm-driven transport, etc.), redissolution in the sediment-water interphase, and anthropogenic activities (waste releases, sediment removal) affect the $^{210}Pb_{ex}$ inventory. In order to fix this problem, different approximations can be applied. A review of several of these models can be found in Appleby and Oldfield [47].

^{210}Po is typically deficient relative to its parent, ^{210}Pb, in the surface ocean due to preferential removal by biota, while it is in near equilibrium or in excess below the surface mixed layer due to rapid regeneration from sinking organic matter [48]; typical concentrations are about 1 mBq/l. The higher microbiological preference in marine systems for polonium over lead has already been shown [7]. Actually, the activity ratio of $^{210}Po/^{210}Pb$ within the water column can vary through a wide range (0.5 to 12) depending on different factors, especially the presence of polonium bioaccumulators such as zooplankton. Polonium can easily be accumulated by macroorganisms in seawater, and its contribution to the total received dose for critically exposed groups (intensive seafood eaters at locations affected by TENORM) was found to be about 2.5 mSv/year; that is, more than twice the present limit established at the European Union [46]. Depending on the species and locations, CF values are in the range of 2200 to 61,000 l/kg for mussels, 2410 to 31,590 l/kg for winkles, and 70 to 2585 l/kg for seaweed. The distribution of the nuclide within the organism depends on the organ. Hence, muscle tissue accumulates it in mussels and the digestive gland accumulates it in winkles. The transport and distribution of ^{210}Po in the aquatic environment and seafood is of special concern because of its impact on humans. These issues are discussed in Chapters 6 and 8, respectively.

4.3.3 TENORM-Related Pollution Cases

Very large amounts of ^{238}U and ^{232}Th series radionuclides have been released to the marine environment during (or after) several no nuclear industrial processes. The European Commission recently finished a study (MARINA II) on the TENORM industries in northern Europe [49]. The total discharges in 1981 were estimated at 65 TBq (^{210}Po and ^{226} Ra) and 32 TBq (^{210}Pb). These activities can enhance the local activity concentrations, however, their effects on the ocean are reduced for two reasons: dilution in seawater [50,51] and binding to sediments, which act as a reservoir for a fraction of the released radioactivity.

A well-known and illustrative example of this sort of scenario is the release of phosphogypsum in southwest Spain either directly or indirectly (via leaching and percolation) from gypsum repository stacks. Hence very important local effects, including drastic radionuclide increases in river water, sediments, and salt marshes, have been reported [52–55]. The effects of tidal washout and self-cleaning processes after reducing the direct releases were also reported [56,57]. Similar recent work reporting the local effects of phosphogypsum deposits and phosphate ore processing and releases can be found for the Red Sea [58], India [59], the U.S. [60], and the Irish Sea [61].

Although several industrial processes are involved in the release of natural radioactive materials to the environment, only phosphate fertilizer production and gas and oil production are considered here as related to direct releases to the ocean. In contrast to the production of phosphate fertilizers, during gas and oil production, radioactivity is released by a single relocation of naturally occurring radioactivity, without any kind of chemical enrichment or separation. Water from the reservoir containing low levels of petroleum is pumped to the surface. The produced water is separated from the oil and either injected into a well or discharged after treatment to surface waters [62]. The average concentration of the radionuclides ^{226}Ra and ^{228}Ra in discharges from all oil-producing platforms in northern Europe and over all the years is estimated at a reference value of 10 Bq/l each; for gas production, the corresponding figures are ^{226}Ra, 10 Bq/l; ^{210}Pb, 5 Bq/l; and ^{228}Ra, 3 Bq/l [49]. The values vary within a very wide range (two to three orders of magnitude), however, depending on local and industrial factors [51,63]. According to Betti et al. [49], the European releases associated with phosphogypsum are decreasing with time, while those associated with gas and oil production are increasing.

4.3.4 ARTIFICIAL RADIONUCLIDES IN THE OCEANIC ECOSYSTEM

Artificial radionuclides are present in the ocean as a result of different anthropogenic activities. Injected radionuclides can return to the troposphere as fallout during the air mass exchange processes at temperate latitudes and the poles, and with special intensity when winter ends and spring begins. Bearing in mind that ocean waters cover approximately two-thirds of the Earth's surface, it clearly shows the relative higher input of fallout radionuclides into the ocean. As there is no air mass mixing between different hemispheres, it can be concluded that the greater proportion of artificial radioactivity from fallout has occurred in the Northern Hemisphere, in agreement with the greater number of nuclear atmospheric tests that have occurred there. It has been calculated that the most affected geographic band is between 40°N and 60°N latitude [1].

The release of radioactive effluents from the nuclear fuel cycle is an extremely important source of artificial radioactivity. These releases act as local sources of a very wide range of radionuclides to the ocean. Quite the opposite of TENORM releases, however, their effects can be felt several thousand miles away from the original source. This is due to the fact that TENORM releases involve naturally occurring radionuclides that after dilution can increase the natural background amounts. In contrast, artificial radionuclides are released to an ecosystem with a low background (associated to fallout); this additional supply can sometimes be easily detected. Additional sources for artificial radioactivity are nuclear accidents and the use of nuclear medicine. There is, however, a lack of knowledge concerning this radioactivity, possibly because its contribution to the environment has been predicted as negligible when compared to the previously mentioned sources.

4.3.4.1 Fissile Materials and Transuranide Activation Products

^{235}U is extensively used as a nuclear fuel for the production of nuclear energy and also for nuclear bombs. With the exception of local contamination episodes related to direct injection of nuclear debris during nuclear atmospheric tests, the variations in uranium isotope ratios are not usually as important as those due to local effluents from enrichment/reprocessing plants. Actually, using uranium as a nuclear fuel requires recycling the uranium as far as possible, and this economical reason ensures that avoiding uranium losses is of special concern. Therefore the injection of enriched/depleted uranium into the oceans has not been enough to cause a global change of natural isotope ratios. As shown below, this is not the case for other radionuclides.

^{239}Pu is possibly the most used fissile material. The low fission efficiency (usually less than 10% of plutonium suffers fission) has introduced and scattered a large amount of this isotope in the environment. Furthermore, ^{240}Pu and ^{241}Pu are generated as activation products during the irradiation of ^{239}Pu. The amounts released by nuclear tests are estimated as 7.8 PBq (^{239}Pu), 5.2 PBq (^{240}Pu), and 170 PBq (^{241}Pu) [15]. The total inventory of plutonium in the ocean has been estimated as 20 PBq [18]. Additional sources such as nuclear fuel reprocessing facilities are important and their contribution has been estimated at approximately 10% of overall plutonium amounts.

Elemental plutonium has been the object of intense surveillance during the nuclear era because of its high toxicity, although its geochemistry is complicated by the fact that four oxidation states (Pu^{3+}, Pu^{4+}, PuO_2^-, PuO_2^{2-}) are possible in seawater [64]. The $^{239+240}Pu$ fallout level concentration in Atlantic Ocean seawater has been estimated to be about 8 µBq/l within the latitude band 25°N to 50°N (3 µBq/l within the band 5°N to 25°N). For the North Pacific, the average in surface waters is about 3 µBq/l [65], and results show no important differences due to latitude in the 5°N to 35°N band. Water column profiles reflect a very characteristic distribution, with a minimum in surface and deep waters and a maximum at an intermediate depth of 250 to 1000 m, which can vary depending on location [66]. This effect is related to the very high reactivity of plutonium; hence, after thorough mixing within the ocean and horizontal diffusion and advection, plutonium is adsorbed onto scavenging particles and flows to the sediment. There are reported differences on profiles in the particulate matter and dissolved fraction of plutonium [65,66].

Besides the local effects due to accidents, there is a very interesting scenario in the Arctic Ocean, where the concentrations of plutonium are much higher than those predicted from fallout and releases from Sellafield (U.K.) and La Hague (France). Hence, two major hypotheses for this plutonium excess are being considered: (1) the local effect from nuclear tests in Novya Zemlia (former USSR), and (2) intake through the Ob and Techa Rivers (Siberia) from reprocessing plants and direct storing of high-radioactivity wastes. It is possible to identify the plutonium origin depending on the ^{238}Pu/^{239,240}Pu isotope ratio. Hence the activity ratio is approximately 0.18 for plutonium originating from fallout and deviates from this ratio for releases from reprocessing plants [67].

The transference of plutonium atoms to the sediments is a very important source for artificial radioactivity in the environment. Hence the released radioactivity remains unfixed within a bottom sink, but acts as a source for redistribution; K_D values of 4.8×10^4 to 5.1×10^4 have been reported in the Kara Sea [68]. This effect could be especially important at those sites where intense and local emissions are occurring, such as the Irish Sea. This is due to the effects of resuspension following tidal and storm episodes, exchange with the pore water, and subsequent transport. Regarding the bioavailability of plutonium, a recent review of the CFs for several transuranides in marine invertebrates was performed by Ryan [69]. The assimilation efficiencies of transuranic elements in marine invertebrates are high compared to vertebrates and mammals in general (from 20×10^4 to 2×10^4). Fish, mollusks, and seaweed have been analyzed for plutonium (and americium) content and the data reflect concentrations of less than 1 mBq/kg, seaweed being the exception, with concentrations of several becquerel per kilogram for *Fucus vesiculosus* [70]. An average CF value of 2.5×10^4 l/kg was reported for microplankton from the Mediterranean Sea by Sanchez-Cabeza et al. [71], being one order of magnitude less for surface mesoplankton. The calculated dose due to seafood consumption in the Irish Sea ranges from 0.09 to 0.37 μSv/year, and this small dose contribution includes the contribution from ^{241}Am.

Elements with high sediment affinity, such as plutonium, have been used to study the ability of sea ice to incorporate, intercept, and transport contaminants in the Arctic Ocean [72]. Furthermore, artificial plutonium can provide a good reference point for dating, as its presence within the sediment should mark deposition after the beginning of the nuclear era.

^{241}Am has also been released with nuclear tests, with inventories of 25 Bq/m^2 in sediments within the band 40°N to 50°N latitude [73]. Direct releases from Sellafield have been determined to be about 940 TBq, and approximately 360 TBq more following the β decay of ^{241}Pu [74]. Usual levels in surface water are in the range of 0.1 to 2.5 μBq/l [75,76], showing a depth profile behavior similar to that of plutonium. Measurements performed in the western Mediterranean Sea and the Strait of Gibraltar show that only about 5% of the initially released ^{241}Am is still present in the water column, reflecting its large affinity for scavenging particles. An additional supply in this region is due to the Palomares (Spain) nuclear accident in 1966, which is reflected in a drastic increase in its activity concentration in seaweeds, from 9 (typical background value) to 240 mBq/kg [77]. The rapid removal of americium from the water column is explained by its affinity for sinking particles, which is even higher than that of plutonium; their corresponding residence times are calculated as about 15 years for plutonium and 3 years for americium. In fact, local impacts have been seen in different areas of the Irish Sea due to releases from Sellafield, as concentrations in seawater three orders of magnitude higher than those due to global fallout have been reported [74]. However, it has been calculated that a greater proportion of americium is rapidly accumulated in sediments only 20 km away from the release point. The sediments inventory for ^{241}Am is quite similar to that of plutonium. The contribution of americium to the Irish seafood consumer is in the range of 1%. Different radionuclides such as curium (^{242}Cm, ^{243}Cm, ^{244}Cm) are also released from reprocessing plants, with a contribution to the average dose rate of less than 0.5%. Even the most affected areas contain a ^{237}Np total inventory in sediments about three orders of magnitude less than those of plutonium and americium [67].

4.3.4.2 Fission Fragments and Other Activation Products

^{90}Sr and ^{137}Cs are among the most representative and most widely studied artificial radionuclides because of their rate of release from global fallout, nuclear fuel reprocessing plants, and different accidents and waste dumping. ^{90}Sr has a fission yield of 5.8%, and its high solubility as Sr^{2+} ion is the origin of its conservative behavior in seawater. According to Aarkrog [15], the total input of ^{90}Sr to the world's oceans has been 380 PBq as global fallout (52% in the Pacific Ocean and 33% in the Atlantic Ocean) and 6.5 PBq from European reprocessing plants (both of them on the Atlantic Ocean), with only 20% being released from La Hague. On the other hand, in the case of ^{137}Cs, the nuclear accident at Chernobyl supplied a small fraction of the total ^{90}Sr to the environment. Their concentrations in seawater vary over a wide range, depending on the location and proximity to nuclear releases or dumping sites and oceanographic factors (water mass circulation). Thus typical concentrations in the North Sea are 2 to 20 mBq/l. In the Sea of Japan, values are in the range of 0.4 to 3.3 mBq/l (average 1.6 mBq/l) and the seawater column profiles show a typical exponential decay with depth [78]. This range of values is comparable to the 0.4 to 1.5 mBq/l range in the Indian Ocean [79]. Similar values were found in Japanese coastal surface waters, although some locations in this area reflected an increase because of the 11 atmospheric nuclear tests performed by China, but showed no effective increase from the Chernobyl accident [80]. The local input of ^{90}Sr in the Pacific Ocean has been estimated to be about 113 PBq, while the corresponding local inventory due to global fallout is about 66 PBq [15]. As more than one ^{90}Sr half-life has occurred since the production peak of the nuclear arms race, we should see a decrease in these elements in seawater (with an effective half-life of 15 years).

The IAEA recommended K_D value is 200 l/kg for pelagic sediments and 10^3 l/kg for coastal plankton, hence low ^{90}Sr amounts in pelagic sediments should be expected. However, some effective removal can be found as a consequence of uptake to biota and coprecipitation of magnesium and calcium in skeleton carbonates and trace amounts have been found in deep sediments [81]. The CFs are in the range of 1 to 2 l/kg for mollusks and fish.

The highly conservative behavior of ^{90}Sr in seawater has been shown (and applied) in oceanographic studies, and it has been estimated that besides the local input, long-distance transport is very important. For example, rivers in Siberia and Canada contribute about 3.2 PBq of ^{90}Sr to the East Greenland Current [15]. This amount is two times higher than that due to released ^{137}Cs from reprocessing plants, even though the released amount is estimated to be six times less. Similar studies have reflected additional inputs of this radionuclide to the Mediterranean Sea, as the calculated inventories (2500 TBq in seawater and 120 TBq in sediments) do not agree with the predictions from global fallout [82].

The global fallout contribution to the total inventory of ^{137}Cs in the ocean was calculated using a ^{137}Cs/^{90}Sr isotope ratio of 1.6, as the total amount of ^{90}Sr is better known [83]. For the European reprocessing plants, 40 PBq were released to the Atlantic Ocean, about 3% from La Hague (English Channel), and the rest from Sellafield (Irish Sea). The total ocean input from the Chernobyl accident released an additional 15 to 20 PBq, with the Baltic Sea being the most contaminated (approximately 4.5 PBq). Typical surface seawater concentrations in the North Sea (including both pre- and post-Chernobyl) are 3.5 to 300 µBq/l. This is partially due to the less conservative behavior of cesium in the sea (K_D approximately 2×10^3 l/kg). Thus ^{137}Cs is found in settling particulate matter, and it can be incorporated into clay minerals by adsorption through ionic exchange. However, the distribution of this nuclide is not homogeneous. Hirose et al. [84] reported concentrations as high as 5 mBq/l within the upper 10 m in the Japan Trench. The depth profiles were fairly typical: exponential decrease with depth, with a level at the bottom (approximately 8000 m) less than 12 µBq/l. Livingstone and Povinec [85] reviewed and improved the databases for cesium distribution, showing a clear concentration distribution such as Baltic Sea > Irish Sea > Black Sea > northeast Atlantic > North Atlantic > Arctic Ocean > Mediterranean Sea > North Pacific > Indian Ocean > Central Pacific; it seems that the outflow from the Black Sea could be the additional source for the excess supply in the Mediterranean Sea.

Because of the large amount of this nuclide released to the environment, it has been the target of increasing interest for the scientific community. Concentrations in Baltic fish in the range of 12 to 22 Bq/kg have been reported [86], while Heldal et al. [87] report concentrations 14 Bq/kg for cod in the Irish Sea. It has been shown that the concentration factor increases within the trophic chain, ranging from 10 (lower levels) to 200 (upper levels, sea mammals). The ingestion of fish and shellfish with high ^{137}Cs concentrations can increase the radiological risk for the affected population. As an estimation of that risk, calculations of the corresponding collective doses can be performed; dividing the collective dose by the affected population, the average individual dose can be calculated. For Mediterranean and Black Sea inhabitants, such a collective dose was calculated as 5 man-Sv [85], compared to 1100 man-Sv for naturally occurring ^{210}Pb.

Two important iodine radioactive isotopes have been released to the environment since the beginning of the nuclear era. ^{131}I is very significant from the radiological point of view, although exposure through the marine environment is not very significant because of its short half-life. In contrast, ^{129}I has both a long half-life and persistence in the marine environment, but low radiological significance. Global fallout is not an important anthropogenic source of ^{129}I; the released amounts from European nuclear fuel plants are some 50 times greater than the amount released by nuclear testing and three orders of magnitude higher than the amount released from Chernobyl. ^{129}I is also naturally occurring. Since the beginning of the nuclear era the $^{129}I/^{127}I$ isotope ratio has increased by approximately two orders of magnitude against the natural values within the upper layers of the ocean. The extraordinarily conservative behavior of this element in the ocean (residence time about 10^5 years) has suggested its use as a very effective water mass tracer, besides its biophylic character [88–90].

Natural background levels of ^3H in surface waters are in the range of 20 to 100 mBq/kg [91]. Fallout-related input is considered the most important anthropogenic source, increasing activity concentrations up to several tenths of a becquerel per liter during the mid-1960s. Certain areas affected by nuclear reprocessing effluents can show a significant increase (up to 2 to 10 Bq/kg). The cycle of tritium in nature is complicated, as the major proportion of effluents is produced as water vapor. Liquid effluents have the form ^3H_2O. Tritium is also very persistent in seawater, and is useful as a radioactive tracer. The ocean inventory for 2000 has been estimated as 13,300 PBq [15]. This isotope can be easily accumulated as organic bound tritium (OBT). CF values have been reported as 2×10^4 for mussels, 300 for seaweed, and 100 for suspended particles and sediment [91]. However, even for critically exposed groups, its radiological significance is very small.

It has been estimated that 94% of natural ^{14}C (1.15×10^{19} Bq) is present in the oceans. ^{14}C is a major contributor to the dose from cosmogenic nuclides (approximately 10 μSv/year). As with tritium, the contribution of ^{14}C to the ocean inventory from nuclear reprocessing plants is reported to be negligible when compared to that from nuclear fallout. Anthropogenic ^{14}C follows the marine carbon cycle, causing deviations in the natural $^{14}C/^{12}C$ isotope ratio. This contribution to the ^{14}C isotope ratio is in agreement with the so-called Suiss effect, that is, a deviation in the natural ratio following intensive fossil fuel burning, which is depleted in ^{14}C [92]. Upper ocean layers show an isotope ratio 4% less than the natural atmospheric ratio, while this depletion reaches 17% in the deep ocean.

A very interesting radionuclide for water mass tracing is ^{99}Tc (fission yield approximately 6%). $^{99}TcO_4$ ion is extremely conservative in an oxidized environment and, as a consequence, it can travel several thousand kilometers from the releasing sources (see below for details). The released amounts from nuclear tests have been estimated at about 140 TBq; as a comparison, the Sellafield releases from 1978 to 1998 directly to the Irish Sea are estimated at about 950 TBq [93]. During the mid-1990s, a new enhanced actinide removal plant (EARP) was opened at the nuclear reprocessing facility of Sellafield. This plant allowed the company to drastically decrease releases of actinides, while increasing the releases of some other nuclides such as [99]Tc. This is reflected in a dramatic increase in technetium releases since 1994. Naturally occurring bioaccumulators such as brown seaweed (especially *Fucus vesiculosus*, CF approximately 10^5 l/kg) have been monitored as radionuclide indicators. An additional interesting issue is the use of brown seaweed to prepare soils before planting: [99]Tc taken up by the seaweed and arising from nuclear reprocessing plants can be released to the ground and become incorporated in plants, increasing the possibility of transference through the trophic chain [94]. Although the radiotoxicity of this nuclide is low, this additional exposure path should be taken into account.

Relatively recent studies on this radionuclide show perfectly how radioactive tracers can be used for oceanographic work. For example, Dahlgaard et al. [95] used a transit time (t) for coastal water masses from La Hague to Kattegat, which is defined as the time from radionuclide release to the sea until its concentration is at its maximum (this detail is necessary as successive tides of this radionuclide suffer certain time and distance effects as a consequence of many oceanographic factors). The transference factor (TF_k; in Bq/m³/TBq/month) is defined as the ratio of the activity concentration at a given time at the sampling location and the activity released t months earlier at the discharge point (which is supposedly known using the data published from the facilities themselves). Finally, a cross correlation can be performed in order to minimize the parameter M with respect to TF_k, defined as [96]:

$$M = \sum_{i,j,k} \left[TF_k \, x\!\left(t_i\right) - y\!\left(t_j\right) \right]^2, \qquad (4.3)$$

where x is the ^{99}Tc discharge (in TBq/month), y is the activity concentration in seawater (in Bq/m³), and $(t_j) - (t_i)$ is the transit time. Using this approach with several restrictions (especially when additional sources of the radionuclide are to be considered), transit times in the range of 15 to 18 months were derived, corresponding to transference factors of 0.045 to 0.072 Bq/m³/TBq/year, showing the sensitivity of the method to water mass mixing. From Sellafield to northern Norway, the corresponding figures were 42 months and 6 Bq/m³/PBq/year [96].

The presence of [125]Sb has been reported as far as the Norway coast, with values similar to those in the English Channel and Irish Sea where this radionuclide is released. A recent example was reported by Bailly du Bois and Guegueniat [97]: 3 to 12 mBq/l were reported for the English Channel and 1.9 to 3.0 mBq/l for the western Norwegian coast. It must be understood that the levels recorded far away from the source location have a different release origin because the travel time is 2 to 3 years from Sellafield and several months less from La Hague. Other radionuclides that can produce a local increase in dose due to their trends to be incorporated into edible tissues of seafood are [65]Zn, [103]Ru, and [60]Co. On the other hand, manganese and iron isotopes are usually incorporated into the sediments.

Several radionuclides such as ^{99}Tc, ^{129}I, ^{137}Cs, and ^{125}Sb can be used as a "footprint" for nuclear waste releases to the North Atlantic Ocean. Hence ^{137}Cs and ^{99}Tc are characteristics of the emissions from Sellafield, although minor amounts are released from La Hague. Exactly the opposite can be said regarding ^{129}I and ^{125}Sb, whose source term is about five times higher than that of Sellafield.

4.4 RADIOACTIVITY IN RAINWATER

4.4.1 INTRODUCTION

With regard to radioactivity, the important parts of the atmosphere are the troposphere and stratosphere. The troposphere extends from the Earth's surface to an altitude of about 11 km. The height depends on the latitude and on the season. The so-called tropopause separates the troposphere from the stratosphere, the next atmospheric region. The stratosphere occupies a band of fairly constant temperature that extends from 11 km to about 30 km. The separation line is imaginary, but it is true that the major part of the atmosphere resides in the troposphere, and the relevant processes and changes governing the weather take place in it. The troposphere and stratosphere are not isolated, and stratospheric circulation patterns lead to air exchanges between the troposphere and stratosphere. This phenomenon is of crucial importance for the transport of radioactivity released from nuclear weapons tests, as will be seen later.

The radioactivity in the troposphere and stratosphere occurs through different mechanisms that will be briefly described. Once the injection occurs, radioactive particles or gases follow the global transport pattern taking place in the atmosphere.

Rainwater helps to remove radioactivity from the troposphere and transport it to the Earth's surface. Rainwater is neither a source nor a sink of radionuclides, but rather a connection between two different environmental compartments: the atmosphere and the surface of the Earth.

Rainwater helps to transport and disseminate radionuclides and therefore shows very well the level of radioactivity in the environment. Thus the study of radioactivity concentrations in rainwater should be included in all surveillance programs. In most cases they include weekly or monthly sampling, which is enough to estimate the level of radioactivity contamination in the environment. In the case of a nuclear accident, the periodicity of sample collecting must change.

Sampling of rainwater is relatively simple. Generally the collection is performed in a container or funnel with a known collecting area. The biggest problem to be solved is the preservation of samples between precipitation periods. This is a relevant problem, especially in dry areas, where the time elapsed between rainfalls is long and the rain volume low. If one is interested in a determination of the atmospheric transport of radionuclides, dry fallout has to be collected separately from rainwater. This fact leads to special collector designs.

4.4.2 THE PRESENCE OF RADIOACTIVITY IN RAINWATER: SOURCES AND PATHWAYS

4.4.2.1 Natural Radioactivity

Primordial radionuclides can be introduced into the atmosphere through several pathways. Radon emanation from the Earth's crust is probably one of the most important ways. The abundance of ^{238}U makes ^{222}Rn emanation the more relevant mechanism. This introduces a wide group of radionuclides into the atmosphere. Fortunately ^{222}Rn emanation also liberates a precious chronological tool, ^{210}Pb. The dating method based on it is well known.

Resuspension from the soil is also an important mechanism. In this way, previously deposited particles contaminated with radioactivity are picked up by the wind and reintroduced into the lower parts of the troposphere. In some cases, rainwater helps to settle these particles back to Earth or simply washes them away by dissolving the radionuclides. Both radon emanation and resuspension processes are especially important for areas with high levels of natural radioactivity, that is, areas where wastes are released from industries that use TENORMs.

Cosmogenic radionuclides are continuously being produced in the atmosphere by the interaction of cosmic radiation with the nuclei present there. They can also be transported by rainwater. A wide variety of cosmogenic nuclides exist. Many of them can be used as specific tracers for different environmental compartments. Examples are ^{14}C, ^{36}Cl, ^{85}Kr, and ^3H, among others. From a radiological viewpoint, the case of ^3H is certainly relevant and special attention will be paid to it in later sections. Unfortunately the majority of cosmogenic nuclides are also produced during nuclear weapons tests and in the nuclear fuel cycle. In fact, this effect masks to a great extent their production by cosmic radiation. So some data about them are discussed in the paragraphs devoted to man-made radionuclides.

4.4.2.2 Man-Made Radioactivity

The proliferation of nuclear tests introduced a large quantity of radioactivity into the atmosphere mainly from the late 1950s to the early 1970s. The released radioactivity was deposited in a local manner either by dry fallout or rainwater. Part of the produced radioactivity was injected into the stratosphere. This amount depends on the power of the weapon. The result of such tests was a global effect. The radioactive material in the stratosphere is more or less homogeneously distributed over the hemisphere where the explosion took place and is reintroduced into the troposphere according to global air circulation patterns and interactions between the stratosphere and troposphere.

Atmospheric releases from normal nuclear fission reactor operations populate the lower parts of the troposphere with radioactive fission or activation products. This produces mostly local contamination effects, but atmospheric emissions from nuclear fuel reprocessing plants can travel long distances before deposition. Today this is the most relevant mechanism by which the nuclear fuel cycle introduces artificial radioactivity to the atmosphere, and consequently to rainwater.

The occurrence of nuclear accidents, of course, masks any other effect, at least temporarily. This was the case with the Chernobyl accident, which contaminated the whole Northern Hemisphere to various degrees. The monitoring of radioactivity in rainwater is a very important tool for detecting contamination and preventing radiological consequences.

4.4.3 LEVELS AND DISTRIBUTION

4.4.3.1 Natural Radioactivity

According to Kathren [92], several pioneering works at the beginning of the 20th century demonstrated the existence of radioactivity in atmospheric air and rainwater. A connection of the observed radioactivity with the emanation of ^{222}Rn due to the presence of ^{226}Ra in the neighboring soils was shown.

Today this is a well-established fact and many works can be found in the literature showing the presence of primordial radionuclides in the atmosphere. The main objective of these documents is the determination of radon isotopes and their descendants in the atmospheric aerosol, since it is very relevant from a radiological viewpoint. Consequently there is not very much literature on the presence and levels of primordial nuclides in rainwater.

Some early works of Sakuragi et al. [98] and Kuroda et al. [99] provided results on uranium concentrations in rainwater samples taken during the spring of 1980 in Fayetteville, Arkansas. They found anomalous ^{234}U/^{238}U and ^{235}U/^{238}U activity ratios that they attributed to the Soviet satellite Cosmos 94, which fell over Canada on January 24, 1978. These authors, together with Essien et al. [100], noted a relevant increase in the ^{238}U concentration in rainwater taken from the same area related to the eruption of Mount St. Helens on May 18, 1980.

The influence of nuclear tests on the concentration of uranium in rainwater was also reported by Matsunami et al. [101], who also found anomalous concentrations in rainwater taken in the southern Pacific Ocean caused by French nuclear testing in 1970 and 1971.

However, in the absence of the events described above, levels of primordial radionuclides in a given area are governed by resuspension effects. This is claimed in A. Martinez-Aguirre et al. [102], where results on uranium isotopes and ^{226}Ra concentrations are given for rainwater collected at Seville, Spain, from 1986 to 1988. The total mass concentration of uranium and the radioactivity concentration of ^{226}Ra in the samples vary widely over time. This, of course, depends in a complicated manner on meteorological factors, especially precipitation rates and wind strength and direction. Thus high precipitation rates are followed by low radioactive concentrations in the atmosphere. Levels of ^{238}U and ^{234}U range from 1 to 10 mBq/l. Their activity ratio is 1.09 ± 0.30, very close to the expected value for natural uranium. According to the authors, this result confirms that the origin of uranium in rainwater is resuspension from surface soils surrounding the town. Concentrations for ^{226}Ra range from 3 to 17 mBq/l, close to those for ^{238}U, although their activity ratio, ^{226}Ra/^{238}U, changes greatly, with a mean value of

2.27 ± 1.22, that is, far from the equilibrium. This also resembles their different behavior in soils, in which uranium can be leached more easily than radon.

The importance of resuspension is very clear in Hirose et al. [103]. The authors found a seasonal trend in the deposition of ^{232}Th over Tsukuba and Nagasaki in Japan. It corresponded to the seasonal cycle of soil dust fallout originating from East Asia. The authors suggest that ^{232}Th can be used as an atmospheric tracer of soil particles originating from the continents.

Finally, a full account of the environmental radioactive impact of nonnuclear industries that use naturally occurring radioactive materials can be found in a special issue of *Journal of Environmental Radioactivity* published in 1996.

4.4.3.2 Man-Made Radioactivity

Contamination of the environment by man-made radioactivity started in July 1945, when the first nuclear weapon was tested at Alamogordo, New Mexico. Certainly the massive global radioactive contamination of the Earth is due to atmospheric nuclear weapons tests. The U.S. and the former Soviet Union carried out programs of atmospheric testing that ended in 1962 when a moratorium was signed by the two superpowers with the agreement of the U.K. France and China did not accept the moratorium and they continued their programs until 1980, when the last atmospheric test took place in China.

Nuclear explosions disseminate many different radionuclides in the atmosphere, the majority of which have very short half-lives. Only a few nuclides remain in the environment after an explosion with relatively long half-lives. These are the ones that play a relevant role from an environmental standpoint. With this in mind, it is very easy to understand why special attention was paid to the determination of ^{137}Cs $(T_{1/2} = 30.1$ years) and ^{90}Sr $(T_{1/2} = 29.1$ years) in atmospheric samples.

The historical time variation of ^{137}Cs and ^{90}Sr in rainwater shows a latitudinal variation, but in general terms it can be observed that activity appeared in rainwater at the beginning of the 1950s, when nuclear tests started, and which, after a maximum in 1963, has steadily decreased. This is the effect of the moratorium of 1962 that followed a time period when nuclear testing reached a maximum. In fact, it is estimated that from 1961 to 1962, the total atmospheric nuclear test yield was about 340 MT, compared with the total yield from 1945 to 1990 of some 545.4 MT.

Rainwater removes radioactivity injected in the troposphere after some 2 or 3 weeks. The radioactivity injected into the stratosphere, after homogenization over the entire hemisphere, is reintroduced into the troposphere through the temperate zones with an average residence time of roughly 1 year.

More recently, other nuclides have been taken into account when studying radioactivity in the atmosphere. Such are the cases for ^{99}Tc $(T_{1/2} = 2.14 \times 10^5$ years), ^{36}Cl $(T_{1/2} = 3.01 \times 10^5$ years), and ^{129}I $(T_{1/2} = 15.7 \times 10^6$ years). It is estimated that 0.14 PBq of ^{99}Tc have been released to the environment from weapons detonations. Because of its very long half-life, it is very difficult to measure. The development of mass spectrometry techniques has facilitated its determination.

There is very little data in the current literature on the content of ^{99}Tc in rainwater. In García-León et al. [104], levels are measured in rainwater in southern Spain from 1984 to 1988. Activity concentrations ranging from 0.009 to 0.18 mBq/l were found and the so-called spring effect — a maximum in the activity transfer from the stratosphere to the troposphere — was found for ^{99}Tc. Some previous data from Texas were published by Attrepp et al. [105]. The combination of both datasets allowed the authors to plot the ^{99}Tc/^{137}Cs activity ratio in the atmosphere. This activity ratio should be about 10^4. However, the observed increase in that activity ratio and the magnitude of the values themselves were used by the authors for the calculation of a residence time of ^{99}Tc in the atmosphere, which was estimated at about 1.6 years. Nevertheless, it is possible that the increase was mainly governed by the influence of atmospheric emissions from nuclear fuel reprocessing plants. More recent measurements by inductively coupled plasma mass spectrometry (ICP-MS) have shown that the level of ^{99}Tc in rainwater is less than 10^1 mBq/l [106].

Some 50,000 kg of ^{129}I has been produced so far by natural processes. Only about 260 kg of this amount is mobile in nature; the remainder is bound to the lithosphere. Nuclear explosions have liberated about 40 kg to the atmosphere. The most important source of ^{129}I is the nuclear fuel reprocessing process. Some 1000 kg has been released to the environment this way, and it is estimated that about 5600 kg are stored in nuclear wastes. The long half-life of ^{129}I has made it very difficult to measure. Today, accelerator mass spectrometry permits its determination in a number of natural compartments. One of them is rainwater.

Little data are available in the literature. In samples taken from southern Spain during 1998 and 1999 [107], levels of 2.2×10^7 to 107.8×10^7 atoms/l were found. These values are typically lower than those measured in central Europe, where levels in the range of 10^8 atoms/l appear for samples collected in Germany and Switzerland during the late 1980s and early 1990s. The difference can be attributed to the longer distance to Spain from the reprocessing plants of Sellafield and La Hague. The influence of such facilities is quite clear in Lopez-Gutierrez et al. [107]. In Lopez-Gutierrez et al., the ^{129}I deposition by rainwater is presented along with the total ^{129}I emissions from La Hague and Sellafield.

Muramatsu and Ohmomo [108] show the influence of the nuclear fuel repro-cessing plant of Tokaimura on rainwater samples taken in its vicinity. Concen-trations up to 100 µBq/l were obtained for ^{129}I in water collected some 2.5 km from the plant, compared with activity levels of 0.5 µBq/l for samples collected 100 km from Tokaimura.

^{36}Cl is also naturally produced in the atmosphere by a nuclear reaction (spallation) consisting of the bombing of atmospheric argon (the target) with natural radiation (the projectile). ^{36}Cl is, at the same time, an activation product that is produced during nuclear weapons tests and during nuclear fuel burning. It is a relevant nuclide for the future of nuclear waste storage, as previously stated. ^{36}Cl cannot be measured by normal radiometric methods. However, accelerator mass spectrometry has provided data on its presence in nature. In the case of rainwater, there is very little data. In Figure 4.2 and Figure 4.3, results are shown

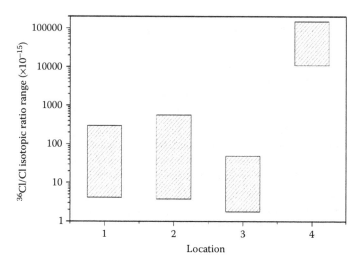

FIGURE 4.2 ^{36}Cl/Cl isotope ratio ranges at different locations and sampling dates. Location 1: Seville (Spain), 1999–2000. Location 2: Maryland (USA), 1991–1993. Location 3: Israel, 1983–1989. Location 4: Long Island, New York (USA), 1957–1960.

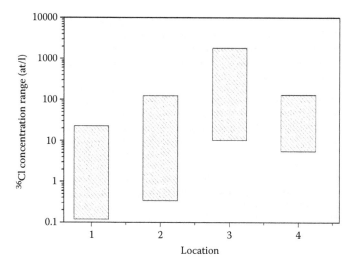

FIGURE 4.3 ^{36}Cl concentration ranges (atm/l) at different locations and sampling dates. Location 1: Seville (Spain), 1999–2000. Location 2: Israel, 1983–1989. Location 3: Long Island, New York (USA), 1957–1960. Location 4: Ontario (Canada); not specified.

from the few works existing in the literature. With the exception of the samples taken from 1957 to 1960, concentrations of ^{36}Cl and isotopic ^{36}Cl/Cl ratios are very similar for all the samples and study periods. Thus observed concentrations were within the range of 0.10 to 130 atoms/l, and observed atom ratios are within the range of 4×10^{15} to 5×10^{4}. The case of the Long Island, New York, samples reflects the influence of nuclear tests in the atmosphere. In fact, the nuclear pulse for ^{36}Cl has already been observed in ice core samples [109], which is in agreement with the previous comments.

The presence of ^{36}Cl in the atmosphere is masked by the input of stable chlorine from the sea. This effect can be observed in Santos et al. [110] for samples collected in Seville, Spain, a town far from nuclear installations. It is very easy to see that for high southwest winds, the ^{36}Cl/Cl ratio decreases. This is due to the introduction of stable chlorine from the sea, since the Atlantic Ocean is located to the southwest. The authors claim to have found a spring effect for ^{36}Cl. This is not surprising, since ^{36}Cl is produced mainly in the stratosphere.

So far the influence of nuclear fuel reprocessing plants on the concentration of ^{36}Cl in rainwater has not been demonstrated. Nevertheless, in all the available articles, the measured total ^{36}Cl deposition is higher than that calculated with cosmic ray production models. This excess can be explained in terms of the recycling of ^{36}Cl from the biosphere as methyl chloride [111]. However, inputs from nuclear plants cannot be ignored.

^{3}H is found in nature mostly as heavy water (HTO), although a small proportion of it is in the form of molecular hydrogen (HT). It is produced by the interaction of cosmic rays with the elements in the upper layers of the atmosphere, and according to Villa [112], the amount of ^{3}H present in the environment for this reason is approximately 1 EBq. Since the beginning of the nuclear era, ^{3}H has been introduced in the environment as a product of fusion or fission nuclear reactions. Through 1982, some 240 EBq has been injected in the atmosphere due to thermonuclear explosions and about 0.056 EBq from fission bombs. Taking into account its half-life of 12.33 years, the amount of ^{3}H to date from this source is about 70 EBq, of which some 40 EBq are present in ocean water. In any case, this amount still masks the cosmogenic ^{3}H. The decline of ^{3}H in the environment can be seen in the measurements of concentrations in rainwater. A very interesting example of this is presented in Rank et al. [113], where the concentration of ^{3}H in rainwater taken in Vienna, Austria, is presented. In 1961 some 500 Bq/kg were observed, compared with the concentration found in 1996 of only 2 Bq/kg. Similar levels were found by Radwan et al. [114] and Baeza et al. [115] in Poland and western Spain, respectively, for samples collected from 1994 to 1996. Concentrations of up to 2 Bq/l, measured in Japan by Okada and Momoshima [116] in 1990, are higher than the previous results, which is consistent with the effect of the general decline of ^{3}H. Nevertheless, care has to be taken when comparing ^{3}H results from different geographical areas. It is well known that the concentrations vary with latitude for the same time period. In fact, Momoshima et al. [117] estimate that the concentration of ^{3}H increases by a factor of two for every 13 degrees of latitude. On the other hand, the proximity of the ocean to the collection point influences the results because it is considered a sink for ^{3}H.

More recent measurements of ^{3}H in rainwater collected at Seville during 2002 showed concentrations in the range of 0.2 to 0.3 Bq/l, which reinforces the decrease of ^{3}H levels in rainwater [118]. The situation in the Southern Hemisphere is similar, although the ^{3}H concentration in rainwater is noticeably lower. This is because there have been fewer nuclear tests in the Southern Hemisphere than in the Northern Hemisphere. As expected, ^{3}H is also produced during nuclear power plant operation. Its annual production increases with time, and according to Villa [112], it will reach some 1.9 EBq/year by 2010. ^{3}H produced in the nuclear industry affects the environment on a more local scale, although the long-range effects of gaseous and liquid tritium releases from Sellafield and La Hague have to be taken into account.

The presence of ^{3}H in the atmosphere is closely related to the operation of nuclear installations. The scientific literature regarding this effect is extensive. An example is the work of Miljevic et al. [119], which presents a complete study of the spatial and temporal distribution of ^{3}H in precipitation and other samples around Belgrade from 1988 to 1997. The annual average ^{3}H concentration ranged from 2.2 to 35.4 Bq/l, decreasing with the distance from the Vinca Institute of Nuclear Sciences, where a heavy water reactor was in operation.

As explained in the previous section, the input of plutonium from nuclear fuel reprocessing plants is clearly less than that from nuclear tests. Very few studies can be found on the concentration of plutonium isotopes in rainwater samples. A very interesting example is provided by Rubio Montero and Martin Sanchez [120]. Rainwater samples collected in Badajoz, in southwest Spain, from 1992 to 1996 contained concentrations from 6.2 to 19 μBq/l of $^{239+240}$Pu.

Nuclear accidents have accompanied the development of the nuclear industry and nuclear research. Sometimes the radioactivity release is a local contamination event. Such are the cases of the Kysthym accident in 1957 in the former Soviet Union, Palomares (Spain) in 1966, and Thule (Greenland) in 1968. The accident at Windscale, in the U.K., can also be included in this group, although a portion of the released radioactivity was detected in western Europe. Nevertheless, the majority of the pollution was deposited in the U.K.

The contamination from other accidents is of global importance. One example is the U.S. satellite SNAP-9, powered by a ^{238}Pu generator, which suffered an accident in 1964 while entering the atmosphere, disseminating about 0.4 PBq of ^{238}Pu in the Southern Hemisphere and about 0.2 PBq in the Northern Hemisphere, changing the expected plutonium isotopic ratio in the environment. The Soviet Cosmos 954 satellite, powered by a nuclear reactor, suffered a similar accident in 1978 when reentering the atmosphere in northern Canada. It is estimated that before the accident the reactor core contained about 3 TBq of ^{90}Sr, 0.2 PBq of ^{131}I, and 3 TBq of ^{137}Cs, of which, 75% was introduced in the upper atmosphere and in this way was globally distributed.

The most important accident to date took place at the Chernobyl nuclear power plant, in the former Soviet Union, on April 26, 1986. Radioactivity was released over 10 days, and according to the United Nations Scientific Committee on the Effects of Atomic Radiation (UNSCEAR) in 1988 and the World Health Organization (WHO) in 1989, the total ^{137}Cs released was 100 PBq. One third of this amount was deposited in the Soviet Union. In addition, 8 PBq of ^{90}Sr and 0.06 PBq of $^{239+240}$Pu were released, with about 90% being deposited in the Soviet Union.

The accident affected virtually the entire Northern Hemisphere and much data exist in the literature on its radioactive impact. In fresh rainwater samples it was possible to measure more than 28 γ-emitting radionuclides. An example can be found in Ballestra et al. [121] for samples taken in Monaco. ^{137}Cs concentrations in rainwater increased by four orders of magnitude because of the accident. The ^{134}Cs/^{137}Cs activity ratio reached a value of about 0.5 in the same samples, giving a unique signal of origin to the radioactivity. $^{239+240}$Pu also increased almost two orders of magnitude in rainwater because of the accident. The authors concluded that about 1400 Bq/m^2 were deposited in the Mediterranean area from the Chernobyl accident, which means an increase of some 30% of the previous total fallout. About 10 mBq/m^2 was found for $^{239+240}$Pu, which is 0.1% of the total from previous nuclear tests.

The arrival of the Chernobyl plume over southern Spain produced an increase in the concentration of ^{137}Cs in rainwater of two orders of magnitude [104]. Aoyama et al. [122] and Hirose et al. [123] provide data on the arrival of γ-emitting and long-lived nuclides over Japan. Sixteen nuclides were identified in the γ spectrum in rainwater samples collected shortly after the accident. The maximum deposition of ^{131}I, some 400 mBq/m^2, took place on May 6–7 as a consequence of 24 mm of rainfall. By the end of May, this deposition decreased by an order of magnitude. The results for plutonium isotopes, which show the range of the Chernobyl contamination, are also interesting. Up to 7 mBq/m^2 was observed at Akita, Japan, for $^{239+240}$Pu. However, the isotopic $^{239+240}$Pu/^{137}Cs ratio was 5×10^6, one order of magnitude less than that found in northern European countries. On the other hand, after careful analysis of precipitation data, Aoyama [124] showed that approximately 10^3 of the cesium isotopes released during the accident reached the stratosphere and thus were homogeneously distributed over the Northern Hemisphere.

Fourteen years after the accident, Papastefanou et al. [125] demonstrated that traces of the Chernobyl plume still remain in dust from the Sahara Desert [125]. The authors found concentrations of ^{137}Cs up to 26.6 Bq/kg in the dust extracted from a colored rain event over Thessalonica, Greece, in April 2000, originating in the Sahara Desert. This shows the relevance of resuspension effects.

4.5 RADIONUCLIDES IN GROUNDWATER

4.5.1 INTRODUCTION

Water appears in nature as a vapor, a liquid, or a solid, and over the entire planet both above the ground surface (surface water) and below it (subsurface water). Continental waters come from precipitation, where it runs off over the land or infiltrates through the subsurface in a chain of processes known as the hydrologic cycle. Not all subsurface water is groundwater; this term is applied to subsurface water flowing into a repository, and therefore flowing under a pressure greater than atmospheric pressure.

Groundwater is only a small fraction of the total water in the world — about 0.6% — but it represents the main source of freshwater. Unfortunately the groundwater below a depth of 0.8 km is saline or is very difficult to extract. The potential useful water for human consumption is estimated to be about 4 million km^3 [126].

Groundwater is contained in geologic formations called aquifers, which are areas that are sufficiently permeable to permit water flow. Sands and gravels are the most common aquifer materials, but igneous and metamorphic rocks can form aquifers if they are fractured and porous. Aquifers can be classified into two types: confined and unconfined. A confined aquifer is a layer of water covered by a relatively impervious material, and, therefore, it is completely filled with groundwater under a pressure greater than atmospheric pressure, without any free water table. Pressure conditions in a confined aquifer are determined by the piezometric surface, which is the surface obtained by connecting equilibrium water levels in tubes (piezometers) penetrating into the confined layer.

An unconfined aquifer is a layer of water without a confining layer on top of the groundwater. This is called the groundwater table (or free surface). The groundwater table height corresponds to the equilibrium water level in a well penetrating the aquifer. The zone between the ground surface and the groundwater table is called the vadose zone or the zone of aeration. It contains water that is held to the soil particles by capillary or cohesion/adhesion forces.

A groundwater pollutant can be defined as any physical, chemical, biological, or radioactive substance contained in groundwater. Pollutants can be introduced to the aqueous system through natural activities such as soil leaching and mixing of waters with different properties, or by human activities such as waste disposal, mining, agricultural operations (mainly the application of fertilizers), urban and industrial effluents, and other activities such as the storage and transport of hazardous materials, interaquifer exchange, and saltwater intrusion.

The agricultural use of fertilizers is the main source of groundwater pollution, including natural radioactive elements. This kind of TENORM contains levels of uranium series radionuclides about 50 times higher than typical soils, and retains a large fraction of its radioactive content in the fertilizer [126–129]. A portion of the radionuclides contained in fertilizers leaches through the soil and can reach the groundwater table [130,131].

The goal of this section is to analyze the behavior of several natural radionuclides in groundwater, the levels found, and some applications for the use of natural radionuclides in the study of the processes involved in the hydrologic behavior of aquifer systems.

4.5.2 RADIONUCLIDE FRACTIONATION IN GROUNDWATER

Natural radionuclides can provide a useful tool for fingerprinting groundwater from different sources that is not provided by elemental concentration data. Isotopic fractionation between groundwater and the substratum is common, and these isotopic signatures can be used to determine previous water-rock interactions. Natural isotopic ratios can thus provide information about the source of the groundwater (e.g., about the recharge area), mixing of different groundwater masses, flow patterns, and water-rock interactions [132,133]. Isotopic studies can provide complementary information about groundwater flow patterns and represent important tools to establish remediation actions and aquifer management policies.

The main uranium series disequilibria are found in the hydrosphere. This is due to the different chemical behavior of each element (including natural radioisotopes) within the aqueous system. However, a certain proportion of radionuclide disequilibria can also be due to physical mechanisms. For example, the activity ratio of $^{235}U/^{238}U$ (being each isotope is the parent of a decay series) is practically constant all over the world (approximately 0.044). On the other hand, the $^{234}U/^{238}U$ activity ratio is frequently found to be far from one (i.e., the radioactive equilibrium condition) in the majority of aqueous systems.

The uranium series disequilibria are usually found in the hydrosphere because of the different mechanisms of water-solid interaction. These fractionations are not only produced between elements because of their different chemical behavior, but the emission of radioactive particles can produce other isotopic fractionation processes. A daughter nuclide can, after the emission of an α particle, be ejected from a solid grain (so-called α recoil). Furthermore, the radioactive particle can damage the crystalline lattice, leaving this zone more active for water leaching.

As ^{238}U is the radionuclide with a greater abundance and presence in nature, it is one of the most useful natural radioisotopes in groundwater studies. It is known that in a closed system (e.g., unweathered rock), all intermediate radionuclides from the same decay series should be expected to be under secular equilibrium after a period of about 1 million years. This fact is based on the half-life of ^{234}U (245,000 years), which is the longest-lived intermediate radionuclide of the ^{238}U series.

The first application of uranium series disequilibrium methods were reported by Rosholt et al. [134] and subsequently by Titayeva et al. [135]. These applications are based on two facts. First, ^{234}U and ^{238}U are usually under secular equilibrium in rocks. However, they are usually far from this condition in aqueous media. Second, natural levels of ^{238}U can vary within a very wide range (10^1 to 10^3 mBq/l) [136]. The combination of these factors is the basis for a very useful geochemical tool.

As previously mentioned, several physical effects can produce a preferential leaching of some daughter radionuclides. This is the reason why different isotopes of the same element can show a different mobility in aqueous media depending on their radioactive or stable nature. Two pathways produce isotopic separation at the water-bedrock interface. The first process is the result of nuclear transformations. This process breaks chemical bonds, causing displacement within the crystal structure and creating microchannels that allow for migration of water molecules into mineral grains. Furthermore, these conditions increase the possibility of autoxidation of the daughter nuclide to a more soluble valence. In this way a daughter nuclide can be more easily dissolved than its parent, allowing its preferential leaching from the bedrock of the aquifer. In addition, α-recoil enables ejection of the daughter nuclide across grain boundaries, irrespective of the existing redox conditions.

These facts are illustrated through the study of uranium isotopes. The solubility of uranium is controlled by its oxidation state. Under reducing conditions, U^{4+} tends to precipitate because it is very insoluble. In contrast, U^{6+} is soluble under oxidizing conditions. Uranium forms several soluble complexes with carbonate, phosphate, and fluoride ions, but can be absorbed onto organic compounds. The most common complex ion in natural waters is the uranyl carbonate ion.

If a decay series radionuclide is selectively dissolved (mobilized) from the surfaces of aquifer rock, disequilibrium is produced in both the aqueous and solid phases. After this process it may precipitate from the solution phase, which is an elemental selective process. Let us now consider a specific decay chain in the aquifer rock. Due to its weaker bond within the lattice, each daughter radionuclide is more inclined to pass into dissolution than its parent. The lattice itself is affected by the radiation energy deposited by the parent nuclide. This increases the effectiveness of leaching processes at this site. In other cases, the α recoil is so high that the displacement is across the solid phase into the water and the result is isotopic disequilibrium, this effect being independent on the site of each nuclide in the radioactive decay series. Thus it may be expected that the degree of disequilibrium relative to ^{238}U increases down the decay chain. However, additional effects such as the chemical behavior of each radioelement and the physicochemical conditions of the water will change this tendency.

Another important aspect influencing the amount of a radionuclide in water is the half-life. Unsupported dissolved species with short half-lives will decay until reaching secular equilibrium with their parents. The initial disequilibrium of other long-lived radionuclides will persist over a time similar to their respective half-lives. When two radionuclides having similar chemical behaviors are considered, such as ^{228}Ra and ^{224}Ra, the shorter-lived species will tend to remain in secular equilibrium with its parents. Hence ^{224}Ra is usually found in equilibrium with ^{228}Th in groundwater.

Uranium and radium are considered soluble species from a geochemical point of view, and typical natural activity concentrations are greater than 1 mBq/l. On the other hand, thorium and protactinium are detected in solution at very low concentrations (less than 10^2 mBq/l), being insoluble in water. Finally, lead, bismuth, and polonium have variable behaviors depending on the water conditions. The short-lived radionuclides are not usually widely dispersed, so their levels are supplied by their parents in solution or by their dissolution from the aquifer rock. Therefore the mobility of each radionuclide depends on its elemental solubility, mode of radiogenesis, and half-life.

The second way for a radionuclide to be dissolved in water is based on the decay of the parent being after a change in the geochemical conditions of the aquifer bedrock. Thereafter its supply is limited by the growth curve of the daughter. For example, the activity concentrations of ^{228}Ra can significantly increase or decrease as a consequence of thorium heterogeneities in the aquifer.

Another aspect to take into account is colloidal transport. These very small particulate materials increase radionuclide mobility and significantly complicate modeling of the transport of pollutants in aquifers. Under some conditions the principal effect is to enhance the apparent "solubility" of some radionuclides, as is the case for thorium isotopes.

4.5.3 SOME APPLICATION CASES

In the following sections, several applications of disequilibrium phenomena to solve real groundwater problems will be discussed. There are two kinds of systems: conservative and nonconservative. In the conservative system, any changes in radionuclide concentrations can be interpreted as the result of the mixing of different water masses, and it is usually applied to waters that have achieved the steady-state conditions between the dissolved and solid material. One of the first applications of this idea was to trace the input of seawater in a cavernous dolomite in south Florida [137]. Considering the constancy of content (3.3 ppb uranium) and the $^{234}U/^{238}U$ activity ratio in seawater, the authors confirm that the cold saline water of a specific zone (called the Boulder Zone) is actually seawater that enters the aquifer, since the uranium concentrations and the activity ratios were within the values of seawater.

The uranium series disequilibria have been widely used to characterize subsurface waters [138,139], being an example of the methodology to plot the $^{234}U/^{238}U$ activity ratio against the inverse of uranium concentration. A specific case is the mixing of water containing relatively high levels of uranium and water containing very low concentrations of uranium. This mixture produces a pattern where the uranium concentration decreases without affecting the $^{234}U/^{238}U$ activity ratio. In contrast, if the leaching processes are dominant, the previous activity ratio will increase linearly with the reciprocal of the uranium concentration.

Another typical application of uranium isotope disequilibria is the location of the redox front in confined aquifers. In the shallow oxidized zone (frequently the recharge area), the uranium content must increase along the flow line so the $^{234}U/^{238}U$ activity ratio is also enhanced as a consequence of the preferential leaching effects. When the water flow reaches the redox front, a high fraction of uranium precipitates (a great decrease in uranium concentration is produced in this zone) and remains in place in a solid state for a long time. However, if conditions are near chemical equilibrium in the redox front, preferential leaching of ^{234}U from previously precipitated material can occur. So along the redox front, and following the direction of water flow, the $^{234}U/^{238}U$ activity ratio can quickly increase. This fact can be applied to identify the redox barrier [136,140]. Activity ratios of 10 or more can sometimes be observed in large confined aquifers with steady-state flow systems. The study developed by Labajo [141] in a detritic aquifer located in southern Spain demonstrated the utility of uranium determinations in different water phases (dissolution and suspended material) to delimit the oxidized areas as well as to locate the main redox barrier.

Uranium and thorium series dissolved radionuclides have been used to relate the sorption and solid phases to basic processes involved in the water flow through a basaltic aquifer: sorption-desorption, dissolution-precipitation, radioactive growth-decay, and α recoil [133,142]. Roback et al. [133] and Luo et al. [142] found very low thorium and radium isotope activity concentrations in groundwater that were two to four orders of magnitude lower than uranium isotope concentrations (0.3 to 3.6 ppb with an average of 1.83 ppb of uranium). The ^{234}U/^{238}U activity ratio is about 1.6 to 3.0. They also demonstrated that disequilibria in the case of short-lived radionuclides had origins in sorption/adsorption processes, while for long-lived isotopes (^{226}Ra, ^{230,232}Th, and ^{234,238}U), distributions were also affected by dissolution and precipitation. As expected, they estimated the highest retardation factors (ratio flow rates of fluid to those of radionuclide dissolved) for thorium (greater than 10^6) and radium (greater than 10^5) due to the fact that these elements have a very high affinity for solid material. Finally, the spatial patterns of activity ratios allow them to identify the preferential flow pathways and the stagnated zones of the aquifer.

The transport of natural radionuclides has also been studied in many contexts, especially in detritic aquifers. Tricca et al. [132] developed a comprehensive study on the transport of uranium, thorium, and radium radionuclides in an unconfined sandy aquifer located in Long Island, New York. The one-dimensional model takes into account transport by advection, weathering, decay, α-recoil, and sorption/desorption at the water-rock interface, describing the evolution of concentrations of several ^{232}Th and ^{238}U radionuclides along the flow path of groundwater. A wide range in ^{238}U activities (within 1 mBq/kg) was observed in the water table. This finding is explained by the high mobility of uranium [143], for which the input in the vadose zone is significant in the aquifer, while the activity concentrations for ^{232}Th were at least two orders of magnitude less than those for ^{238}U. The isotopic composition of uranium indicated the dominant component of the recoil rate in relation to the weathering rate.

In contrast, the high dispersion found in ^{238}U activity concentrations in aquifer waters reflects the different compositions of vadose zones. In sandy aquifers, thorium is saturated in the water under oxidizing conditions so that the weathering input is irreversibly precipitating onto surfaces of both rocks and suspension particles. However, it is usually found that under reducing conditions, uranium tends to precipitate and thorium activities in solution are much higher, with the thorium/uranium ratio in solutions being near that found in rock [132,141]. In general, the activities of thorium isotopes indicate a very low desorption, reflecting that its mean residence time in the rock surface is about 1,000 years, while in the water it is only about 1 hour. The importance of these works is that, in general, the distribution of naturally occurring radionuclides can be used to calculate values for transport parameters that can be applied to the transport of anthropogenic pollutant nuclides.

The study by Zhu [144] combines radiocarbon dating and hydraulic data to estimate the water recharge rate in a groundwater aquifer located in the Black Mesa basin (Arizona), which is an important source of drinking water. The ^{14}C ages of groundwater are first corrected for the effects of chemical reactions; thereafter, recharge rates are calibrated to observed ^{14}C ages using a numerical ^{14}C transport and flow model. In this work it is supposed that the calibration of the flow model to a distribution of ages is equivalent to calibrating the model to a lumped average of advective velocities. In general, flow models calibrated using hydraulic properties alone produce velocity predictions that can be grossly inaccurate or carry large uncertainties. Therefore simultaneous calibration to ages and heads is valuable for the development of contaminant transport models, which typically take velocity fields from the flow model as input. There, velocities are often the most important factor to determine the direction and rate of contaminant transport.

Besides the previously mentioned range of applications of natural radionuclide disequilibrium, it is possible to find several studies producing unsatisfactory results. For example, Kronfeld et al. [145] studied the waters of the Avon Valley, Nova Scotia, employing uranium disequilibrium as a hydrologic tool to trace water flow or delineate areas where water bodies are mixed. However, this method was not efficacious, as the waters of this system are predominantly influenced by the weathering conditions.

A recent application is the use of natural analogs in radionuclide transport studies. In essence, this philosophy tries to examine the occurrence of materials or processes similar to those found in, or caused by, a repository [146,147]. In most disposal concepts, the main way to bring radionuclides from the repository to the environment is groundwater transport. Natural analogs can include both natural and man-made materials, provided the processes affecting them are natural. This kind of study provides information on both near-field processes and radionuclide migration in the far field and biosphere. Many studies have been made of natural systems with characteristics analogous to those of interest for radionuclide transport modeling in both fractured and intact crystalline rock. The principal targets were the identification of significant physical and chemical processes able to enhance or retard radionuclide migration, and to develop conceptual models for safety assessments of rock processes [148].

In relation to the pollution of groundwater by man-made radionuclides, the migration study of ^{90}Sr and ^{137}Cs from soil to aquifer in the Chernobyl pilot site is of special interest [149,150]. The study site is 2.5 km southwest of the Chernobyl nuclear power plant, known as Red Forest, where radioactive wastes from the accident were deposited a few meters deep. The source term of the radionuclides in the environment consists of a heterogeneous mixture of soil with fuel particles containing a total activity of about 10^{12} Bq for both ^{137}Cs and ^{90}Sr. The underlying aquifer has been seriously affected by leachates containing high levels of these isotopes that penetrated the unsaturated layer and have reached the water table for the last 20 years. ^{90}Sr concentrations in subsurface waters have been measured at between 10×10^3 and 13×10^3 Bq/l and the pollution plume spreads over a few tens of meters downstream. The hydrologic study indicates that ^{90}Sr migration velocity in the aeolian sand aquifer underlying the waste site is retarded by sorption to about 9% of the real groundwater flow velocity. This very low retardation/adsorption capacity is also explained by the quartz composition of these sands and by competition for adsorption of the calcium ions contained in the solution plume leached from the wastes.

One of the most common applications of radionuclides is groundwater dating using natural radionuclides. Terminology for groundwaters that are older than "modern" is important because of the implications for recharge. Fossil groundwaters have been recharged in the past by meteorological processes that no longer prevail. However, paleogroundwaters in many regional flow systems may be old simply because of their low velocities and long flow paths, and may actually receive modern inputs in the recharge environment. None of these effects addresses the aspect of induced recharge under the stress of exploitation. While most paleogroundwaters are not part of active flow systems, heavy pumping can potentially induce flow from adjacent aquitards, poorly connected aquifers, or surface water sources.

Dating old groundwater begins with the determination that they are tritium free, and so have no modern component. Tritium-free groundwater can be considered submodern (recharged more than 50 years ago) or older and have not incorporated any significant amount of modern water during discharge. The only absolute, albeit indirect, dating techniques for groundwater involve the decay (or in-growth) of long-lived radionuclides. By far the most routinely applied is ^{14}C, which is transported as dissolved inorganic carbon (DIC) or dissolved organic carbon (DOC).

Different geochemical techniques for dating (e.g., the extent of water-rock interaction or the degree of salinization) are also important, but not quantitative. The groundwater flow system hydrodynamic characteristics are useful in estimating subsurface mean residence times. It is important to note that one technique alone can be misleading if applied without an understanding of the geochemical and hydrodynamic processes in the aquifer. A collaboration of methodologies is the best approach.

Radiocarbon dating is based on measuring the loss of the parent radionuclide (^{14}C) in a given sample. This assumes two key features of the system. First, it is assumed that the initial concentration of the parent is known and has remained constant in the past. Second, the system is assumed closed to subsequent gains or losses of the parent, except through radioactive decay. But through time, the reaction and evolution of the carbonate system strongly dilute the initial ^{14}C activity in dissolved inorganic carbon. The result is an artificial "aging" of groundwater by dilution of ^{14}C. Several attempts to overcome these problems have been made over the past 30 years and a number of possible correction procedures have been presented by different authors.

4.6 RADIOACTIVITY IN DRINKING WATER

4.6.1 INTRODUCTION

The presence of radioactivity in drinking water is a potential health risk. Consumption represents a possible mode of ingestion of radioactivity. In many places the population drinks water directly from the source, such as well water and bottled mineral water. Depending on the bedrock of the area where the water comes from, its radioactive content will be more or less relevant. This has to be assessed. Even when the water is purified in a treatment plant, radioactivity has to be monitored, since the efficiency of purification processes varies with the chemical element. Routine monitoring of drinking water is a common practice in developed countries and water sampling is a fairly simple process.

4.6.2 The Presence of Radioactivity in Drinking Water

4.6.2.1 Natural Radioactivity

Primordial radionuclides are present in drinking water to a certain degree, especially in well water or mineral water. The most relevant of these nuclides for radiological protection are ^{226}Ra and ^{222}Rn.

The presence of ^{226}Ra in water depends on the water's origin. For well or mineral water, it depends on the content of ^{238}U in the solids of the aquifer where the water is stored. The geochemical characteristics of the aquifer determine the dissolution of radium from the solids into the water. ^{226}Ra is known to be removed by the treatment of water in purification plants. In many cases, however, well water is not purified before consumption, and mineral water is directly bottled without any previous treatment. ^{222}Rn is a daughter of ^{226}Ra and its presence in water depends on several variables, including temperature and pressure, and the behavior of its parent in the water. It seems that water transport instead of diffusion from rocks is the primary control in the dynamics of radon in water. Obviously the amount of ^{226}Ra and ^{222}Rn in the water depends on the geological characteristics of the bedrock, and it is known that granite areas produce highly contaminated waters.

^{3}H is another key nuclide in drinking water. After its production in the atmosphere, the formed heavy water (HTO) molecules can be introduced into water reservoirs and aquifers. The concentration of ^{3}H in well or mineral water depends on the water's age. In fact, closed aquifers have water with a very low ^{3}H content.

4.6.2.2 Man-Made Radioactivity

Man-made radioactivity can enter into water reservoirs through several pathways. Rainwater containing artificial radioactivity can directly or indirectly feed aquifers or other reservoirs. In this way, nuclear weapons tests and the nuclear industry can introduce man-made radioactivity into drinking water. Nuclear accidents have also produced contamination of drinking water.

In principle, the purification processes in water treatment plants remove the majority of nuclides. However, in some cases this is not enough to avoid their ingestion by the public.

4.6.2.3 Levels

4.6.2.3.1 Natural Radioactivity
The concentrations of ^{226}Ra in drinking water are highly variable. Early works showed that water supplies from wells in the U.S. can produce tap water with

some 180 Bq/m^3 of ^{226}Ra [92]. Potable water can contain relevant concentrations of ^{222}Rn. About one fourth of the water in the U.S. contains more than 7×10^4 Bq/m^3 ^{222}Rn, and in some cases concentrations of 3.7×10^5 Bq/m^3 can be found [92]. It is interesting to note that the domestic use of potable water can release dissolved ^{222}Rn into the air, provoking high indoor concentrations.

^{222}Rn concentrations up to about 800 Bq/l are observed in Austrian drinking water samples in granitic areas [151]. For these waters, 0.5 Bq/l of ^{226}Ra have been measured.

In Brazil, 452 water supplies were analyzed for ^{226}Ra and ^{222}Rn by de Oliveira et al. [152], ranging from 2.2 to 235 mBq/l and 0.40 to 315 Bq/l, respectively. Erlandsson et al. [153] found high ^{222}Rn concentrations in Swedish well water of more than 700 Bq/l, associated with leakage from layers of volcanic origin. A study of municipal water supply systems and private wells in Poland showed that on average the concentration of ^{222}Rn is around 5.3 kBq/m^3, with a maximum of 38.3 kBq/m^3 [154].

Bottled mineral waters were studied in Brazil for ^{228}Ra, ^{226}Ra, and ^{210}Pb, with weighted means of 0.097, 0.027, and 0.066 Bq/l, respectively. In Spain, Dueñas et al. [155] observed concentrations of ^{226}Ra of up to 600 mBq/l (with a geometric mean of 12 mBq/l) in bottled mineral water. As for ^{222}Rn, results show a maximum of 52 Bq/l, with a geometric mean of 0.22 mBq/l.

Also in Spain, Collado et al. [156] determined the levels of ^{224}Ra and ^{226}Ra in bottled mineral water. The typical ^{226}Ra content for most of the analyzed trademarks were a few millibecquerels per liter, but one of them had a level of 260 mBq/l. The majority of the measured samples had levels of ^{224}Ra less than the minimum detectable activity (MDA) (i.e., 0.5 to 1 mBq/l), depending on the sample size. A maximum ^{224}Ra activity of 11 mBq/l was found for the sample with a higher ^{226}Ra concentration. In the same work, results for tap water collected at Seville were also presented. A level of 1.3 mBq/l was found for ^{226}Ra, while the concentration for ^{224}Ra is less than 1.4 mBq/l. According to this article, the efficiency of radium removal by water treatment plants is very close to 100%.

A very interesting work is that presented by Gäfvert et al. [157]. They studied the presence of natural and artificial radioactivity in drinking water in southern Sweden and the efficiency of the purification process for several relevant radio-nuclides. The authors found that a combination of $Al_2(SO_4)_3$ and $FeCl_3$ floccula-tion followed by a filtration process is 85% efficient for the removal of uranium isotopes and more than 90% efficient for thorium isotopes and polonium. The authors found concentrations of 0.16, 0.004, 0.013, 0.11, and 0.65 µBq/l for ^{238}U, ^{232}Th, ^{230}Th, ^{228}Th, and ^{210}Po, respectively, in the purified water.

As mentioned above, ^{3}H in Spanish mineral waters was measured by Villa and Manjon [118], with observed concentration ranges of 0.2 to 0.5 Bq/l. The authors used an enrichment process to prepare the ^{3}H samples, thus they got a very low limit of detection. In spite of this, some samples with concentrations below this limit were found. It reveals that the waters came from aquifers con-taining old water with practically no input of ^{3}H from the atmosphere.

Tap water samples collected in Seville, Spain, during 2002 were also analyzed. Levels of 0.15 to 0.47 Bq/l were observed. In general, these values are lower than ^{3}H concentrations measured in previous years at other places all over the globe. The decrease detected is related to the general lowering of ^{3}H concentrations in water in the absence of new inputs from nuclear activities.

4.6.2.3.2 Man-Made Radioactivity

Fission products appeared in drinking water at the beginning of the nuclear era. Of course, the presence of radioactive elements in drinking water is very dependent on the efficiency of purification methods. As time has passed, purification methodologies have improved. Monitoring drinking water for artificial radionuclides is the usual practice in developed countries. For instance, the European Union established a network system years ago to control the radioactivity in key samples all over Europe. ^{3}H, ^{90}Sr, and ^{137}Cs are systematically monitored in drinking water.

Typical ^{137}Cs activities of about 10 mBq/l were generally found in the analyzed samples collected before the Chernobyl accident. However, the effect of the input from this event was clearly evident, especially for samples from northern Europe, where levels up to 10^1 Bq/l were observed.

As for ^{90}Sr, levels are slightly more variable among collection sites. Nevertheless, concentrations lie in the range of 10^2 Bq/l. The influence of the Chernobyl accident was also noted for ^{90}Sr, as the concentration of this isotope increased to more than three times its usual level.

^{3}H is another key nuclide in this network. Concentrations are systematically below the reporting level of 100 Bq/l, with values close to 1 Bq/l. This is in agreement with previous data from Villa and Manjon [118]. There, lower ^{3}H concentrations were observed in samples collected during 2002. The reason for this effect is that a general decrease in the concentration of ^{3}H in water is expected because of its half-life.

In the work of Gäfvert et al. [157], it was found that the purification process is more than 95% efficient for plutonium, with $^{239+240}$Pu concentrations in the range of 0.65 µBq/l. Nevertheless, the process seems to be inefficient for the removal of ^{90}Sr, ^{226}Ra, and ^{137}Cs. This fact is not important in normal situations, but it is extremely relevant in the case of accidental releases of radioactivity that reach water reservoirs.

4.6.3 DOSE ASSESSMENT

A nonnegligible radiation dose can be received by the ingestion of drinking water with a high radioactive content. This is especially relevant in the case of ^{222}Rn and ^{226}Ra. In the articles cited above, dose estimations were made by using the obtained concentrations and the conversion factors (dose equivalents per unit activity) published by UNSCEAR [73] and International Commission on Radiological Protection (ICRP) [158].

Of course, the calculations depend on the assumed annual water consumption. This quantity is fairly close to 2 l/day. With this in mind, average doses from ^{226}Ra of about 26 µSv/year are obtained, with a maximum of 100 µSv/year in Spain. Regarding ^{222}Rn, an average value of 43 µSv/year and a maximum of 170 µSv/year were calculated.

In Brazil, the results are different, as can be seen in Godoy et al. [159]. Estimations were done for the consumption of mineral waters from different areas of Brazil and on the basis of the measured concentrations of ^{222}Rn and ^{226}Ra. Some of the doses in this reference are certainly relevant compared to the normal exposure to natural radioactivity, which is on average 2.4 mSv/year according to UNSCEAR [73].

REFERENCES

1. Eisenbud, M. and Gessell, T.F., *Environmental Radioactivity: From Natural, Industrial, and Military Sources*, 3rd ed., Academic Press, New York, 1987.
2. Monte, L., Brittain, J.E., Hakanson, L., Heling, R., Smith, J.T., and Zheleznyak, M., Review and assessment of models used to predict the fate of radionuclides in lakes, *J. Environ. Radioactiv.*, 69, 177, 2003.
3. Palmer, M.R. and Edmond, J.M., Uranium in river water, *Geochim. Cosmochim. Acta*, 57, 4947, 1993.
4. Schmidt, S., Investigations of dissolved uranium content in the watershed of Seine river (France), *J. Environ. Radioactiv.*, 78, 1, 2005.
5. Broecker, W.S., *Chemical Oceanography*, Harcourt Brace Jovanovich, New York, 1974.
6. Mangini, A. and Dominik, G., Late quaternary sapropel on the Mediterranean ridge: U-budget and evidences for low sedimentation rates, *Sediment. Geol.*, 23, 113, 1979.
7. Turekian, K.K. and Cochran, J.K., Determination of marine chronologies using natural radionuclides, in *Chemical Oceanography*, 2nd ed., Vol. 7, Riley, J.P. and Chester, R., eds., Academic Press, New York, 313, 1974.
8. Dunk, R.M., Mills, R.A., and Jenkins, W.J., A reevaluation of the oceanic uranium budget for the Holocene, *Chem. Geol.*, 190, 45, 2002.
9. Porcelli, D., Andersson, P.S., Wasserburg, G.J., Ingri, J., and Baskaran, M., The importance of colloids and mires for the transport of uranium isotopes through the Kalix River watershed and Baltic Sea, *Geochim. Cosmochim. Acta*, 61, 4095, 1997.
10. Spalding, R.F. and Sachett, W.M., Uranium in run-off from the Gulf of Nexuci distributive province: anomalous concentration, *Science*, 175, 629, 1972.
11. Borole, D.V., Krishnaswami, S., and Somayajulu, B.L.K., Investigations of dissolved uranium, silicon, and particulate trace elements in estuaries, *Estuar. Coast. Mar. Sci.*, 5, 743, 1977.
12. Scott, M.R., The chemistry of U- and Th-series nuclides in rivers, in Ivanovich, M. and Harmon, R.S., eds., *Uranium-Series Disequilibrium: Applications to Earth, Marine, and Environmental Sciences*, 2nd ed., Clarendon Press, Oxford, 1992.
13. Li, Y.-H., Mathieu, G.G., Biscaye, P., and Simpson, H.J., The flux of Ra-226 from estuarine and continental shelf sediments, *Earth Planet. Sci. Lett.*, 37, 237, 1977.

14. Bolivar, J.P., Garcia-Tenorio, R., Mas, J.L., and Vaca, F., Radioactive impact in sediments from an estuarine system affected by industrial releases, *Environ. Int.*, 27, 639, 2002.

15. Aarkrog, A., Input of anthropogenic radionuclides into the world ocean, *Deep Sea Res. II*, 50, 2597, 2003.

16. Eriksson, M., Holm, E., Roos, P., and Dahlgaard, H., Distribution and flux of Pu-238, Pu-239, Pu-240, Am-241, Cs-137 and Pb-210 to high arctic lakes in the Thule district (Greenland), *J. Environ. Radioactiv.*, 75, 285, 2005.

17. Pujol, L.L. and Sanchez-Cabeza, J.A., Use of tritium to predict soluble pollutants transport in Ebro River waters (Spain), *Environ. Pollut.*, 108, 257, 2000.

18. Lee, S.H., La Rosa, J.J., Levy-Palomo, I., Oregioni, B., Pham, M.K., Povinec, P.P., and Wyse, E., Recent inputs and budgets of ^{90}Sr, ^{137}Cs, ^{239,240}Pu and ^{241}Am in the northwest Mediterranean Sea, *Deep Sea Res. II*, 50, 2817, 2003.

19. Kryshev, I.I, Romanov, G.N., Chumichev, V.B., Sazykina, T.G., Isaeva, L.N., and Ivanitskaya, M.V., Radioecological consequences of radioactive discharges into the Techa River on the southern Urals, *J. Environ. Radioactiv.*, 38, 195, 1998.

20. Aldridge, J.N., Kershaw, P., Brown, J., McCubbin, D., Leonard, K.S., and Young, E.F., Transport of plutonium (239/240Pu) and caesium (137Cs) in the Irish Sea: comparison between observations and results from sediment and contaminant transport modelling, *Cont. Shelf Res.*, 23, 869, 2003.

21. Periañez, R., Modelling the physico-chemical speciation of plutonium in the eastern Irish Sea: a further development, *J. Environ. Radioactiv.*, 62, 263, 2002.

22. Samuelsson, C., Natural radioactivity, in *Radioecology. Lectures in Environmental Radioactivity*, Holm, E., ed., World Scientific Publishing, Singapore, 1994.

23. Tsabaris, C. and Ballas, D., On line gamma-ray spectrometry at open sea, *Appl. Radiat. Isot.*, 62, 83, 2005,

24. Alam, M.N., Chowdhury, M.I., Kamal, M., Ghose, S., Matin, A.K.M.A., and Ferdousi, G.S.M., Radionuclide concentrations in mussels collected from the southern coast of Bangladesh – cultivation on ropes from floating rafts, *J. Environ. Radioactiv.*, 47, 201, 2000.

25. Ivanovich, M. and Harmon, R.S., eds., *Uranium-Series Disequilibrium: Applications to Earth, Marine, and Environmental Sciences*, 2nd ed., Clarendon Press, Oxford, 1992.

26. Bourdon, B., Henderson, G.M., Lundstrom, C.C., and Turner, S.P., eds., *Reviews in mineralogy and geochemistry*, Vol. 52, *Uranium-Series Geochemistry*, Mineralogical Society of America, Chantilly, VA, 2004.

27. Chen, J.H., Edwards, R.L., and Wasserburg, G.J., U-238,U-234 and Th-232 in seawater, *Earth Planet. Sci. Lett.*, 80, 241, 1986.

28. Robinson, L., Belshaw, N.S., and Henderson, G.M., U and Th concentrations and isotope ratios in modern carbonates and waters from the Bahamas, *Geochim. Cosmochim. Acta*, 68, 1777, 2004.

29. Rengarajan, R., Sarin, M.M., and Krishnaswami, S., Uranium in the Arabian Sea: role of denitrification in controlling its distribution, *Oceanol. Acta*, 26, 687, 2003.

30. Delanghe, D., Bard, E., and Hamelin, B., New TIMS constraints on the uranium-238 and uranium-234 in seawaters from the main ocean basins and the Mediterranean Sea, *Mar. Chem.*, 80, 79, 2002.

31. McDonald, P., Baxter, S.M., and Scott, E.M., Technological enhancement of natural radionuclides in the marine environment, *J. Environ. Radioactiv.*, 32, 67, 1996.

32. Huh, C., Moore, W.S., and Kadko, D.C., Oceanic 232Th: a reconnaissance and implications of global distribution from manganese nodules, *Geochim. Cosmochim. Acta*, 53, 1163, 1989.

33. Balakrishnaa, K., Shankar, R., Sarin, M.M., and Manjunatha, B.R., Distribution of U-Th nuclides in the riverine and coastal environments of the tropical southwest coast of India, *J. Environ. Radioactiv.*, 57, 21, 2001.

34. Chase, R.F., Anderson, R.F., Fleisher, M.Q., and Kubik, P.W, Scavenging of 230Th, 231Pa and 10Be in the Southern Ocean (SW Pacific sector): the importance of particle flux, particle composition and advection, *Deep Sea Res. II*, 50, 739, 2003.

35. Nozaki, Y., Zhang, J., and Takeda, A., 210Pb and 210Po in the equatorial Pacific and the Bering Sea: the effects of biological productivity and boundary scavenging, *Deep Sea Res. II*, 44, 2203, 1997.

36. Martin, P., Hancock, G.J., Johnston, A., and Murray, A.S., Natural-series radionuclides in traditional north Australian Aboriginal foods, *J. Environ. Radioactiv.*, 40, 37, 1998.

37. Scholz, D., Mangini, A., and Felis, T., U-series dating of diagenetically altered fossil reef corals, *Earth Planet. Sci. Lett.*, 218, 1633, 2004.

38. Thompson, W.G., Spiegelman, M.W., Goldstein, S.L., and Speed, R.C., An open-system model for U-series age determinations of fossil corals, *Earth Planet. Sci. Lett.*, 210, 365, 2003.

39. Moore, W.S., Large groundwater inputs to coastal waters revealed by 226Ra enrichments, *Nature*, 380, 612, 1998.

40. Ishikawa, Y., Kagaya, H., and Saga, K., Biomagnication of 7Be, 234Th, and 228Ra in marine organisms near the northern Pacic coast of Japan, *J. Environ. Radioactiv.*, 76, 103, 2004.

41. Narayana, Y., Radhakrishna, A.P., Somashekarappa, H.M., Karunakara, N., Balakrishna, K.M., and Siddappa, K., Distribution of some natural and artificial radionuclides in the environment of coastal Karnataka of south India, *J. Environ. Radioactiv.*, 28, 113, 1995.

42. Rutgers van der Loeff, M.M., Kühne, S., Wahsner, M., Höltzen, H., Frank, M., Ekwurzel, B., Mensch, M., and Rachold, V., 228Ra and 226Ra in the Kara and Laptev seas, *Cont. Shelf Res.*, 23, 113, 2003.

43. Moore, W.S., Determining coastal mixing rates using radium isotopes, *Cont. Shelf Res.*, 20, 1993, 2000.

44. Broecker, W.S. and Peng, T.-H., *Tracers in the Sea*, Lamont-Doherty Geological Observatory, Palisades, New York, 1992.

45. International Atomic Energy Agency, *Sediment Kd's and Concentration Factors for Radionuclides in the Marine Environment*, Technical Report no. 247, International Atomic Energy Agency, Vienna.

46. McDonald, P., Cook, G.T., Baxter, M.S., Thompson, J.C., The terrestrial distribution of artificial radioactivity in south-west Scotland, *Sci. Total Environ.*, 111, 59, 1992.

47. Appleby, P.G. and Oldfield, F., Applications of lead-210 to sedimentation studies, in *Uranium-Series Disequilibrium: Applications to Earth, Marine, and Environmental Sciences*, 2nd ed., Ivanovich, M. and Harmon, R.S., eds., Clarendon Press, Oxford, 1992.

48. Kim, G., Large deficiency of polonium in the oligotrophic ocean's interior, *Earth Planet. Sci. Lett.*, 192, 15, 2001.

49. Betti, M., Aldave de las Heras, L., Janssens, A., Henrich, E., Hunter, G., Gerchikov, M., Dutton, M., van Weers, A.W., Nielsen, S., Simmomds, J., Bexon, A., Sazykina, T., Results of the European Commission MARINA II study: part II — effects of discharges of naturally occurring radioactive material, *J. Environ. Radioactiv.*, 74, 255, 2004.

50. Bolivar, J.P., García-Tenorio, R., and García-León, M., Radioecological study of an estuarine system located in the south of Spain, *Water Res.*, 34, 2941, 2000.

51. Jerez Vegueria, S.F., Godoy, J.M., and Miekeley, N., Environmental impact studies of barium and radium discharges by produced waters from the "Bacia de Campos" oil-field offshore platforms, Brazil, *J. Environ. Radioactiv.*, 62, 29, 2002.

52. Martinez-Aguirre, A. and García-León, M., Radioactive impact of phosphate ore processing in a wet marshland in southwestern Spain, *J. Environ. Radioactiv.*, 34, 45, 1997.

53. Bolivar, J.P., Garcia-Tenorio, R., Mas, J.L., and Vaca, F., Radioactive impacts in sediments from an estuarine system affected by industrial wastes releases, *Environ. Int.*, 27, 639, 2002.

54. Bolivar, J.P., García-Tenorio, R., and García-León, M., Enhancement of natural radioactivity in soils and salt-marshes surrounding a non-nuclear industrial complex, *Sci. Total Environ.*, 173/174, 25, 1995.

55. Aguado, J.L., Bolivar, J.P., and García-Tenorio, R., Sequential extraction of [226]Ra in sediments from an estuary affected historically by anthropogenic inputs of natural radionuclides, *J. Environ. Radioactiv.*, 74, 117, 2004.

56. Periañez, R., Abril, J.M., and García-León, M., Modelling the dispersion of non-conservative radionuclides in tidal waters — part 1: conceptual and mathematical model, *J. Environ. Radioactiv.*, 31, 127, 1996.

57. Absi, A., Villa, M., Moreno, H.P., Manjon, G., and Perianez, R., Self-cleaning in an estuarine area formerly affected by [226]Ra anthropogenic enhancements, *Sci. Total Environ.*, 329, 183, 2004.

58. El Mamoney, M.H. and Khater, A.E.M., Environmental characterization and radio-ecological impacts of non-nuclear industries on the Red Sea coast, *J. Environ. Radioactiv.*, 73, 151, 2004.

59. Haridasan, P.P., Paul, A.C., and Desai, M.V.M., Natural radionuclides in the aquatic environment of a phosphogypsum disposal area, *J. Environ. Radioactiv.*, 53, 155, 2001.

60. Burnett, W.C. and Elzerman, A.W., Nuclide migration and the environmental radiochemistry of Florida phosphogypsum, *J. Environ. Radioactiv.*, 27, 2001.

61. Poole, A.J., Allington, D.J., and Denoon, D.C., Temporal and spatial survey of dissolved [226]Ra in coastal waters of the eastern Irish Sea, *Sci. Total Environ.*, 168, 233, 1995.

62. Røe Utvik, T.I., Chemical characterisation of produced water from four offshore oil production platforms in the North Sea, *Chemosphere*, 39, 2593, 1999.

63. Shawky, S., Amer, H., Nada, A.A., El-Maksoud, T.M., and Ibrahiem, N.M., Characteristics of NORM in the oil industry from eastern and western deserts of Egypt, *Appl. Radiat. Isot.*, 55, 135, 2001.

64. Silver, G.L., Plutonium oxidation states in seawater, *Appl. Radiat. Isot.*, 55, 589, 2001.

65. Hirose, K., Aoyama, M., Miyao, T., and Igarashi, Y., Plutonium in seawaters of the western North Pacific, *J. Radioanal. Nucl. Chem.*, 248, 771, 2001

66. Lee, S.H., Gastaud, J., Povinec, P.P., Hong, G.-H., Kim, S.-H., Chung, C.-S., Lee, K.-W., and Pettersson, H.B.L., Distribution of plutonium and americium in the marginal seas of the northwest Pacic Ocean, *Deep Sea Res. II*, 50,2727, 2003.

67. Kuwabara, J., Yamamoto, M., Oikawa, S., Komura, K., and Assinder, D.J., Measurements of ^{99}Tc, ^{137}Cs, ^{237}Np, Pu isotopes and ^{241}Am in sediment cores from intertidal coastal and estuarine regions in the Irish Sea, *J. Radioanal. Nucl. Chem.*, 240, 593, 1999.

68. Carroll, J., Boisson, F., Teyssie, J.-L., King, S.E., Krosshavn, M., Carroll, M.L., Fowler, S.W., Povinec, P.P., and Baxter, M.S., Distribution coefficients (Kd's) for use in risk assessment models of the Kara Sea, *Appl. Radiat. Isot.*, 51, 121, 1999.

69. Ryan, T.P., Transuranic biokinetic parameters for marine invertebrates — a review, *Environ. Int.*, 28, 83, 2002.

70. Ryan, T.P., Dowdall, A.M., Long, S., Smith, V., Pollard, D., and Cunningham, J.D., Plutonium and americium in fish, shellfish and seaweed in the Irish environment and their contribution to dose, *J. Environ. Radioactiv.*, 44, 349, 1999.

71. Sanchez-Cabeza, J.A., Merino, J., Masque, P., Mitchell, P.I., Vintro, L.L., Schell, W.R., Cross, L., and Calbet, A., Concentrations of plutonium and americium in plankton from the western Mediterranean Sea, *Sci. Total Environ.*, 311, 233, 2003.

72. Masque, P., Cochran, J.K., Hebbeln, D., Hirschberg, D.J., Dethleff, D., and Winkler, A., The role of sea ice in the fate of contaminants in the Artic Ocean: plutonium atom ratios in the Fram Strait, *Environ. Sci. Technol.*, 37, 4848, 2003.

73. United Nations Scientific Committee on the Effects of Atomic Radiation (UNSCEAR), *Exposure from Natural Sources of Radiation*, United Nations, New York, 1993.

74. Hunt, G.J., Smith, B.D., and Campling, W.C., Recent changes in liquid radioactive waste discharges from Sellafield to the Irish Sea: monitoring of the environmental consequences and radiological implications, *Radiat. Prot. Dosim.*, 75, 149, 1998.

75. Lee, S.H., Gastaud, J., La Rosa, J.J., Liong Wee Kwong, L., Povinec, P.P., Wyse, E., Fifield, L.K., Hausladen, P.A., di Tada, M.L., and Santos, G.M., Analysis of plutonium isotopes in marine samples by radiometric, ICP-MS and AMS techniques, *J. Radioanal. Nucl. Chem.*, 254, 757, 2001.

76. Leon Vintro, L., Mitchell, P.I., Condren, O.M., Downes, A.B., Papucci, C., and Delfanti, R., Vertical and horizontal fluxes of plutonium and americium in the western Mediterranean and the Strait of Gibraltar, *Sci. Total Environ.*, 237-238, 77, 1999.

77. Manjon, G. and Garcia Leon, M., The presence of man-made radionuclides in the marine environment in the South of Spain, *J. Environ. Radioactiv.*, 28, 171, 1995.

78. Ito, T., Povinec, P.P., Togawa, O., and Hirose, K, Temporal and spatial variations of anthropogenic radionuclides in Japan Sea waters, *Deep Sea Res. II*, 50, 2701, 2003.

79. Povinec, P.P., Delfanti, R., Gastaud, J., La Rosa, J., Morgenstern, U., Oregioni, B., Pham, M.K., Salvi, S., and Top, Z., Anthropogenic radionuclides in Indian Ocean surface waters — the Indian Ocean transect 1998, *Deep Sea Res. II*, 50, 2751, 2003

80. Ikeuchi, Y., Temporal variations of 90Sr and 137Cs concentrations in Japanese coastal surface seawater and sediments from 1974 to 1998, *Deep Sea Res. II*, 50, 2713, 2003.

81. Mulsow, S., Povinec, P.P., Somayajulu, B.L.K., Oregioni, B., Liong Wee Kwong, L., Gastaud, J., Top, Z., and Morgenstern, U., Temporal (3H) and spatial variations of 90Sr, 239,240Pu and 241Am in the Arabian Sea: GEOSECS Stations revisited, *Deep Sea Res.*, 50, 2761, 2003.

82. Lee, S.H., La Rosa, J.J., Levy-Palomo, I., Oregioni, B., Pham, M.K., Povinec, P.P., and Wyse, E., Recent inputs and budgets of 90Sr, 137Cs, 239,240Pu and 241Am in the northwest Mediterranean Sea, *Deep Sea Research*, 50, 2817, 2003.

83. Aarkrog, A., Dahlgaard, H., and Nielsen, S.P., Marine radioactivity in the Arctic: a retrospect of environmental studies in Greenland waters with emphasis on transport of 90Sr and 137Cs with the East Greenland Current, *Sci. Total Environ.*, 237, 143, 1999.

84. Hirose, K., Amano, H., Baxter, M.S., Chaykovskaya, E., Chumichev, V.B., Hong, G.H., Isogai, K., Kim, C.K., Kim, S.H., Miyao, T., Morimoto, T., Nikitin, A., Oda, K., Pettersson, H.B.L., Povinec, P.P., Seto, Y., Tkalin, A., Togawa, O., and Veletova, N.K, Anthropogenic radionuclides in seawater in the East Sea/Japan Sea: results of the first stage of the Japanese-Korean-Russian expedition, *J. Environ. Radioactiv.*, 43,1, 1999.

85. Livingstone, H. and Povinec, P., Anthropogenic marine radioactivity, *Ocean Coast. Manage.*, 43, 687, 2000.

86. Holm, E., Source and distribution of anthropogenic radionuclides in the marine environment, in *Radioecology. Lectures in Environmental Radioactivity*, Holm, E., ed., World Scientific Publishing, Singapore, 1994.

87. Heldal, H.E., Føyn, L., and Varskog, P., Bioaccumulation of 137Cs in pelagic food webs in the Norwegian and Barents Seas, *J. Environ. Radioactiv.*, 65, 177, 2003.

88. Raisbeck, G.M., Yiou, F., Zhou, Z.Q., and Kilius, L.R., 129I from nuclear fuel reprocessing facilities at Sellafield (U.K.) and La Hague (France): potential as an oceanographic tracer, *J. Mar. Syst.*, 6, 561, 1994.

89. Hou, X., Dahlgaard, H., and Nielsen, S.P., Chemical speciation analysis of 129I in seawater and a preliminary investigation to use it as a tracer for geochemical cycle study of stable iodine, *Mar. Chem.*, 74, 145, 2001.

90. Cooper, L.W., Hong, G.H., Beasley, T.M., and Grebmeier, J.M., Iodine-129 concentrations in marginal seas of the North Pacific and Pacific-influenced waters of the Arctic Ocean, *Mar. Pollut. Bull.*, 42, 1347, 2001.

91. McCubbin, D., Leonard, K.S., Bailey, T.A., Williams, J., and Tossell, P., Incorporation of organic tritium (3H) by marine organisms and sediments in the Severn Estuary/Bristol Channel (UK), *Mar. Poll. Bull.*, 42, 852, 2001.

92. Kathren, R.L., *Radioactivity in the Environment: Sources, Distribution and Surveillance*, Harwood Academic, New York, 1986.

93. Kershaw, P.J., McCubbin, D., and Leonard, K.S., Continuing contamination of North Atlantic and Artic waters by Sellafield radionuclides, *Sci. Total Environ.*, 237/238, 119, 1999.

94. Webster, S., Salt, C.A., and Howard, B.J., Sea-to-land transfer of technetium-99 through the use of contaminated seaweed as an agricultural soil conditioner, *J. Environ. Radioactiv.*, 70, 127, 2003.

95. Dahlgaard, H., Bergan, T.D.S., and Christensen, G.C., Technetium-99 and caesium-137 time series at the Norwegian coast monitored by the brown alga *Fucus vesiculosus*, *Radioprotection – Colloques*, 32, 353, 1997.

96. Brown, J.E., Kolstad, A.L., Brungot, A.L., Lind, B., Rudjord, A.L., Strand, P., and Føyn, L., Levels of ^{99}Tc in seawater and biota samples from Norwegian coastal waters and adjacent seas, *Mar. Pollut. Bull.*, 38, 560, 1999.

97. Bailly du Bois, P. and Guegueniat, P., Quantitative assessment of dissolved radiotracers in the English Channel: sources, average impact of La Hague reprocessing plant and conservative behaviour (1983, 1986, 1988, 1994), *Cont. Shelf Res.*, 19, 1977, 1999.

98. Sakuragi, Y., Meason, J.L., and Kuroda, P.K., Uranium and plutonium isotopes in the atmosphere, *J. Geophys. Res.*, 88, 3718, 1983.

99. Kuroda, P.K., Essien, I.O., and Sandoval, D.N., Fallout of uranium isotopes from the 1980 eruption of Mount St. Helens, *J. Radioanal. Nucl. Chem.*, 84, 23, 1984.

100. Essien, Y., Sandoval, N., and Kuroda, P.K., Deposition of excess amount of natural U from the atmosphere, *Health Phys.*, 48, 325, 1985.

101. Matsunami, T., Mizohata, A., Mamuro, T., and Tsujimoto, T., Detection of uranium in rain water from nuclear explosions, *Hoken Butsuri*, 13, 193, 1983.

102. Martinez-Aguirre, A., Moron, M.C., and Garcia-Leon, M., Measurements of U-isotopes and Ra-isotopes in rainwater samples, *J. Radioanal. Nucl. Chem.* 152, 37-46, 1991.

103. Hirose, K., Honda, T., Yagishita, S., Igarashi, Y., Aoyama, M., Deposition behaviors of ^{210}Pb, ^{7}Be and thorium isotopes observed in Tsukuba and Nagasaki, Japan, *Atmos. Environ.*, 38, 6601, 2004.

104. Garcia-Leon, M., Manjon, G., and Sanchez-Angulo, C.I., "^{99}Tc/^{137}Cs Activity Ratios in Rainwater Samples Collected in the South of Spain," *J. Environ. Radiat.*, 20, 49, 1993.

105. Attrep, M., Enochs, J.A., and Broz, L.D., Atmospheric technetium-99, *Environ. Sci. Technol.*, 5, 344, 1971.

106. Mas, J.L., Garcia-Leon, M., and Bolivar, J.P., Technetium-99 detection in water samples by ICP-MS, *Radiochim. Acta*, 92, 39, 2004.

107. Lopez-Gutierrez, J.M., Garcia Leon, M., Schnabel C., Suter, M., Synal H.A., Szidat, S., Wet and dry deposition of I-129 in Seville (Spain) measured by accelerator mass spectrometry, *J. Environ. Radioactiv.*, 55, 269, 2001.

108. Muramatsu, Y. and Ohmomo, Y., I-129 and I-127 in environmental samples collected from Tokaimura, Ibaraki, Japan, *Sci. Total Environ.*, 48, 33, 1986.

109. Synal, H.-A., Wagner, M.J.M., Dittrich-Hannen, B., Suter, M., Schotterer, U., Increase of 129I in the environment, *Nucl. Instrum. Meth. B*, 113, 490, 1996.

110. Santos Arevalo, F.J., Lopez Gutierrez, J.M., Garcia Leon, M., Schnabel, C., Synal, H.A., Suter, M., Analysis of ^{36}Cl in atmospheric samples of Seville (Spain) by AMS, *Nucl. Instrum. Meth. B*, 223, 501, 2004.

111. Blinov, A., Massonet, S., Sachsenhauser, H., San Sion, C., Lazarev V., Beer, J., Synal, H.A., Kaba, M., Masarik, J., and Nolte, E., An excess of Cl-36 in modern atmospheric precipitation, *Nucl. Instrum. Meth. B*, 172, 537, 2000.

112. Villa, M., Técnicas experimentales para la medida por centelleo líquido de la actividad de emisores beta en el medio ambiente, PhD dissertation, University of Seville, 2004 [in Spanish].

113. Rank, D., Rajner, V., and Lust, V., Österriechisches Forschungs-und Prüfzentrum Arsenal Ges. M.b.H., Vienna, 1997.

114. Radwan, I., Pietrzak-Flis, Z., and Wardaszko, T., Tritium in surface waters, tap water and in precipitation in Poland during the 1994–1999 period, *J. Radioanal. Nucl. Chem.*, 247, 71, 2001.

115. Baeza, A., Garcia, E., and Miro, C., A procedure for the determination of very low activity levels of tritium in water samples, *J. Radioanal. Nucl. Chem.*, 241, 93, 1999.

116. Okada, S. and Momoshima, N., Overview of tritium-characteristics, sources and problems, *Health Phys.*, 65, 595, 1993.

117. Momoshima, N., Momoshima, N., Tfahafa, P.I., Okai, T., and Takashima, Y., "Measurements of Tritium in Forest Soil" in *Liquid Scintillation Spectrometry*, Noakes, J., Schönhofer, F., and Polach, H.A., eds., University of Arizona, Tucson, AZ, 1993.

118. Villa, M. and Manjon, G., Low-level measurements of tritium in water, *Appl. Radiat. Isot.*, 61, 319, 2004.

119. Miljevic, N., Sipka, V., Zujic, A., and Golobocanin, D., Tritium around the Vinca Institute of Nuclear Sciences, *J. Environ. Radioactiv.*, 48, 303, 2000.

120. Rubio Montero, M.P. and Martin Sanchez, A., Activity of 239+240Pu and 238Pu in atmospheric deposits, *Appl. Radiat. Isot.*, 55, 97, 2001.

121. Ballestra, S., Gastaud, J., and Lopez, J., "Radiochemical Procedures Used at IAEA-ILMR Monaco for Measuring Artificial Radionuclides Resulting from the Chernobyl Accident" in *Low-level measurements of man-made radionuclides in the environment: proceedings of the Second International Summer School, La Rábida, Huelva, Spain, 25 June to 6 July 1990*, Garcia-Leon, M. and Madurga, G., eds., World Scientific Publishing, Singapore, 1991.

122. Aoyama, M., Hirose, K., and Sugimura, Y., Deposition of gamma-emitting nuclides in Japan after the reactor-IV accident at Chernobyl, *J. Radioanal. Nucl. Chem.*, 116, 291, 1987.

123. Hirose, K., Takatani, S., and Aoyama, M., Deposition of Sr-90 and plutonium isotopes derived from the Chernobyl accident in Japan, *J. Radioanal. Nucl. Chem.*, 182, 349, 1994.

124. Aoyama, M., Evidence of stratospheric fallout of cesium isotopes from the Chernobyl accident, *Geophys. Res. Lett.*, 15, 327, 1988.

125. Papastefanou, C., Manolopoulou, M., Stoulos, S., Ioannidou, A., and Gerasopoulos, E., Coloured rain dust from Sahara Desert is still radioactive, *J. Environ. Radiat.*, 55, 109, 2001.

126. Bouwer, H., *Groundwater Hydrology*, McGraw-Hill, New York, 1978.

127. Rutherford, P.M., Dudas, M.J., and Samek, R.A., Environmental impact of phosphogypsum, *Sci. Total Environ.*, 149, 1, 1994.

128. Bolivar, J.P., Garcia-Tenorio, R., and Mas, J.L., Radioactivity of phosphogypsum in south-west of Spain, *Radiat. Prot. Dosim.*, 76, 185, 1998.

129. El-Bahi, S.M., El-Dine, N.W., El-Shershaby, A., and Sroor, A., Elemental analysis of Egyptian phosphate fertilizer components, *Health Phys.*, 86, 303, 2004.

130. Guzman, E.T.R., Alberich, M.V.E., and Regil, E.O., Uranium and phosphate behavior in the vadose zone of a fertilized corn field, *J. Radioanal. Nucl. Chem.*, 254, 509, 2002.

131. El-Mrabet, R. et al., Phosphogypsum amendment effect on radionuclide content in drainage water and marsh soils from southwestern Spain, *J. Environ. Qual.*, 32, 1262, 2002.

132. Tricca, A., Wasserburg, G.J., Porcelli, D., and Baskaran, M., The transport of U- and Th-series nuclides in a sandy unconfined aquifer, *Geochim. Cosmochim. Acta*, 65, 1187, 2001.

133. Roback, R.C., Johnson, T.M., McLing, T.L., Murrell, M.T., Luo, S., and Ku, T.-L., Uranium isotopic evidence for groundwater chemical evolution and flow patterns in the eastern Snake River Plain aquifer, Idaho, *Geol. Soc. Am. Bull.*, 113, 1133, 2001.

134. Rosholt, J.N., Shields, W.R., and Garner, E.L., Isotopic fractionation of uranium in sandstone, *Science*, 139, 224, 1963.

135. Titayeva, N.A., Orlova, A.V., Karpushina, T.I., and Nikulin, V.I., Behaviour of uranium and thorium isotopes in crystalline rocks and surface waters in a cold wet climate, *Geochem. Int.*, 7–8, 1146, 1973.

136. Osmond, J.K. and Cowart, J.B., Groundwater, in *Uranium-Series Disequilibrium: Applications to Earth, Marine, and Environmental Sciences*, 2nd ed., Ivanovich, M. and Harmon, R.S., eds., Clarendon Press, Oxford, 1992.

137. Cowart, J.B., Kaufman, M.I., and Osmond, J.K., Uranium-isotope variations in groundwaters of the Floridian aquifer and Boulder Zone of south Florida, *J. Hydrol.*, 36, 161, 1978.

138. Gascoyne, M., Miller, N.H., and Neymark, L.A., Uranium-series disequilibrium in tuffs from Yucca Mountain, Nevada, as evidence of pore-fluid flow over last million years. *Appl. Geochem.*, 17, 781, 2002.

139. Chu, T.C. and Wang, J.J., Radioactive disequilibrium of uranium and thorium nuclide series in hot spring and river water from Peitou Hot Spring Basin in Taipei, *J. Nucl. Radiochem. Sci.*, 1, 5, 2000.

140. Osmond, J.K. and Cowart, J.B., The theory and uses of natural uranium isotopic variations in hydrology, *Atom. Energy Rev.*, 14, 621, 1976.

141. Labajo, J., Natural radionuclides in Doñana National Park and its surroundings, PhD dissertation, University of Seville, 2003 [in Spanish].

142. Luo, S., Ku, T.L., Roback, R., Murrell, M., and McLing, T.L., In-situ radionuclide transport and preferential groundwater flows at INEEL (Idaho): decay-series disequilibrium studies, *Geochim. Cosmochim. Acta*, 64, 867, 2000.

143. Langmuir, D., *Aqueous Environmental Geochemistry*, Prentice Hall, New York, 1997.

144. Zhu, C., Estimate of recharge from radiocarbon dating of groundwater and numerical flow and transport modelling, *Water Resourc. Res.*, 36, 2607, 2000.

145. Kronfeld, J., Godfrey-Smith, D.I., Johannessen, D., and Zentilli, M., Uranium series isotopes in the Avon Valley, Nova Scotia. *J. Environ. Radioactiv.*, 73, 335, 2004.

146. Come, B. and Chapman, N.A., *Natural Analogues in Radioactive Waste Disposal*, Graham & Trotman, London, 1987.

147. Smellie, J.A., Karlsson, F., and Alexander, W.R., Natural analogues studies: present status and performance assessment implications, *J. Contam. Hydrol.*, 26, 3, 1997.

148. International Atomic Energy Agency, *Use of Natural Analogues to Support Radionuclide Transport Models for Deep Geological Repositories for Long Lived Radioactive Wastes*, Technical Document no. 1109, International Atomic Energy Agency, Vienna, Austria, 1999.

149. Kashparov, V.A., Oughton, D.H., Zvarich, S.I., Protsak, V.P., and Levchuk, S.E., Kinetics of fuel particle weathering and ^{90}Sr mobility in the Chernobyl 30-km exclusion zone, *Health Phys.*, 76, 251, 1999.

150. Dewiere, L., Grenier, C., Ahamdach, N., Bugai, D., and Kashparov, V., ^{90}Sr migration to the geo-sphere from a waste burial in the Chernobyl exclusion zone, *J. Environ. Radioactiv.*, 74, 139, 2004.

151. Schönhofer, F., in *Low-Level Measurements of Radioactivity in the Environment: Techniques and Applications*, Garcia-Leon, M. and Garcia-Tenorio, R., eds., World Scientific Publishing, Singapore, 1994.

152. de Oliveira, J., Mazzilli, B.P., Sampa, M.H., and Bambalas, E., Natural radionuclides in drinking water supplies of São Paulo State, Brazil and consequent population doses, *J. Environ. Radioactiv.*, 53, 99, 2001.
153. Erlandsson, B., Jakobsson, B., and Jönsson, G., Studies of the radon concentration in drinking water from the horst Soderasen in southern Sweden, *J. Environ. Radioactiv.*, 53, 145, 2001.
154. Zalewski, M., Karpinska, M., Mnich, Z., Kapala, J., and Zalewski, P., Study of 222Rn concentrations in drinking water in the north-eastern hydroregions of Poland, *J. Environ. Radioactiv.*, 53, 167, 2001.
155. Dueñas, C., Fernandez, M.C., Carretero, J., Liger, E., and Canete, S., Ra-226 and Rn-222 concentrations and doses in bottled waters in Spain, *J. Environ. Radioactiv.*, 45, 283, 1999.
156. Collado, G.M., Romero, I.V., Gonzalez, H.P.M., Garcia-Balmaseda, R.G.-T., Garcia Leon, M., Determination of Ra-226 and Ra-224 in drinking waters by liquid scintillation counting, *Appl. Radiat. Isot.*, 48, 535, 1997.
157. Gäfvert, T., Ellmark, C., and Holm, E., Removal of radionuclides at a waterworks, *J. Environ. Radioactiv.*, 63, 105, 2002.
158. International Commission on Radiological Protection, Age-dependent doses to members of the public from intake of radionuclides: Part 2. Ingestion dose coefficients. A report of a Task Group of Committee 2 of the International Commission on Radiological Protection, *Ann ICRP*, 23, 1, 1993.
159. Godoy, J.M., Amaral, E., and Godoy, L., Natural radionuclides in Brazilian mineral water and consequent doses to the population, *J. Environ. Radioactiv.*, 53, 175, 2001.

5 Radionuclide Concentrations in Soils

Guillermo Manjón Collado

CONTENTS

5.1   INTRODUCTION

Long-lived radionuclides can easily be studied in zones not affected by recent (days) nuclear accidents. This is one of the reasons that short-lived radionuclides are not included in this chapter. Two different origins of long-lived radionuclides in soils can be considered. First, artificial radionuclides are transuranic elements (plutonium isotopes) and long-lived fission products (^{137}Cs, ^{90}Sr). In both cases, the presence in the environment of these kinds of radionuclides is due to nuclear weapons tests or the nuclear power industry.

Next, natural radionuclides are radionuclides belonging to the three natural decay chains (^{238}U, ^{235}U, ^{232}Th), ^{40}K, and cosmogenic radioisotopes (^{3}H, ^{7}Be, ^{14}C). In the case of natural decay chains, radioelements might be inside the silicon dioxide crystals in soils. A fraction of the radon (gas) can be transferred from soils into the atmosphere by emanation. Then, ^{222}Rn decays in ^{210}Pb, which falls back, associated with aerosols, onto the Earth's surface.

On the other hand, artificial radionuclides are stored in the stratosphere and fall to the Earth's surface according to atmospheric dynamics. Artificial and cosmogenic radionuclides and ^{210}Pb are typical fallout radionuclides that are being deposited.

In this chapter, the behavior of radionuclides in soils is studied. The main characteristics of the mentioned radionuclides are analyzed, experimental procedures are exhaustively discussed, and obtained data are analyzed.

The study of the behavior of radionuclides has been divided into four items. First, the fractionation of radionuclides in soils is considered, according to the soil fraction (soil solution, organic matter, residual) associated with the radionuclides. Second, radionuclide migration along the soil profile is studied. Third, the role of microorganisms is presented (e.g., in the remediation of contaminated soil). Finally, radionuclide bioavailability and transfer into plants is considered. Knowledge of the behavior of radionuclides in soil can lead to countermeasures in case of soil contamination.

Finally, some scientific and social applications of radionuclide concentration measurements in soils, such as dose assessment, earthquake prediction through radon measurements, and dating of soil cores and erosion, are explained.

5.2 BEHAVIOR OF LONG-LIVED RADIONUCLIDES IN SOIL

If the scientific literature is reviewed, environmental studies on the presence of radionuclide concentrations include in-depth discussions of the fractionation, vertical distribution, the influence of microorganisms, and the soil to plant transfer of radionuclides. Fewer articles can be found on the behavior of long-lived radionuclides in soil.

Factors influencing the behavior of radionuclides in soils are mainly the chemical properties of the radioelement and the characteristics of the soil, including mineral composition, organic matter content, and chemical reaction milieu [1]. Other factors also affecting the behavior of radionuclides in soil are rainfall amounts, temperature, and soil management. Finally, the pH value is an important parameter controlling the kinetics of elements in soil and consequently the kinetics of radionuclides. In order to understand the mobility of radionuclides in soil, it is important to study the inorganic and organic composition of soils. The presence of inorganic matter (clay minerals and oxides) can cause processes of sorption and complexation. On the other hand, biological activity can increase radioelement mobility.

Radionuclides can be absorbed by some mineral fractions of the soil (silt and clay fractions). The main minerals in these fractions are smectite, illite, vermiculite, chlorite, allophone, and imogolite. Other contributors to the absorption process are the oxides and hydroxides of silica, aluminum, iron, and manganese. Soils with a high content of illite, smectite, vermiculite, or mica within the clay fraction absorb large amounts of cations due to their intrinsic negative charge [1]. On the other hand, anions can be absorbed by aluminum and iron oxides at pH values in the range of 8 to 9. Water-soluble anionic compounds such as phosphate, selenite, molybdate, and arsenate can be absorbed by the formation of stable complexes and the exchange of ligands with aluminum and iron oxides. The presence of organic matter reduces anion absorption.

Organic matter is extremely heterogeneous and consists of organic acids, lipids, lignin, and fulvic and humic acids. The number of interactions and reactions of radionuclides with organic matter is high. These processes are affected by the pH and the cation concentration in soil.

The dynamics of soil water, as well as the texture and structure of soil, have a direct impact on radionuclide speciation. Chemically unchanged substances can be partially transferred through water flow, whereas slow infiltration favors interaction with the soil matrix and soil solution.

5.2.1 FRACTIONATION

The speciation of the soils, based on a sequential extraction protocol used by Krouglov et al. [2], was applied by Baeza et al. [3], to samples collected in La Bazagona and Muñoveros, Extremadura (western Spain). These authors have considered different fractions in a soil as follows:

- Exchangeable fraction: Dried samples of soil are treated with NH_4OAc, where the exchangeable fraction is dissolved.
- Dilute acid soluble fraction: The solid residue is attacked with 1M HCl, where the dilute acid soluble fraction is dissolved. This fraction is bound to organic matter.
- Concentrated acid extractable acid fraction: The solid residue obtained in the last step is attacked with 6M HCl at boiling temperature. This fraction is bound to carbonates and oxides (iron or manganese).
- Residual fraction: This is the final residue. This is the fraction more strongly bound to the soil matrix.

However, five fractions may be observed in the sequential extraction. Thus Blanco et al. [4] compare two classical experimental procedures [5,6] that consider five different fractions in soils: exchangeable fraction, fraction bound to organic matter, fraction bound to carbonates, fraction bound to iron and manganese oxides, and residual fraction. In this work, the residual fractions were totally dissolved by HNO_3/HF digestion under pressure using a microwave oven. Table 5.1 shows the main steps of both procedures.

These two methods were checked by measuring isotopes of radium, uranium, and thorium. In the conclusion of this work, the authors found that the method of Schultz et al. [6] improves some of the defects recognized in the method of Tessier et al. [5]. For this reason, the method of Schultz et al. is usually applied in studies of the behavior of radionuclides in soil [7]. However, the unsystematic nature of the differences in results does not permit a direct comparison of the historical results obtained by both methods [7].

TABLE 5.1
Sequential Extraction Processes According to the Methods of Tessier et al.
[5] and Schultz et al. [6]

Fraction	Reagents	
	Method of Tessier et al. [5]	Method of Schultz et al. [6]
Exchangeable	1M MgCl$_2$ pH 7, 1 h, room temperature	0.4M MgCl$_2$ pH 5, 1 h, room temperature
Organic matter	(1) 0.02M HNO$_3$ + H$_2$O$_2$ 30%, pH 2, 2 h, 85°C (2) H$_2$O$_2$ 30%, pH 2, 3 h, 85°C (3) 3.2M NH$_4$OAc in HNO$_3$ 20%, 30 min, room temperature	NaOCl 5–6%, pH 7.5, 2 × 0.5 h, 96°C
Carbonates	1M NaAc, pH 5 (HOAc), 5 h, room temperature	1M NaAc in 25% HAc, pH 4, 2 × 2 h, room temperature
Oxides (iron or manganese)	0.04M NH$_2$OH·HCl in 25% HOAc, pH 2, 6 h, 96°C	0.04M, NH$_2$OH·HCl, pH 2 (HNO$_3$), 5 h, room temperature

The distribution of radionuclides in soil can be studied using particle size fractions [8]. In this case, soil samples are homogenized and different particle size fractions are separated by physical procedures [9] such as sieving and settling. Usually the sample depth must be large enough to collect all the artificial radionuclides deposited in the soil in order to establish the total amount of fallout in an area.

For such a study, three size fractions must be considered: the sand-size fraction (larger than 63 μm), the silt-size fraction (2 to 63 μm), and the clay-size fraction (smaller than 2 μm). In the work of Spezzano [8], seven types of soils from the same area (Viverone Lake in southwest Italy) were studied. In this case, the physical and chemical characteristics of the different soils were determined in order to discuss the different behavior of ^{137}Cs from global fallout and ^{137}Cs from the Chernobyl accident. Table 5.2 shows the results obtained. In this work, organic matter was determined by the Walkley and Black method [10,11], cation exchange capacity by the BaCl$_2$-triethanolamine method, and pH (in 0.1M KCl, 1:2 solid:liquid ratio) following standard methods [12].

Soil bulk densities (in kg/m^3) are evaluated by dividing the mass of dried soil sample by the volume of the soil core. The concentration of the most abundant element was determined by microwave digestion of the soil using high-purity reagents and Teflon vessels, and analysis by atomic absorption spectrometry [8]. Soluble and exchangeable cesium was determined by extraction with 1M NH$_4$Ac at pH 7 (1:20 solid:liquid ratio, 24 h equilibration).

Table 5.3 shows the concentrations of ^{137}Cs for each size fraction of the studied soils (corrected for decay to May 1986). In this table the strong binding of ^{137}Cs to clay minerals is easily observed.

TABLE 5.2
Chemical and Physical Characteristics in Soil [8]

Land Use	Woodland	Peat Bog	Cultivated	Pasture
Bulk density (kg/m³)	1650	700	1440	1350
pH (0.1M KCl)	3.63	4.24	4.72	4.07
Organic carbon (%)	1.4	18	3.0	2.9
CEC (mEq/kg)	28	499	148	112
Clay (<2 μm) (%)	15	9	30	16
Silt (2–63 μm) (%)	47	62	61	57
Sand (>63 μm) (%)	38	29	9	27
Na (g/kg)	14.4	6.5	9.8	12.3
K (g/kg)	9.2	9.4	16.4	11.6
Ca (g/kg)	5.6	3.9	3.3	5.2
Mg (g/kg)	14.2	16.8	25.7	28.6

TABLE 5.3
Concentrations of ^{137}Cs (in Bq/kg) in the Particle Size Fractions of the Investigated Soils (Corrected for Decay to May 1986) [8]

Land Use	Woodland	Peat Bog	Cultivated	Pasture
Clay (<2 μm)	303 ± 10	578 ± 17	788 ± 20	265 ± 9
Silt (2–63 μm)	32 ± 3	271 ± 11	122 ± 6	63 ± 4
Sand (>63 μm)	7 ± 1	130 ± 11	67 ± 4	16 ± 2

5.2.2 VERTICAL DISTRIBUTION

The information obtained by a fractionation analysis of radionuclides in soil can be very useful for designing predictive models or to decide realistic countermeasures. In addition, several horizons or layers are usually examined due to their quite different physicochemical properties [13]. Thus three organic horizons are easily distinguished: Of1 (litter, only slightly decomposed), Of2 (fragmented litter, partially decomposed by fermentation processes), and Oh (well-humified organic matter). The mineral soil horizons that can be analyzed are Aeh (0 to 5 cm), Alh (5 to 10 cm), Al (10 to 36 cm), and Bt (36 to 50 cm) [14]. This method was applied to soil collected in a spruce forest 50 km northwest of Munich, Germany. However, these horizons are different in other works. Actually these horizons can be separately studied for a better understanding of radionuclide behavior and the deepest layer can be neglected if artificial radionuclide fallout is the objective of the work [13].

TABLE 5.4
Physicochemical Properties of a Forest Soil in Different Layers [13]

Horizon	Depth (cm)	pH (CaCl$_2$)	Organic Carbon (%)	Clay (%)
		Organic Layer		
Of1	7–4.5	3.2	49	
Of2	4.5–2	3.2	49	
Oh	2–0	2.9	40	
		Mineral Soil		
Aeh	0–5	3.2	2.8	19
Alh	5–10	3.6	1.3	21
Al	10–40	3.9	0.9	28

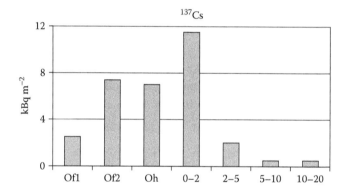

FIGURE 5.1 Total activity of ^{137}Cs per unit area in the various soil layers. For the organic layers, the name of the horizons is given. Within the mineral soil, the depth is given in centimeters [13].

In general, physicochemical properties of soil samples are analyzed. Table 5.4 shows some of these properties and results obtained in a forest soil [13]. Other parameters such as density, cation exchange capacity, and exchangeable cations are also determined. Before the sequential analysis, the air-dried soil of each layer is usually sieved to 2 mm for the removal of stones and roots.

Figure 5.1 shows the results obtained by Bunzl et al. [13] in a study of ^{137}Cs distribution in a soil profile. The total amount of ^{137}Cs in this soil is due to global fallout and the Chernobyl accident. The Chernobyl contribution was determined through the ^{134}Cs/^{137}Cs activity ratio. The highest ^{137}Cs activity was determined in the first mineral soil layer (0 to 2 cm).

The percentage of ^{137}Cs (means of five soil cores) found after sequential extraction (method of Tessier et al. [5]) in fractions I to V in the seven layers of soil is presented in Figure 5.2. It is clear that radiocesium is mainly bound to

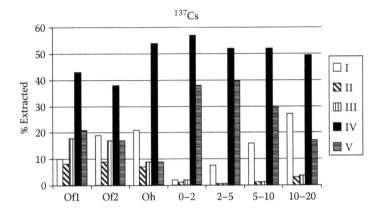

FIGURE 5.2 Percentage of [137]Cs (means from five plots in a spruce stand) found for the various soil layers in five fractions according to Tessier et al.'s [5] method: I, readily exchangeable; II, bound to sesquioxides; III, bound to organic matter; IV, persistently bound; V, residual. For the organic layers, the names of the horizons are given. Within the mineral soil, the depth is given in centimeters [13].

fraction IV (40 to 60%), but the presence of ^{137}Cs in the residual fraction is also important in mineral soil layers. The percentage in fraction I increases with depth for the mineral soil layers and the amounts in fraction II and III are negligible. The corresponding values decrease with the depth in fraction V. If we consider the organic layers, ^{137}Cs is bound to fraction IV.

If a short-term fallout of radionuclides is deposited onto the surface of a soil as a pulse, a typical fast-moving tail is observed in soil layers below the peak concentration. This phenomenon can be explained by assuming that either the hydraulic properties of the soil or the sorption properties of the soil, or both, exhibit a horizontal variability. This fact can be demonstrated by Monte Carlo calculations, assuming a convection-dispersion model [14].

For example, we have the case of the zone close to the Chernobyl nuclear power plant. The soil in this zone was affected by a pulse of contamination of artificial radionuclides (e.g., ^{137}Cs). A typical study of the vertical distribution and migration of radionuclides was published by Bossew et al. [15]. The sampling site was located in the exclusion zone of the Chernobyl nuclear power plant and is shown in Figure 5.3. According to this map, a ^{137}Cs deposition of 2 to 4 MBq/m² is estimated.

Figure 5.4 shows the shape of a ^{137}Cs profile in an undisturbed soil sample. The maximum of ^{137}Cs and the shapes observed in all the samples analyzed in this work were quite different in spite of the close proximity of the sampling sites (10 m).

The apparent migration velocity, v (in cm/year), and the apparent dispersion coefficient, D (in cm²/year), were selected as migration parameters. These parameters were evaluated by fitting the ^{137}Cs profiles to a Gauss-type function. The apparent migration velocity ranged from 0.14 to 0.22 cm/year and the apparent

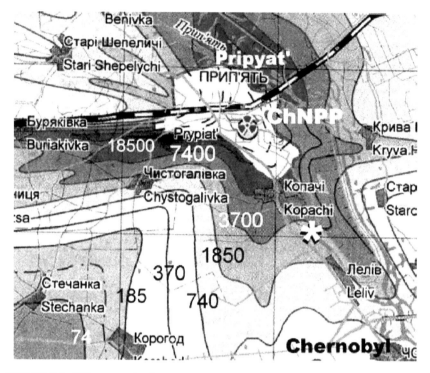

FIGURE 5.3 ^{137}Cs contamination map of the area around the Chernobyl nuclear power plant [61] with contamination isolines in kBq/m². The location of the investigation site is marked with an asterisk [15].

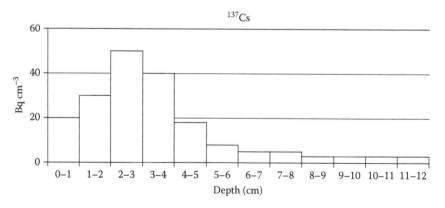

FIGURE 5.4 Vertical distribution of ^{137}Cs in a soil core collected in the exclusion area of Chernobyl nuclear power plant in 2000 [15].

dispersion coefficient ranged from 0.04 to 0.07 cm²/year. The uncertainties of the fitted parameters ranged from less than 1% to 10% for v and less than 5% to 35% for D. This study was extended to other fallout radionuclides and migration parameters. There are essentially three mobility groups. Strontium, cesium, cobalt, antimony, niobium, and plutonium show low mobility, americium is more mobile, and europium is the most mobile of all the investigated elements. This is explained by the different interactions between soils (sorption) and elements.

Fujiyoshi and Sawamura [16] studied the vertical distribution in soils of natural radionuclides (^{40}K, ^{226}Ra, ^{210}Pb). In the case of natural radionuclides, the geological characteristics of the soil are very important in order to determine the vertical distribution and the total content. For instance, the vertical distribution of ^{40}K is related to biological activity (root uptake of nutrients). Profiles of ^{226}Ra can be used to determine a possible heterogeneity within a soil horizon. ^{210}Pb is probably the most interesting natural radionuclide because of its double natural origin in the soil profile. ^{210}Pb is a radionuclide daughter of ^{222}Rn (gas), which is in the atmosphere as a result of emanation from the soil surface. Then a fraction (unsupported) of ^{210}Pb in the soil is derived from the atmosphere via fallout or wet deposition. The origin of the other natural fraction (supported) is the activity of ^{226}Ra in the soil profile. The remaining ^{210}Pb is anthropogenic (e.g., from the combustion of fossil fuels) [16].

A profile of the $^{210}Pb/^{226}Ra$ activity ratio is plotted against depth in Figure 5.5 [16]. A peak in the $^{210}Pb/^{226}Ra$ activity ratio is at a depth of 32 cm. This depth corresponds to a time in the 18th century. This fact could be related to the progressive clearing started in the 17th century, but the discussion is not closed.

Humic substances such as humic acid (HA) and fulvic acid (FA) are a fraction of the organic matter in a soil. These have a high affinity for actinide and lanthanide metal ions in a terrestrial system. Chung et al. [17] investigated the possibility of retaining fallout radionuclides in an organic matter-rich soil of Jeju Island, Korea. In order to simulate the behavior of actinide metals, Eu(III) was used as a tracer. Synchronous fluorescence spectroscopy (SyFS) was used to characterize the Eu(III) binding to humic substances. The element composition of HA and FA (carbon, hydrogen, nitrogen, and sulfur) was determined by a combustion method.

The amounts of humic substances extracted from the soil samples at different depths are shown in Table 5.5. The results show that HA and FA are distributed

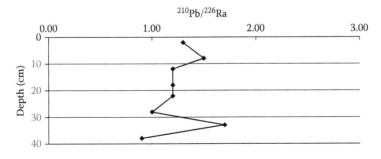

FIGURE 5.5 Profiles of the activity ratio of $^{210}Pb/^{226}Ra$ with soil depth in a 95-year-old Tharandt coniferous forest [16].

TABLE 5.5

$^{239+240}$Pu Activity Concentration, Amount of Humic Acid (HA) and Fulvic Acid (FA) Extracted from Soil Samples (100 g) at Different Depths [17]

Depth (cm)	$^{239+240}$Pu (Bq/kg)	Humic Acid (g/100g soil)	Fulvic Acid (g/100 g soil)	FA/HA (g/g)
0–5	5.1	2.14	1.04	0.49
5–10	6.2	1.50	0.99	0.66
10–15	2.8	1.72	1.10	0.64
15–20	1.3	1.39	0.95	0.68
20–25	0.2	0.57	0.63	1.11

into the deep soil, while the ratio of FA/HA tends to slightly increase across the soil depth. The increased ratio of FA/HA may be ascribed to the higher mobility of FA due to its low molecular weight, high acidic functional group content, and relatively high solubility [18]. In order to better understand the effects of soil humic substances on radionuclide distribution, the physicochemical and binding properties of humic substances with Eu(III) were further characterized. The stability of the complexes tends to increase as the soil depth increases, and HA has a slightly stronger binding ability to the Eu(III) ions than FA.

Conclusions of this work are

- The increased ratio of FA/HA with soil depth may be caused by the solubility and mobility of FA with high acidic functional group contents and low metal ion loading.
- The high solubility of FA compared to HA was also confirmed by elemental analysis (the high oxygen/carbon ratio), direct pH titration results, and ^{13}C nuclear magnetic resonance (NMR) spectral analysis (high carboxylic carbon contents). The basic information for the soil humic substances in this work may be useful in understanding and modeling the radionuclide (actinides) transport in the soil layer.

5.2.3 INFLUENCE OF MICROORGANISMS ON THE BEHAVIOR OF RADIONUCLIDES

The presence of microorganisms (bacteria) can change the behavior of radionuclides in soil, mainly by reduction reactions that change the oxidation state of an element. As an example, the case of ^{99}Tc, which is a fission product of ^{235}U or ^{239}Pu, is discussed. Its long half-life (2.1×10^5 years) makes the presence of ^{99}Tc in the environment a certainty for a long time.

The behavior of technetium in the environment (soil) mainly depends on its chemical form. The pertechnetate form (TcO_4, Tc(VII)) is highly soluble and mobile in the environment. Moreover, this chemical form is readily available to plants. In contrast, Tc(IV) is insoluble and immobile because of the strong sorption of this species by solid materials, and it is not readily available to plants.

The reduction of Tc(VII) to Tc(IV) is caused by bacteria such as *Shewanella putrefaciens* [19], *Geobacter sulfurreducens* [20], and some sulfate-reducing bacteria [21] under strict anaerobic conditions. In addition to the technetium reduction, *Geobacter metallireducens* produces insoluble technetium precipitate. These technetium-reducing anaerobic bacteria are often found in soils under waterlogged conditions (e.g., paddy fields) [22]. The presence of such technetium-reducing anaerobic bacteria in paddy soils raises the expectations of reduction and precipitation of technetium in the water covering these soils.

Microorganisms have an impact on the geochemical cycles of various metals. Thus technetium-insolubilizing microorganisms can affect the behavior of other metal elements. Ishii et al. [23] recently published a study demonstrating insoluble technetium formation in the surface water covering paddy fields and determining microbial contributions to technetium insolubilization as a first step toward knowing the behavior of technetium in an agricultural environment. In addition, the insolubilization of other trace elements was studied using a multitracer to search for elements that behave similar to technetium. Multitracers ensure efficient acquisition of information on the behavior of various metal ions using radioactive tracers (^{46}Sc, ^{58}Co, ^{65}Zn, ^{75}Se, ^{83}Rb, ^{85}Sr, ^{88}Y, ^{95}Nb, ^{139}Ce, ^{143}Pm, ^{153}Gd, ^{173}Lu, ^{175}Hf, and ^{183}Re) in the same sample under identical conditions [23].

Figure 5.6 shows a photograph of an untreated gray lowland sample (P38) of surface water after staining with SYBR Gold (a nucleic acid fluorescence dye). Most of the SYBR Gold-positive particles were characterized as spheres and rods; a few inorganic particles were also observed. Particles other than microbiological

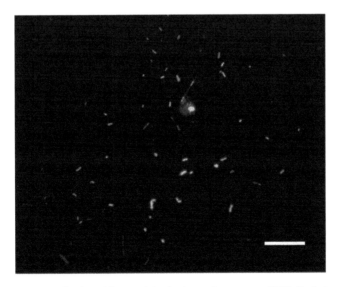

FIGURE 5.6 SYBR Gold-positive particles in the surface water of P38. Scale bar = 20 μm [23].

cells could be discriminated from cell particles by their shapes and fluorescence color. In addition to the inorganic particles, the numbers of protozoa and algae were also negligible. The microscopic observations indicated that the microbial components in the surface water sample were mainly fungi and bacteria. It was not possible to distinguish between fungi and bacteria by microscope observations, but the presence of fungal cells was confirmed by the formation of characteristic fungal colonies on an agar plate (data not shown).

Russell et al. [24] studied the effect of microbial sulfate reduction on the adsorption of ^{137}Cs in soils from different regions in Australia. The main result of this work was that the process of bacterial sulfate reduction substantially decreased the adsorption of ^{137}Cs in arid and tropical soils of Australia. This work started from a well-documented ability of sulfate-reducing bacteria to catalyze the removal of radionuclides from a soil solution by the production of hydrogen sulfide and alteration of the redox potential [25]. Russell et al. [24] studied the effect of the activity of such bacteria on the adsorption of ^{137}Cs in different soil types from different climates.

Analyzed samples were collected from an arid area of Australia (central northern South Australia) and from a tropical area. In the tropical area, two types of soils, a sandy loam (Blain) and a clay loam (Tippera), were collected from the Douglas Daly Research Farm in the Northern Territory of Australia. The climate of this region is monsoonal, and crops of mung and sorghum were grown over the wet season from December to April.

When sulfate-reducing bacteria were added to the assays under conditions allowing sulfate reduction, less ^{137}Cs adsorption was observed in all soils, but the effect was more pronounced in tropical samples than in the arid samples (Figure 5.7). Sulfate reduction resulted in a decrease in adsorption in Tippera soils from 90% to 50%, and by more than half an order of magnitude in Blain soils. The implication of these results for tropical soils contaminated with radionuclides such as

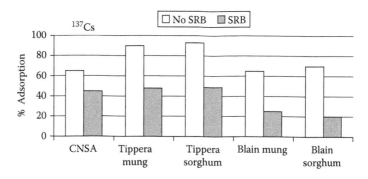

FIGURE 5.7 Effect of sulfate-reducing bacteria on the adsorption of ^{137}Cs in different soils. Open bars represent adsorption in treatments containing soil without sulfate-reducing bacteria; striped bars represent adsorption to soil in the presence of sulfate-reducing bacteria. Mung and sorghum were the crops grown in the tropical soils investigated [24].

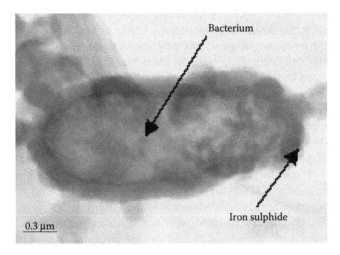

FIGURE 5.8 A sulfate-reducing bacterium covered with iron sulfide and isolated from a soil sample [26].

^{137}Cs is that microbial activity can result in the transfer of radionuclides from the soil to other organisms through increased bioavailability [24].

Abdelouasa et al. [26] published an exhaustive research work about the microbial effect of technetium reduction in organic matter-rich soils. In this work, the concentration of technetium in the presence of sulfate-reducing bacteria (Figure 5.8) was experimentally studied. The conclusion of this experiment was that anaerobic microorganisms such as metal- and sulfate-reducing bacteria play a major role in technetium immobilization in organic matter-rich subsurface environments if oxygen access is limited.

Another article describes a series of experiments from 1990 to 1995. These experiments were undertaken to investigate the type of microbial attack on hot particles and the specific characteristics of the mitospore fungi [27]. The main purpose of this investigation was to study the accumulation of radionuclides in different fungi and their ability to destroy the surfaces of explosion particles.

In both the Chernobyl accident and nuclear weapons detonations, part of the released radioactivity is in the form of agglomerates, so-called hot particles, which show a behavior in the environment that is quite different from the activity released in gaseous or aerosol form. Due to their different dissolution characteristics in the environment, they are of concern for the long-term behavior of deposited radionuclides as a function of the two fallout types, especially in zones where there was a significant fraction deposited in the form of hot particles, such as in the 30 km exclusion zone around the Chernobyl nuclear power plant or the site of nuclear weapons testing.

The long-term behavior is mainly controlled by the solubility of the hot particles and their dissolution by environmental effects. Since the solubility of these particles is generally low, their dissolution by *Micromycetes* mycelium is one of the forms of long-term change in the solution properties. Therefore the investigation of the biological activity of *Micromycetes* overgrowing on radioactive hot particles in the 30-km zone around the Chernobyl nuclear power plant and from nuclear weapons test sites, and their ability to destroy these particles and consequentially to accumulate (absorb) the radionuclides is of great interest.

The objects of the investigation were five species of mitosporic fungi (eight strains) from a collection at the Institute of Microbiology and Virology of the National Academy of Science of Ukraine [27]. In this work, hot particles and radioactive samples (milled hot particles) were used.

The radioactive material contained ^{60}Co, ^{90}Sr, ^{137}Cs, ^{152}Eu, ^{154}Eu, ^{155}Eu, ^{241}Am, and ^{239}Pu. Explosion particles were isolated in 1993–1994 on the test sites of the nuclear (1949) and thermonuclear (1953) explosions at the Semipalatinsk test site (in what is now Kazakhstan).

Cultivation using radioactive samples (milled hot particles) was as follows: The *Micromycetes* were cultivated on a two-layered agar medium. The lower layer contained a mixture of soil (1.5 g), radioactive sample, and Chapek's agar medium (10 ml); the upper layer of the medium contained the soil semiagar (7 ml), which was prepared with the addition of a soil extract (50 ml/l of the medium). Specially processed sterile nylon strainers (with pore sizes of 25 μm and 16 μm) were placed on the surface of this medium. The fungi were inoculated by injection in the center of the net. The same system with a two-layer medium but without the radioactive sample and without fungi served as controls.

All investigated species of the mitospore fungi were allowed to grow in the presence of the explosion particles, and biomass accumulation of *Cladosporium cladosporioides* and *Penicillium roseo-purpureum* species showed an inverse dependency on the activity of the explosion particles. After 15 to 25 days of cultivation, the fungal mycelium overgrew the particles.

Prolonged contact of the fungal mycelium with the surface of the particles probably stimulated mechanical and fermentative destruction of the explosion particles (the latter may be caused by the fungal exometabolites). Figure 5.9, obtained by electron microscopy, proves the significant weathering effect on the particle surfaces.

The authors suggest that the destruction of the radioactive particle matrix by the fungi is achieved by two processes:

- A combined one that includes overgrowing and mechanical destruction of the particles by the fungal mycelium with the simultaneous action of its exometabolites to dissolve the particles. This mechanism seems to be valid, especially for those fungi that are able to directionally grow toward a low-intensity radiation source [27].
- Destruction solely by fungal exometabolites without contact of the fungal mycelium and the radioactive particle.

Finally, the authors say radionuclide accumulation in the solid nutrient medium (agar medium) may occur mainly due to the destruction of the radioactive materials by the exometabolites of the respective fungi. For a better understanding

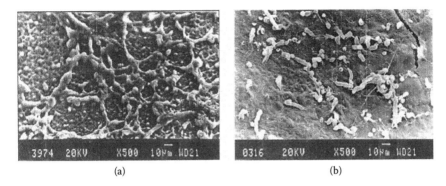

(a)   (b)

FIGURE 5.9 Surface of particle 7-1 before and after interaction with *Cladosporium sphaerospermum* 60: (a) before interaction; (b) after interaction [27].

of these processes, several experiments were conducted with artificially milled hot particles. Milling increased the calculated surface of the particles approximately 30- to 100-fold.

The presence of microorganisms can remove natural radionuclides such as uranium. A recent example is the research published by Lee et al. [28]. They studied the effects of the bacterium *Acidithiobacillus ferrooxidants* in the presence of initial Fe^{2+}, nutrient medium, and pyrite. Black shale taken in the Deokpyeong area in Korea, which contains 349 mg/kg of uranium, was used in this experiment. The main conclusion of this experiment was that nutrient addition to the solution in which the bacterium and Fe^{2+} were present resulted in no significant increase in the extent of uranium leaching relative to the Fe^{2+}-bearing oligotrophic condition. The results might be due to the natural supply of inorganic nutrients to the cells from the soil matrix.

5.2.4 Soil to Plant Transfer and Bioavailability of Radionuclides

A significant part of the radionuclides released into the environment, for example, after a nuclear accident, is likely to be available for sorption on the soil matrix (i.e., clay and humus structures that are in equilibrium with the soil solution). Radionuclides in the soil solution constitute a pool available for root uptake. This pool of radionuclides is also available for downward migration within the soil profile. From a radiological protection point of view, the migration depth of radionuclides in the soil plays an important role in decreasing the external dose rates from contaminated soils. The mobility of radionuclides in the soil is an important factor in designing soil decontamination strategies involving techniques such as electrokinetic remediation and phytoremediation.

Jouve et al. [29] presented a new method of absorption of the soil solution based on the process of soaking. This soaking was thought to operate in similar conditions as the uptake of water by plants via capillary tension and osmotic pressure.

Two series of experiments were set up to evaluate the various methods. In the first series, three methods were compared: immiscible displacement of the soil solution [30], the batch method [31], and a new method of absorption of the soil solution using a polyacrylamide. In the second series of experiments, the batch method was replaced by the two-compartment centrifuge method [32].

The sample pretreatment was as follows. Soil samples were air dried and sieved at 2.5 mm. The saturation amount of water in the soil was assessed using a container filled with 10 g of dry soil to which water was added to fill the visible microdips at the soil surface. The volume of the added water was assumed to represent 100% of saturation. Then a 100 g sample of each soil type was contaminated using a solution of 600 kBq of ^{134}Cs and 60 kBq of ^{85}Sr in distilled water, with specific activities of 0.18 and 8.8 Bq/µg for ^{134}Cs and ^{85}Sr, respectively. These solutions were poured on the soil sample at a volume of 120% of saturation for each soil type in order to ensure homogeneous contamination of the sample. After drying at room temperature, the soil was manually mixed and divided into 10 subsamples of 10 g.

The new method proposed by the authors was as follows [29]. Each subsample was placed in a 5-cm polyethylene box and moisturized with distilled water at 70% of saturation. A 47-mm cellulose acetate membrane (Millipore) was placed on the soil surface. A 0.45-µm membrane was used for the experiments. A 2-cm disk of absorbent polymer was placed on the filter membrane. The polymer is composed of an anionic reticulated polyacrylamide resin, the electric charge of which is neutralized by sodium ions. The polymer disk is composed of angular particles with a maximum size of 2 to 3 mm. These particles are sandwiched between two paper sheets to form a 0.25 m × 3 m mat as used in substrates for hydroponic cultures (SODETRA, La Baronne, Biot, France). The 2-cm disks were stamped out of the mats using a trenchant still cylinder. Disks having a weight of 1 ± 0.2 g were selected for the experiments. A 2-cm-diameter lead disk, 0.5 cm thick, was placed on the polyacrylamide disks to press them against the filter and to ensure close contact between the soil and the absorbent. The polyethylene box was then tightly closed to avoid the evaporation of water from the system and prevent subsequent measurement bias on the weight of the absorbed water, which was determined by differential weighing (Figure 5.10). After about 16 h of absorption, the polyacrylamide disks were placed in a 5 cm × 1 cm cylindrical box and subjected to γ spectrometry. K_d is expressed as the ratio of the radioactivity in the soil (in Bq/g) and in the extracted solution (in Bq/ml).

The new method is likely to provide a good picture of the behavior of cesium in a soil-soil solution system, but the three above-mentioned methods are not satisfactory to reflect the availability of strontium for root uptake, K_d probably not being the best assessment parameter. Moreover, the new method was easy to implement compared to the tested methods, yielding better reproducibility of the measurements.

Denys et al. [33] investigated the availability of ^{99}Tc in undisturbed soil cores. The accumulation of ^{99}Tc occurs mainly in leaves, where the pertechnetate may be reduced by the photosynthetic apparatus, and consequently transfer to grains or kernels is low. However, most of the experiments carried out to assess soil to

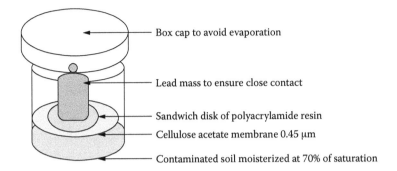

FIGURE 5.10 Diagrammatic description of the new method.

plant transfer of ^{99}Tc do not take into account the possible downward movement of the radionuclide.

Because of its high mobility, this movement was shown to be significant in soils such as podzols, and even similar to that of a nonreactive water tracer. Moreover, the leaching of ^{99}Tc might be different among soils in response to the soil structure. As a consequence, downward transfer of ^{99}Tc into zones not available to plant roots might significantly affect the soil to plant transfer of the radionuclide estimated with small closed systems (i.e., hydroponic or pot experiments).

In this work, the fate of ^{99}TcO$_4$ and the competition between root absorption and leaching processes in cultivated undisturbed soil cores was examined. Also, the uptake of ^{99}TcO$_4$ during crop growth in drained cores was compared to pot experiments in which no leaching occurred in order to validate pot assessments of the transfer factor, which is the ratio of specific activities in plant parts and soil (in Bq/kg dry weight of plant parts divided by the Bq/kg dry weight of soil). Irrigated maize (*Zea mays* L.) was grown on a series of undisturbed soil cores from three soil types differing in their chemical and physical properties (e.g., water movement properties). Each core was equipped at its bottom with a leaching water collector, allowing quantification of drainage and ^{99}Tc leaching.

Undisturbed soil cores (50 cm × 50 cm) were sampled from three agricultural soils with differing physical and chemical properties: a clayey Rendzic Leptosol (R), a clayey Fluvic Cambisol (F), and a sandy-loamy Dystric Cambisol (D), obtained from the Bure site, in northeast France (French laboratory for the study of deep underground nuclear waste disposal). The length of the tubes allowed inclusion of the Ap horizon (0 to 20 cm) and the upper part of the B horizon (20 to 45 cm). Cores were sampled by slowly pushing the tubes into the ground with a shovel with appropriate precautions to avoid anisotropic pressure constraints. Three cores were sampled for each soil type.

Two periods could be distinguished according to the evolution of the cumulative quantity of leached water with time:

- From day 0 to day 107 (contamination to harvest) for both R and F soils, the volume of leached water increased just after soil contamination

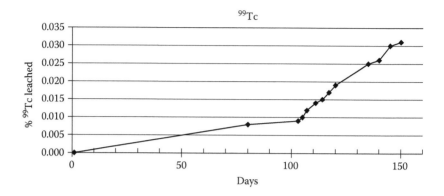

FIGURE 5.11 Cumulative fraction of ^{99}Tc leached through the Dystric Cambisol for a core (three cores were analyzed) [33].

and remained constant (plateau on Figure 5.11). For the D soil, only one leaching event was recorded during this period, just after contamination of the core.

- From day 108 to day 150 (after harvest) relatively high leaching rates through the three soils were observed. The quantity increased with time and closely followed the profile of the water input.

The activities of ^{99}Tc in maize were broadly similar between soils, although high variability was observed within each soil type.

The authors calculated an effective uptake of ^{99}Tc in leaves and grains. The effective uptake reached 70% of the input in the leaves and was not significantly different among soils. These results confirmed those obtained from pot experiments, even though leaching was allowed to occur in "close-to-reality" hydraulic conditions. As a consequence, it was concluded that pot experiments are an adequate surrogate for more complex "close-to-reality" experimental systems for measuring transfer factors.

Chen et al. [34] studied the accumulation of [238]U, [226]Ra, and [232]Th by some local vegetables and other common crops. The radioactive waste (e.g., tailings) produced by uranium mining activities contains a series of long-lived radionuclides, such as uranium, radium, and thorium isotopes. Although soil to plant transfer of such radionuclides has been studied in other areas, data are still very sparse in China, especially about the environmental radiological effect of uranium mining activities. The objective of this work was to investigate the uptake and soil to plant transfer factors of radionuclides ([238]U, [226]Ra and [232]Th) in uranium mining impacted soils in southeastern China, where uranium mine tailings have been used as landfill materials. Slightly elevated concentrations of these radionuclides were detected in some of the soils as well as soil-derived foodstuffs. However, very little information is available about the source of the pollution.

To prepare soil tailings mixtures, the tailings were thoroughly mixed with the soil in a ratio of 1:10 (soil I) and 1:5 (soil II) according to the weight. Nine plant species, including local vegetables, were selected for this investigation, including broad bean (*Vicia faba*), Chinese mustard (*Brassica chinensis*), India mustard (*Brassica juncea*), lupine (*Lupinus albus*), corn (*Zea mays*), chickpea (*Cicer arietinum*), tobacco (*Nicotiana tobacum*), ryegrass (*Lolium perenne*), and clover (*Trifolium pratense*). Nitrogen, phosphorus, and potassium were applied as essential nutrients in the form of a solution to each pot at the rate of 0.2 g N/kg soil as $(NH_4)_2SO_4$, 0.15 g P_2O_5/kg as $CaHPO_4$, and 0.125 g K/kg as KCl.

After 3 months of growth, the shoots and roots of the plants were sampled and washed with water; soil samples from each pot were also collected. The mean transfer factors for ^{238}U of the plant shoots in soil I and soil II are shown Figure 5.12.

The transfer factors for different plants are larger in soil I. The transfer factors (TFs) for the plant shoots and roots, which are the ratios of activity concentration in plant parts and soil (in Bq kg^{-1} dry weight plant part divided by Bq kg^{-1} dry weight soil) [37], ranged from 0.005 to 0.037, and from 0.042 to 0.39, respectively. This was generally in agreement with values for plants grown in contaminated soils reported in Vera Tome et al. [35]. Statistical analysis revealed a difference in uranium transfer from soils to plants ($p < 0.05$) (Figure 5.12). Differences in uranium transfer factors would be expected due to the different characteristics of the plants. However, relatively small variations were found between the plants. Among the plant species, the highest transfer factors (0.037 and 0.037 for soil I and soil II, respectively) for ^{238}U were found for lupine shoots. In contrast, Chinese mustard shoots exhibited the lowest transfer factors (0.006 and 0.005 for soil I and soil II, respectively). Among these nine plant species with their natural metabolic differences, the difference in mean ^{238}U transfer factors were found to vary by a factor of about seven.

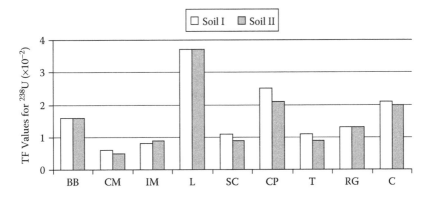

FIGURE 5.12 Transfer factors for ^{238}U of various plant shoots grown in soil I and soil II. Bars with the same letters in the same soil tailings mixture are not significantly different at $p < 0.05$. BB, broad bean; CM, Chinese mustard; IM, Indian mustard; L, lupine; SC, sweet corn; CP, chickpea; T, tobacco; RG, ryegrass; C, clover [34].

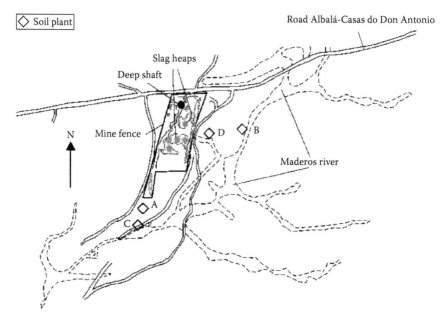

FIGURE 5.13 Map (scale 1:5000) of the area in which the mine is located. The sampling points for the different soil and plant samples are marked [35].

For the other radionuclides, the observed ranges of transfer factor values for ^{232}Th tended to be about one order of magnitude lower than that for ^{238}U and ^{226}Ra. In all cases, ryegrass and clover exhibited relative higher uptake of ^{226}Ra and ^{232}Th than other plants.

A Mediterranean environment was studied by Vera Tome et al. [35]. In this work, the transfer factors for natural uranium isotopes (^{238}U and ^{234}U), thorium isotopes (^{232}Th, ^{230}Th, and ^{228}Th), and ^{226}Ra were obtained for plant samples growing in granitic and alluvial soils around a unused uranium mine called "Los Ratones," located in the Extremadura region in southwest Spain, which covers an area of approximately 2.3 km². This mine was used from 1960 to 1974 and restoration work was performed in 1998–1999. The study area's geology is principally granitic. A map is shown in Figure 5.13.

The characteristics of the contamination in this area can be described by the mean activity concentration values (in Bq/kg) in the affected area: 10,924, 10,900, 10,075, and 5,289 for ^{238}U, ^{234}U, ^{230}Th, and ^{226}Ra, respectively, in soil samples, and 1,050, 1,060, 768, and 1,141 for the same radionuclides in plant samples. In the nonaffected area, the mean activity concentration values (in Bq/kg) were 184, 190, 234, and 251 for ^{238}U, ^{234}U, ^{230}Th, and ^{226}Ra, respectively, in soil samples, and 28, 29, 31, and 80 in plant samples.

The soils of this zone are essentially an altered granitic type. The soil texture (see Table 5.6) shows very few differences in the percentages of the different

TABLE 5.6
Mean Values of the Granulometric Analysis (in Percentages) of the Soil Samples at the Different Sampling Points (Four Samples for Each Site). The weight loss by ignition (LOI) (%) mean values are also shown [35].

Sampling Point	Particle Size (mm)					LOI (%)
	1.000–2.000	0.505–1.000	0.130–0.505	0.068–0.130	<0.068	
A	16.3	22.4	36.1	12.3	13.0	8.5
B	5.5	16.5	48.3	16.5	13.2	6.2
C	9.5	23.1	37.6	14.8	15.1	9.1
D	13.7	24.2	39.6	11.6	10.9	12.1

particle size fractions between the sampling points. Table 5.6 also gives the weight loss by ignition.

The same points were chosen for plant sampling (see Figure 5.13). The plants are principally grass-pasture (Fabaceae, Poaceae, Asteraceae, etc.). The distribution of these types of plants over the total study area is such that a homogeneous distribution can be considered a good approximation.

Table 5.7 lists the transfer factor values obtained in this work for each radionuclide studied at the different sampling points. They were obtained as the mean value of the activity concentrations of each radionuclide in soil and pasture samples from four sampling campaigns. The mean transfer factors and ranges for each radionuclide are also given.

Both transfer factors for the uranium radioisotopes (^{238}U and ^{234}U) are similar. Likewise, the transfer factors for ^{232}Th and ^{230}Th are also comparable. However, the transfer factors determined for ^{228}Th are clearly higher than the ones calculated

TABLE 5.7
Transfer Factor Values for Uranium and Thorium Isotopes and ^{226}Ra at the Different Sampling Points (Four Samples for Each Site). The transfer factor mean values and the ranges for each radionuclide considering all the points are also shown [35].

Radionuclide	Sampling Points				All Points	
	A	B	C	D	Mean Value	Range
^{238}U	0.076	0.053	0.072	0.069	0.067	0.020–0.250
^{234}U	0.089	0.057	0.075	0.070	0.072	0.021–0.252
^{232}Th	0.048	0.051	0.089	0.051	0.058	0.013–0.270
^{230}Th	0.071	0.049	0.081	0.037	0.056	0.08–0.249
^{228}Th	1.27	1.07	2.63	2.05	1.65	0.517–4.31
^{226}Ra	0.128	0.237	0.137	0.190	0.17	0.097–0.504

for other thorium isotopes. This fact can be easily explained by the intake of [228]Ra (progenitor of [228]Th) and the uptake of [228]Th itself [35].

Vera Tome et al. [35] also determined transfer factors for stable elements (boron, carbon, calcium, chlorine, cobalt, copper, iron, hydrogen, potassium, magnesium, manganese, molybdenum, nitrogen, oxygen, phosphorus, sulfur, silicon, and zinc). For this, an inductively coupled plasma (ICP) technique using a Perkin-Elmer emission spectrometer was used. Thus the authors were able to observe strong similarities between [226]Ra and some essential elements (calcium, manganese, and phosphorus), which confirms the preferential uptake of this radionuclide, in contrast to uranium and thorium isotopes.

Transfer factors corresponding to artificial radionuclides discharged from the nuclear fuel processing plant at Sellafield (Seascale, U.K.) were determined by Copplestone et al. [36]. In this work, actinide radionuclides and radiocesium were analyzed.

This site is characterized by sand dunes lying to the west of Sellafield, close to where a low-level liquid waste discharge pipeline enters the sea (Figure 5.14). The dunes form a narrow corridor, up to 50 m wide, that runs parallel to the coastline for about 2 km. The River Ehen (as shown in Figure 5.14) separates the dunes from nearby agricultural land. Vegetation covers more than 90% of the sand dunes, the community being dominated by red fescue (*Festuca rubra*) and marram grass (*Ammophila arenaria*). The almost neutral soil is skeletal in pedological terms and consists mainly of subangular and rounded sand particles in the size range 0.2 to 2 mm, with little organic matter (52%).

Two transects, 50 m × 4 m, were marked out approximately 5 m apart, as shown in Figure 5.14. The front transect (forward transect) along the seaward side of the dunes was dominated by *A. arenaria*, while the back transect (rare transect) was in a slightly more sheltered position on the landward side. The vegetation cover here was dominated by *F. rubra*.

Transfer factors (TFs), which are the ratios of activity concentration in vegetation (in Bq kg[-1] dry weight plant) divided by activity concentration in soil (in Bq kg[-1] dry weight soil) [34], were determined for *A. arenaria* and *F. rubra* and the results are presented in Table 5.8. According to the authors, the transfer factors for each species along the two transects remained reasonably consistent. *A. arenaria* values from the forward transect range from 0.086 to 0.097 for [238]Pu and from 0.050 to 0.055 for [239+240]Pu. However, the data indicate that there are differences in the transfer factors between the two species for the actinides. For example, along the front transect, the [238]Pu values decline to between 0.019 and 0.065 for *F. rubra* compared to the *A. arenaria* values reported above. The transfer factors are also much higher than expected if root uptake is the dominant mechanism for the soil to plant transfer of radionuclide contamination. The transfer factors for ^{137}Cs range between 0.04 and 1.4 and are comparable with other studies.

The concentration factors for the two species of vegetation were higher than expected if root uptake was the exclusive transfer mechanism. This reflects the

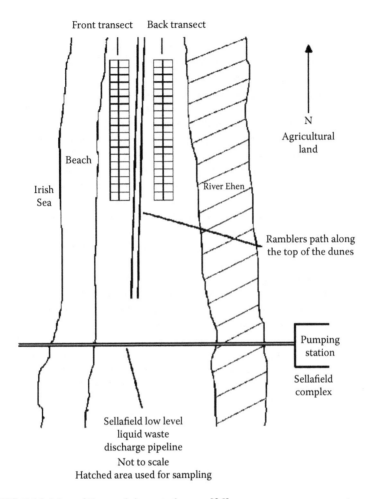

FIGURE 5.14 Map of the sand dune study area [36].

generally low level of transfer of radionuclides from the rooting substrate to the plant and the dominant influence of external contamination adhering to the plant foliage.

The study of the bioavailability of radionuclides in agricultural soils was developed from another point of view by El-Mrabet et al. [37]. The objective of this work was the radionuclide enrichment of soil, drainage water, and crops in an agricultural practice where phosphogypsum application was made to increase the fertility of the soil. Phosphogypsum contains a high proportion of $CaSO_4 \cdot 2H_2O$, which is an efficient amendment that has been widely used in the saline-sodic marsh soils of southwest Spain [38].

Phosphogypsum is the main waste product in the production of phosphoric acid and phosphate fertilizers. The raw material is phosphate rock, which usually contains high activity concentrations (in Bq/kg) of natural radionuclides. In the

TABLE 5.8
Transfer Factors for Samples of *A. arenaria* and *F. rubra* [36]

Month/Transect	^{137}Cs	^{238}Pu	$^{239+240}$Pu	^{241}Am
A. arenaria				
Forward transect				
May 1993	0.113	0.097	0.055	0.212
January 1994	0.091	0.094	0.050	0.171
September 1994	0.050	0.086	0.050	0.061
Rear transect				
May 1993	0.047	0.055	0.046	0.118
January 1994	0.061	0.054	0.046	0.136
September 1994	0.038	0.025	0.022	0.056
F. rubra				
Forward transect				
May 1993	0.102	0.039	0.028	0.099
January 1994	0.122	0.065	0.056	0.145
September 1994	0.080	0.019	0.016	0.039
Rear transect				
May 1993	0.060	0.057	0.030	0.074
January 1994	0.097	0.060	0.057	0.104
September 1994	0.137	0.018	0.015	0.025

case of factories in Huelva (southwest Spain), typical activity concentrations of natural radionuclides (^{238}U, ^{226}Ra, ^{210}Pb (^{210}Po)) in raw material range from 700 to 1000 Bq/kg [39]. For this reason, the use of phosphogypsum in soil amendments is strongly regulated in the U.S. [40] in order to prevent environmental and health risks.

The experimental site in the study of El-Mrabet et al. [37] was located in Marismas de Lebrija, in the reclaimed marsh soils of the estuarine region of the Guadalquivir River (southwest Spain). The grain size distribution of soils with depth is presented in Table 5.9.

For the study, three similar plots were divided in four zones. A different treatment was applied to each zone in the three plots. These treatments were (1) control (no amendment), (2) 13 Mg/ha of phosphogypsum, (3) 26 Mg/ha of phosphogypsum, and (4) 30 Mg/ha of manure. Sugar beet (*Beta vulgaris* L. cv. *saccharifera* Alef.) was cultivated in the first crop under sprinkler irrigation and cotton was cultivated in the second crop under furrow irrigation. Fertilizer was applied to all plots at preplant. Rain, irrigation, and drainage events were registered, and regular sampling of drainage water was manually done after every rain or irrigation event during the cropping season. Table 5.10 shows the activity concentration of natural radionuclides in the products used in the study.

TABLE 5.9
Grain Size Distribution of Soils
with Depth [37]

| Depth (cm) | g/kg | | | Type |
	Sand	Silt	Clay	
0–30	60	258	685	Clay
30–60	182	365	460	Clay
60–90	122	395	485	Clay
90–120	280	364	410	Clay

TABLE 5.10
Activity Concentration (in Bq/kg) in Products Applied to Soil
in the Study [37]

Product	^{226}Ra	^{238}U	^{232}Th	^{234}Th
Superphosphate	130 ± 85	590	486	760 ± 180
Ammonium phosphate	Not detected	496	9.0	660 ± 150
Phosphogypsum	510 ± 40	700–1000	700–1000	65 ± 19
Manure	Not detected	Not reported	Not reported	Not detected

The conclusions of this work are

- The application of phosphogypsum as a soil amendment does not produce any significant increase in natural radionuclide concentrations in treated soils, even after two consecutive treatments.
- Drainage waters were not affected by phosphogypsum amendments with different treatments (control, phosphogypsum, and manure amendments).
- The plant uptake of natural radionuclides was mainly related to the natural pool of soils, since the amounts applied in amendments and fertilizers were negligible.

5.3 RADIOACTIVE CONTAMINATION AND COUNTERMEASURES

Soil contamination by radionuclides and possible countermeasures have been recently reviewed by Zhu and Shaw [41]. On average, 79% of the radiation to which humans are exposed is from natural sources, 19% is from medical applications, and the remaining 2% is from fallout of weapons tests and the nuclear power industry [42]. However, these last activities have introduced large amounts

TABLE 5.11
Characteristics of the Radionuclides That Occur in the Major Radioactive Contaminations in Soils [41]

Radioisotope	Half-life (Years)	Radiation	Main Occurrence
^{14}C	5.7×10^3	β⁻	Natural and nuclear reactor
^{40}K	1.3×10^9	β⁻	Natural
^{90}Sr	28	β⁻	Nuclear reactor
^{134}Cs	2	β⁻, γ	Nuclear reactor
^{137}Cs	30	β⁻, γ	Nuclear reactor
^{239}Pu	2.4×10^4	α, γ	Nuclear reactor

of artificial radionuclides such as ^{90}Sr, ^{137}Cs, and ^{99}Tc and actinides (plutonium isotopes, ^{241}Am). These radionuclides, once deposited in soils, are taken up by plants and may be distributed in the food chain.

The nuclear power industry may increase its contribution in the future because of the scarcity of fossil fuels and to reduce the global warming process. Routine and accidental events could cause local or regional contamination that could be considered a risk for environment or human health. Because of this, remediation of contamination in soil is becoming an important aspect of radiological protection. The main radionuclides involved in radioactive studies in soils are listed in Table 5.11.

The behavior of radionuclides in soil is similar to the stable isotopes of each element, however, radionuclides can be considered an ultratrace element if the stable isotope is not present in the soil. The physical and chemical properties of each element, as well as the physical and chemical characteristics of the soil and other factors such as climate and vegetation must also be considered.

Understanding the physical and chemical processes involved in soil to plant transfer is important. Moreover, information about the intake of radionuclides by plants is primarily used for radiological assessment and research. Currently the European Union is developing a database on the uptake of radionuclides by plants from the soil.

The ultimate remediation of radionuclide-contaminated soils could be to remove surface layers from the affected site and to treat the soil with various dispersing and chelating chemicals [43]. This method can be applied only in small contaminated areas. Removing and transporting soil is difficult in terms of equipment and manpower, and is very costly. In 1966, after an aircraft accident, a conventional explosion of two thermonuclear bombs released high levels of actinide radioisotopes into the soil of Palomares (southeast Spain). The remediation applied was the removal and transport of vegetation and the first layers of contaminated soil.

Because of the prohibitive costs of these countermeasures and the small scale of remediation, alternative methods have been proposed. In the case of contamination of a forest, it is possible to apply the following countermeasures in order to reduce the level of contamination [44]:

- Spraying contaminated canopies with detergents or other cleaning agents.
- Defoliation and removal of fallen leaves.
- Clear-cutting and removal of the timber.
- Plowing after clear-cutting and prior to planting.
- Scraping and removal of the surface layer.

However, these countermeasures have never been used.

Agriculture soil contamination is probably the most relevant event because radionuclides could reach humans via the food chain. The application of mineral and chemical adsorbents to soils is intended to reduce the phytoavailability of radionuclides in the soil. Natural and synthetic zeolites are some of the best candidates for this purpose. Ammonium-ferric-hexacyano-ferrate(II) is another chemical that is believed to have great potential.

The application of fertilizers to soils induces both chemical and biological changes that affect the overall transfer of radionuclides from the soil to plants. Zhu [45] developed some experiments and demonstrated unequivocally that increasing the external potassium concentration dramatically reduces the influx rates of radiocesium into both spring wheat and broad bean plants (Figure 5.15).

If soils are contaminated with significant amounts of radionuclides, bioremediation is emerging as an alternative to some of the energy-intensive and high-cost soil cleaning methods discussed above. Fungi are a major component of the soil microflora, particularly in acid soils, and play a critical role in the soil's ecological functions. High radiocesium activities have been reported in the fruiting bodies

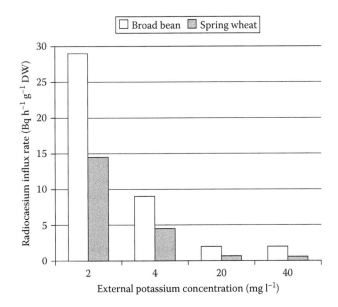

FIGURE 5.15 The effect of external potassium concentrations on the influx rates of radiocesium into plant roots 56 days after transplanting [41].

TABLE 5.12
Soil-Fungus Transfer Factors and Available Transfer Factors for ^{137}Cs, ^{90}Sr, [40]K, and [226]Ra [3]

Species/Site	Transfer Factor				Available Transfer Factor			
	[137]Cs	[40]K	[226]Ra	[90]Sr	[137]Cs	[40]K	[226]Ra	[90]Sr
	La Bazagona							
Lactarius deliciosus	1.7–5.0	0.8–0.9	0.03–0.12	0.4	7–20	70–68	0.03–1.2	0.5
	Muñoveros							
Hebeloma cylindrosporum	33–55	1.6–1.8	0.22	1.44	330–550	56–65	1.7	2.03
Tricholoma sp.	3–10	0.9–1.6	1.3	0.5–1.18	30–104	34–58	11 ± 11	1.7

of a number of fungal species. Based on the bioaccumulation of radionuclides by soil fungi, it might be interesting to explore the possibility of using fungi to "lock up" the radionuclides (radiocesium in particular) in surface soil layers so as to reduce soil migration and groundwater pollution [41].

The soil-mushroom transfer factor for a given radionuclide is usually defined as the ratio of the activity of this radionuclide in the fruiting bodies and that in the soil [46]. Alternatively, Baeza et al. [47] suggest the use of an available transfer factor, where the activity of a radionuclide in the soil is corrected by its available fraction. Table 5.12 lists the results obtained by Baeza et al. [47] in species of mushrooms collected in Extremadura. According to these results, the most efficiently transferred radionuclide was ^{137}Cs, followed by [40]K, ^{90}Sr, and [226]Ra. In this study, the highest transfer factors were for *Hebeloma cylindrosporum*, the genus *Tricholoma*, and *Lactarius deliciosus*.

As can be seen in Table 5.12, the [40]K available transfer factor presents a greater increase than the other radionuclides. It is also remarkable that all the fungus species have a high available transfer factor for [40]K. This seems to indicate that potassium is indeed essential for fungi [47].

Finally, phytoextraction of radionuclides from soils is another possibility for soil remediation. Researchers are looking for plants with sufficient uptake to increase the extraction of radionuclides from contaminated soils. For instance, Lasat et al. [48] identified redroot pigweed (*Amaranthus retroflexus*) as an effective accumulator of radiocesium.

5.4 SCIENTIFIC AND SOCIAL APPLICATIONS

5.4.1 Dose Assessment

An estimation of dose assessment from the activity concentration of γ emitters can be obtained in soils. Quindos et al. [49] calculated conversion factors from becquerels per kilogram (Bq/kg) into nanograys per hour (nGy/h) by experimental fieldwork. The device chosen was the Mini-Instruments Environmental Monitor type 6-80, with an energy compensated Geiger-Müller tube, MC-71. The results of the measurements of the absorbed dose rate in air are reported in units of nGy/h. All the values given are for dose rates from terrestrial γ rays 1 m above the ground and exclude any contribution from either cosmic rays or instrument background.

According to Quindos et al. [49], the laboratory measurements of the concentrations of ^{40}K, ^{214}Pb, ^{214}Bi, ^{208}Tl, ^{228}Ac, ^{212}Pb, and ^{212}Bi in soil samples were taken from the same places where the *in situ* measurements were made. Four sets of surface soil samples were randomly collected at distances of 0, 2, 4, and 7 m from the *in situ* detector. Soil samples corresponded to a 15-cm-diameter soil core taken at a depth of 20 cm. The concentrations of radionuclides in the soil samples were determined by γ spectrometry employing a coaxial HPGe crystal of 59% efficiency. In total, more than 1500 "*in situ*" and "in lab" measurements were made and the results are shown in Table 5.13.

The conditions of the fieldwork experiments are essential in order to obtain good agreement, as in Table 5.13. The main reason to take into account the experimental conditions is that several factors influence the value of the exposure rates from a typical natural γ field. Basically exposure rates measured 1 m above the soil surface have their origin in radionuclides within the first few centimeters of soil, with a relative contribution of 50% coming from sources in the first 10 cm

TABLE 5.13

Dose Conversion Factors for Different Radionuclides Given in the Literature and As Derived from Experimental Data in Quindos et al. [49]

	Dose Conversion Factors (nGy/h per Bq/kg)			
Nuclide	Saito and Jacob [63]	Beck et al. [64]	Clouvas et al. [65]	Quindos et al. [49]
		^{232}Th series		
^{228}Ac	0.22	0.28	0.19	0.21
^{212}Bi	0.027	0.021	0.024	0.025
^{208}Tl	0.33	0.32	0.30	0.32
^{212}Pb	0.028	0.021	0.019	0.026
Total	0.60	0.67	0.54	0.58
		^{238}U series		
^{214}Pb	0.05	0.05	0.04	0.11
^{226}Ra	0.0012		0.0010	
^{214}Bi	0.40	0.38	0.36	0.35
Total	0.46	0.43	0.40	0.46
^{40}K	0.042	0.042	0.040	0.043

and almost 80% from the first 25 cm. Soil moisture, the presence of radon, and ground roughness are the most important factors that influence exposure rates [49].

The main conclusion of Quindos et al. [49] is that the estimation of exposure rates obtained from measurements of radioactivity concentrations in soils, using theoretical conversion factors, is more advantageous than the *in situ* γ measurements, not only from an economic aspect, but also because the exposure rates are well defined under normal error intervals when appropriate experimental conditions are used.

A typical dose assessment was developed by Colmenero et al. [50]. In this case the annual effective dose rate (in nSv/h) was evaluated from the activity concentration (in Bq/kg) of the radioactive series and the ^{40}K in soils [51].

The research was based on the possible increase in the concentration of some natural radionuclides in soil, water, and even in the airborne dust in the State of Chihuahua, Mexico, due to human activities. The mining of uranium in this region started in the early 1970s and lasted until 1983, while the processing of uranium into a concentrate was performed by Uranium of Mexico (URAMEX). Both sites are located close to the city of Aldama, Chihuahua, Mexico (approximately 20,000 inhabitants).

The results of the γ spectrometry of soil samples from the Aldama area show that the zone nearest to the old URAMEX plant exhibits some soil surface contamination that becomes less evident with distance, until it reaches an average value that may be attributed to the features of the soil in this region (Figure 5.16).

5.4.2 Radon in Soil and Earthquakes

Zmazek et al. [52] published an exhaustive work about the anomalies in radon emanation from soils caused by earthquakes. This methodology is tedious and sometimes inconclusive. First, there is an inverse relationship between radon exhalation and barometric pressure [53]. A decrease in barometric pressure, considering other environmental variables constant, generally causes an increase in radon exhalation from the soil surface. Other environmental variables are soil temperature, air temperature, and rainfall which cause a seasonal pattern in soil exhalation.

So radon concentrations can be predicted on the basis of environmental data (air and soil temperature, barometric pressure, rainfall) during seismically nonactive periods. However, prediction is significantly worsened during a seismically active period. For that, regression (or function approximation) and other statistical methods were used by the authors [52] to predict radon concentrations.

Figure 5.17 shows radon exhalation anomalies related to earthquakes using average seasonal data. R_D is defined as the radius of the zone where precursory phenomena related to earthquakes may be manifested [54] and R_E is the distance between the epicenter and the measuring site. The studied area was located around Krko (eastern Slovenia). Average radon concentrations were calculated for spring, summer, fall, and winter. The periods when radon concentrations deviate by more than ± 1, ± 1.5, and ± 2 from the related seasonal value were considered radon anomalies possibly caused by earthquake events and not by meteorological parameters.

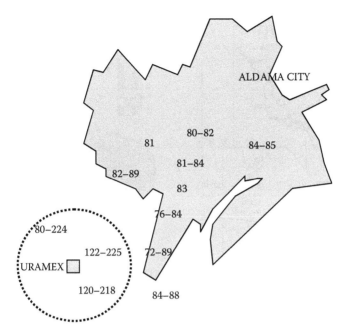

FIGURE 5.16 Map of Aldama, Chihuahua, Mexico, with the annual effective dose rate (in nSv/h), in black, superimposed. The area around the former URAMEX uranium processing plant is remarked by the circle. These results were evaluated using activity concentrations in 30 soil samples [50].

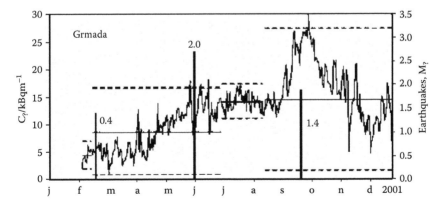

FIGURE 5.17 Time run of daily average radon concentrations in soil gas, C_{Rn}, at the Grmada station. Numbers attached to the earthquake bars are R_E/R_D values [54]. Full lines represent average radon concentrations (for definitions of seasons, see the text), while dashed lines indicate ±2 deviation from the seasonal average value. Radon anomalies are C_{Rn} values outside the ±2 region [52].

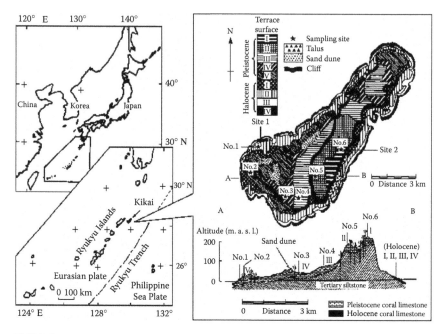

FIGURE 5.18 Schematic location map of the study area and soil sampling sites of Kikai Island. Modified from [62].

5.4.3 DATING

Maejima et al. [55] worked on the application of [10]Be to date soils. Soil samples were taken from six soil profiles (Figure 5.18) consisting of Initial Rendzina-like soil (core 1), Rendzina-like soil (core 2), Brown Rendzina-like soil (core 3), Terra fusca-like soil (core 4), Terra rossa-like soil (core 5), and intergraded between Terra rossa-like soil and red-yellow soil (core 6).

[10]Be was extracted from 1 g of soil (less than 1-mm fraction) in every analysis. Soil aliquot was dissolved in concentrated HNO_3-HF-$HClO_4$ solution. [9]Be as $BeSO_4$ was added and evaporated to dryness. The beryllium fraction was isolated by cation and anion exchange. Then NH_4-NH_3OH was added and $Be(OH)_2$ was precipitated. Hydroxide was ignited to BeO at 850°C for 15 min, mixed with silver powder, and pressed into a copper cathode. [10]Be concentrations were measured using the Microanalysis Laboratory–Tandem Accelerator System (MALT-AMS) at the University of Tokyo, Japan. Moreover, before adding [9]Be carrier, approximately 1 g of soil was analyzed by inductively coupled plasma mass spectrometry (ICP-MS) to obtain the [9]Be content of the soil.

There is a positive correlation between the clay content (less than 2-μm fraction) and [10]Be concentrations. The presence of [10]Be in soils is due to rainfall. This radionuclide infiltrates humid climate soils and is adsorbed tightly onto clay materials so that its content (in atoms/cm^2) increases with soil age. Therefore if the [10]Be content since the initiation of soil formation and the average annual

TABLE 5.14
Estimated Age (×10³ Years) of Soils on the Raised Coral Reef Terraces of Kikai Island [55]

		Soil Age		
		Topographic	¹⁰Be	
Soil Core	Age of Coral	Position	No Erosion	Erosion
1	3.5–5.2	3.5–3.9	>8	>8
2	35–45	35–40	>18	>20
3	50–60	50–55	>56	>68
4	80	70–80	>127	>143
5	100	95–100	>136	>158
6	125	120–125	>102	>119

deposition rate of ^{10}Be (in atoms/cm^2/year) are known, then the age of the soil can be determined. The results must be corrected for the loss of ^{10}Be by leaching or erosion from the soil.

Dating by the described method was compared with other estimations published in the literature. This comparison is shown in Table 5.14. Here ">" was used to indicate the minimum soil age. In the case of soil core 2, a loss of ^{10}Be by leaching or erosion could cause an underestimation of soil age.

5.4.4 TRACERS IN SOIL EROSION

According to the review published by Zapata [56], nuclear methods can be applied to erosion assessment. By artificially labeling soil particles with an appropriate radionuclide, both the extent and source of soil loss can be determined. Gamma emitters have mainly been applied in these studies (^{59}Fe, ^{46}Sc, ^{110}Ag, ^{198}Au, ^{137}Cs, ^{51}Cr); however, other techniques involve the use of a number of environmental radionuclides such as fallout ^{137}Cs, natural ^{210}Pb, cosmogenic ^{7}Be, and others ($^{239+240}$Pu, ^{14}C, ^{32}Si, ^{26}Al, ^{36}Cl).

However, ^{137}Cs is the most widely used radionuclide in soil erosion and sedimentation research because of its high affinity for fine particles, its relatively long half-life, its relative ease of measurement, and the well-defined temporal pattern of fallout input [57].

The assessment of the loss or deposition of radionuclides in soil is usually made by comparing the average total content (in Bq/m^2) of the area to the measured content at individual sampling points. Where sample contents are lower than the local reference content, loss of cesium-labeled soil and therefore erosion can be inferred. Similarly sample contents in excess of the reference level are indicative of the addition of cesium-labeled soil by deposition [56].

Other environmental radionuclides, including unsupported ^{210}Pb and ^{7}Be, have attracted much less attention, but there is increasing evidence that they offer considerable potential for use in soil erosion investigations, both individually or complementary to [137]Cs [56]. [210]Pb is derived from [222]Rn, which can remain in soil or can be partially exhaled from soil into the atmosphere. Once in the atmosphere, [222]Rn decays in ^{210}Pb, which is immediately adsorbed by aerosol and falls onto the soil surface. For that, ^{210}Pb is not in equilibrium with [226]Ra ([222]Rn) in the soil. The fraction of ^{210}Pb in equilibrium with [226]Ra is called supported and the fraction associated to fallout is called unsupported.

We can consider the unsupported fraction as a fallout radionuclide fraction, and it is possible to apply a technique to study erosion in a similar way as in the case of [137]Cs. The global distribution of fallout ^{210}Pb is unknown. However, the few data might indicate greater deposition flux over the land than over the ocean, and lower deposition over the western margins of continental land masses due to the predominant west to east trajectory of air mass movement. Appleby and Oldfield [58] report an average deposition flux for the world of 118 Bq/m²/year, in a range of 50 to 150 Bq/m²/year.

A procedure to test the use of unsupported ^{210}Pb for quantifying long-term rates (about 100 years) of soil redistribution associated with cultivated land was published by Walling et al. [59]. The main steps of such a procedure are (Figure 5.19):

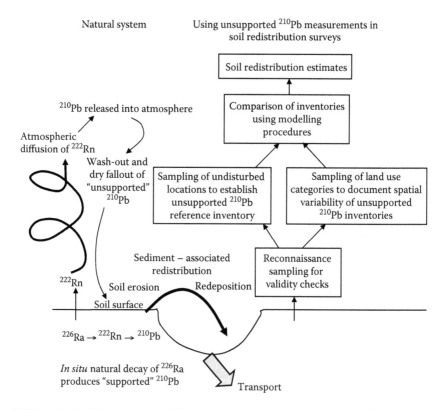

FIGURE 5.19 Using unsupported ^{210}Pb measurements to estimate soil erosion and deposition rates [59].

1. Determination of unsupported ^{210}Pb activity and contents in a few cores in order to test the validity of the procedure. Moreover, the exponential distribution of ^{210}Pb activity with depth in undisturbed soils must be confirmed.
2. Collection of soil cores from an undisturbed area with minimal slope and no evidence of erosion or deposition to establish the unsupported ^{210}Pb reference contents.
3. Collection of soil cores to obtain the unsupported ^{210}Pb content in cultivated and uncultivated land.
4. Estimation of erosion or deposition rates for the sampling points by comparing their measured unsupported ^{210}Pb inventories with the local reference contents and using a theoretical conversion model to convert the values for the percentage decrease or increase of contents to equivalent estimates of the erosion or deposition rates.

A typical profile found in an undisturbed soil (a) is shown in Figure 5.20 [59]. In this case, the unsupported ^{210}Pb concentration exhibits a peak at the surface and an approximate exponential decline with depth. In contrast, the

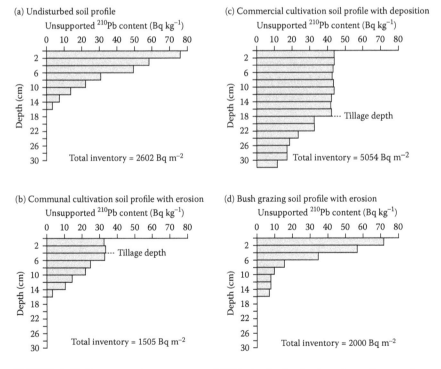

FIGURE 5.20 Representative unsupported ^{210}Pb depth distributions for soil cores from the study catchment [59].

unsupported ^{210}Pb concentration in a core collected in a cultivated soil (Figure 5.20 (b and c)) from communal and commercial areas are essentially uniform throughout the plough layer, reflecting the mixing caused by tillage. However, the total content in both cores is clearly different from the reference value. Thus the total content for soil core (b) in Figure 5.20 is 42% lower than the content measured for the undisturbed soil, indicating erosion. In contrast, the total content for soil (c) is almost double the reference value (soil (a)), indicating significant deposition. Soil (d) was collected in a grazing area. Here, unsupported ^{210}Pb declines exponentially. This confirms that this soil has not been mixed by cultivation. The total content for this soil core is 23% lower than the corresponding value for the undisturbed soil (a), indicating losses of material.

^{7}Be is produced naturally in the upper atmosphere by cosmic ray spallation of nitrogen and oxygen. This radionuclide is immediately associated to aerosol after a nuclear reaction. Subsequent deposition onto the land occurs as both dry and wet fallout. In most environments, ^{7}Be fallout reaching the soil surface will be rapidly and strongly fixed by the surface soil [60]. The short half-life of ^{7}Be ($T_{1/2} = 53.3$ days) and the similar behavior to ^{137}Cs create the potential for its use in tracing the short-term behavior of sediment in marine and lacustrine systems. However, there have been a few attempts to use ^{7}Be as a tracer in soil erosion investigations.

The principles involved in using ^{7}Be to document rates and patterns of soil redistribution are essentially the same as those employed for ^{137}Cs and described above for unsupported ^{210}Pb. Blake et al. [61] have confirmed the potential for using ^{7}Be as a tracer in soil erosion investigations. According to the authors, ^{7}Be offers a valuable complement to ^{137}Cs and unsupported ^{210}Pb to estimate rates of soil distribution associated with individual erosion events or short periods.

REFERENCES

1. Koch-Steindl, H. and Pröhl, G., Considerations on the behaviour of long-lived radionuclides in the soil, *Radiat. Environ. Biophys.*, 40, 93, 2001.
2. Krouglov, S.V., Kurinov, A.D., and Alexakhin, R.M., Chemical fractionation of ^{90}Sr, ^{106}Ru, ^{137}Cs and ^{144}Ce in Chernobyl-contaminated soils: an evolution in the course of time., *J. Environ. Radioactiv.*, 38, 59, 1998.
3. Baeza, A., Guillen, J., and Bernedo, J.M., Soil-fungi transfer coefficients: importance of the location of mycelium in soil and of the differential availability of radionuclides in soil fractions, *J. Environ. Radioactiv.*, 81, 89, 2005.
4. Blanco, P., Vera Tome, F., and Lozano, J.C., Sequential extraction for radionuclide fractionation in soil samples: a comparative study, *Appl. Radiat. Isot.*, 61, 345, 2004.
5. Tessier, A., Campbell, P.G.C., and Bisson, M., Sequential extraction procedure for the speciation of particulate trace metals, *Anal. Chem.*, 51, 844–850, 1979.
6. Schultz, M.K., Burnett, W., and Inn, K.G.W., Evaluation of a sequential extraction method for determining actinide fractionation in soils and sediments. *J. Environ. Radioactiv.*, 40, 155, 1998.

7. Blanco, P., Vera Tome, F., and Lozano, J.C., Fractionation of natural radionuclides in soils from a uranium mineralized area in the south-west of Spain, *J. Environ. Radioactiv.*, 79, 315, 2005.

8. Spezzano, P. Distribution of pre- and post-Chernobyl radiocaesium with particle size fractions of soils, *J. Environ. Radioactiv.*, 83, 117, 2005.

9. Livens, F.R. and Baxter, M.S., Particle size and radionuclide levels in some West Cumbrian soils, *Sci. Total Environ.*, 70, 1, 1988.

10. Walkley, A., Black, I.A., 1934. An examination of the Degtjareff method for determining soil organic matter and a proposed modification of the chromic acid titration method, *Soil Sci.*, 37, 29–38.

11. Nelson, D.W., Sommers, L.E., 1982. Total carbon, organic carbon, and organic matter. In *Methods of Soil Analysis. Part II, 2nd ed.*, Page, A.L., Miller, R.H., Kenney, D.R. (Eds.), American Society of Agronomy, Madison, WI, USA, pp. 539–580.

12. Italian Ministry of Agriculture and Forestry, Metodi uficiali di analisi chimica del suolo, Decree 11 May 1992, *Supplemento ordinario alla Gazzetta Uficiale della Repubblica Italiana* no. 121, 25 May 1992.

13. Bunzl, K., Kracke, W., Schimmack, W., and Zelle, L., Forms of fallout ^{137}Cs and [239+240]Pu in successive horizons of a forest soil, *J. Environ. Radioactiv.*, 39, 55, 1998.

14. Bunzl, K., Migration of fallout-radionuclides in the soil: effect of non-uniformity of the sorption properties on the activity-depth profiles, *Radiat. Environ. Biophys.*, 40, 237, 2001.

15. Bossew, P., Gastberger, M., Gohla, H., Hofer, P., and Hubmer, A., Vertical distribution of radionuclides in soil of a grassland site in Chernobyl exclusion zone, *J. Environ. Radioactiv.*, 73, 87, 2004.

16. Fujiyoshi, R. and Sawamura, S., Mesoscale variability of vertical profiles of environmental radionuclides (K, Ra, Pb and Cs) in temperate forest soils in Germany, *Sci. Total Environ.*, 320, 177, 2004.

17. Chung, K.H., Choi, G.S., Shin, H.S., and Lee, C.W., Vertical distribution and characteristics of soil humic substances affecting radionuclide distribution, *J. Environ. Radioactiv.*, 79, 369, 2005.

18. Stevenson, F.J., Geochemistry of soil humic substances, in *Humic Substances in Soil, Sediment and Water*, Aiken, G.R., McKnight, D.M., Wershaw, R.L., and MacCarthy, P., eds., John Wiley & Sons, New York, 1985.

19. Lloyd, J.R. and Macaskie, L.E., A novel phosphorimager-based technique for monitoring the microbial reduction of technetium, *Appl. Environ. Microbiol.* 62, 578, 1996.

20. Lloyd, J.R., Sole, V.A., Van Praagh, C.V.G., and Lovley, D.R., Direct and Fe(II)-mediated reduction of technetium by Fe(III)-reducing bacteria, *Appl. Environ. Microbiol.*, 66, 3743, 2000.

21. De Luca, G., De Philip, P., Dermoun, Z., Rousset, M., and Vermeglio, A., Reduction of technetium(VII) by *Desulfovibrio fructosovorans* is mediated by the nickel-iron hydrogenase, *Appl. Environ. Microbiol.* 67, 4583, 2001.

22. Dianou, D. and Traore, A.S., Sulfate-reducing bacterial population in some lowland paddy field soils of Brukina Faso (West Africa), *Microbes Environ.*, 15, 41, 2000.

23. Ishii, N., Tagami, K., Enomoto, S., and Uchida, S., Influence of microorganisms on the behaviour of technetium and other elements in paddy soil surface water, *J. Environ. Radioactiv.*, 77, 369, 2004.

24. Russell, R.A., Holden, P.J., Payne, T.E., and McOrist, G.D., The effect of sulfate-reducing bacteria on adsorption of ^{137}Cs by soils from arid and tropical regions, *J. Environ. Radioactiv.*, 74, 151, 2004.

25. Lloyd, J.R. and Macaskie, L.E., Bioremediation of radionuclide-containing waste-waters, in *Environmental Metal-Microbe Interactions*, Lovely, D.R., ed., ASM Press, Washington, DC, 2000.

26. Abdelouasa, A., Grambowa, B., Fattahia, M., Andres, Y., and Leclerc-Cessa, E., Microbial reduction of ^{99}Tc in organic matter-rich soils, *Sci. Total Environ.*, 336, 255, 2005.

27. Zhdanova, N.N., Redchits, T.I., Zheltonozhsky, V.A., Sadovnikov, L.V., Gerzabek, M.H., Olsson, S., Strebl, F., and Mück, K., Accumulation of radionuclides from radioactive substrata by some micromycetes, *J. Environ. Radioactiv.*, 67, 119, 2003.

28. Lee, J.-U., Kim, S.-M., Kim, K.-W., and Kim, I.S., Microbial removal of uranium in uranium-bearing black shale, *Chemosphere*, 59, 147, 2005.

29. Jouve, A., Lejeune, M., and Rey, J., A new method for determining the bioavailability of radionuclides in the soil solution, *J. Environ. Radioactiv.*, 43, 277, 1999.

30. Mubarak, A. and Olsen, R.A., Immiscible displacement of the soil solution by centrifugation, *Soil Sci. Soc. Am. J.*, 40, 329, 1976.

31. Benes, P., Stamberg, K., and Stegmann, R., Study of the kinetics of the interaction of Cs-137 and Sr-85 with soils using batch method: methodological problems, *Radiochim. Acta*, 66/67, 315, 1994.

32. Davies, B.E. and Davies, R.I., A simple centrifugation method for obtaining small samples of soil solution, *Nature*, 198, 216, 1963.

33. Denys, S., Echevarria, G., Florentin, L., Leclerc-Cessac, E., and Morel, J.-L., Availability of ^{99}Tc in undisturbed soil cores, *J. Environ. Radioactiv.*, 70, 115, 2003.

34. Chen, S.B., Zhu, Y.G., and Hu, Q.H., Soil to plant transfer of [238]U, [226]Ra and [232]Th on a uranium mining-impacted soil from south-eastern China, *J. Environ. Radioactiv.*, 82, 223, 2005.

35. Vera Tomé, F., Blanco Rodriguez, M.P., and Lozano, J.C., Soil-to-plant transfer factors for natural radionuclides and stable elements in a Mediterranean area, *J. Environ. Radioactiv.*, 65, 161, 2003.

36. Copplestone, D., Johnson, M.S., and Jones, S.R., Behaviour and transport of radionuclides in soil and vegetation of a sand dune ecosystem, *J. Environ. Radioactiv.*, 55, 93, 2001.

37. El-Mrabet, R., Abril, J.-M., Periáñez, R., Manjon, G., Garcia-Tenorio, R., Delgado, A., and Andreu, L., Phosphogypsum amendment effect on radionuclide content in drainage water and marsh soils from southwestern Spain, *J. Environ. Qual.*, 32, 1262, 2003.

38. Dominguez, R., del Campillo, M.C., Peña, F., and Delgado, A., Effect of soil properties and reclamation practices on phosphorus dynamics in reclaimed calcareous marsh soils from the Guadalquivir Valley, SW Spain, *Arid Land Res. Manage.*, 15, 203, 2001.

39. Bolivar, J.P., Garcia-Tenorio, R., and Garcia-Leon, M., Radioactive impact of some phosphogypsum piles in soils and salt marshes evaluated by γ-ray spectrometry, *Appl. Radiat. Isot.*, 47(9/10), 1069–1075, 1996.

40. U.S. Environmental Protection Agency, Potential uses of phosphogypsum and associated risks: background information document, EPA 402-R92-002, U.S. Environmental Protection Agency, Washington, DC, 1992.

41. Zhu, Y.G. and Shaw, G., Soil contamination with radionuclides and potential remediation, *Chemosphere*, 41, 121, 2000.
42. Wild, A., *Soil and the Environment*, Cambridge University Press, Cambridge, 1993.
43. Entry, J.A., Vance, N.A., Hamilton, M.A., Zabowsky, D., Watrud, L.S., and Adriano, D.C., Phytoremediation of soil contaminated with low concentrations radionuclides, *Water Air Soil Pollut.*, 88, 167, 1996.
44. Guillitte, O., Tikhomirov, F.A., Shaw, G., and Vetrov, V., Principles and practices of countermeasures to be carried out following radioactive contamination of forest areas, *Sci. Total Environ.*, 157, 399, 1994.
45. Zhu, Y.G., Effect of potassium supply on the uptake radiocaesium by crops, Ph.D. dissertation, University of London, London, UK, 1998.
46. Shutov, V.N., Bruk, G.Y., Basalaea, L.N., Vasilevitskiy, V.A., Ivanova, N.P., and Kaplun, I.S., The role of mushrooms and berries in the formation of internal exposure doses to the population of Russia after the Chernobyl accident, *Radiat. Prot. Dosim.*, 67, 55, 1996.
47. Baeza, A., Guillen, J., and Bernedo M., Soil-fungi transfer coefficients: importance of the location of mycelium in soil and of the differential availability of radionuclides in soil fractions, *J. Environ. Radioactiv.*, 81, 89, 2005.
48. Lasat, M.M., Ebbs, S.D., and Kochian, L.V., Phytoremediation of a radiocaesium-contaminated soil: evaluation of cesium-137 bioaccumulation in the shoots of three plant species, *J. Environ. Qual.*, 27, 165, 1998.
49. Quindos, L.S., Fernandez, P.L., Rodenas, C., Gomez-Arozamena, J., and Arteche, J., Conversion factors for external gamma dose derived from natural radionuclides in soils, *J. Environ. Radioactiv.*, 71, 139, 2004.
50. Colmenero Sujo, L., Montero Cabrera, M.E., Villalba, L., Renteria Villalobos, M., Torres Moye, E., Garcia-Leon, M., Garcia-Tenorio, R., Mireles Garcia, F., Herrera Peraza, E.F., and Sanchez Aroche, D., Uranium-238 and thorium-232 series concentrations in soil, radon-222 indoor and drinking water concentrations and dose assessment in the city of Aldama, Chihuahua, Mexico, *J. Environ. Radioactiv.*, 77, 205, 2004.
51. United Nations Scientific Committee on the Effect of Atomic Radiation, *Sources and Effects of Ionizing Radiation, Annex A: Dose Assessment Methodologies*, United Nations Scientific Committee on the Effect of Atomic Radiation, New York, 2000.
52. Zmazek, B., Zivcic, M., Todorovski, L., Dûeroski, S., Vaupoti, J., and Kobal, I., Radon in soil gas: how to identify anomalies caused by earthquakes, *Appl. Geochem.*, 20, 1106–1119, 2005.
53. Klusman, R.W. and Webster, J.D., Preliminary analysis of meteorological and seasonal influences on crustal gas emission relevant to earthquake prediction, *Bull. Seismol. Soc. Am.*, 71, 211, 1981.
54. Dobrovolsky, I.P., Zubkov, S.I., and Miachkin, V.I., Estimation of the size of earthquake preparation zones, *Pure Appl. Geophys.*, 117, 1025, 1979.
55. Maejima, Y. Matsuzaki, H., and Higashi, T., Application of cosmogenic [10]Be to dating soils on the raised coral reef terraces of Kikai Island, southwest Japan, *Geoderma*, 126, 389, 2005.
56. Zapata, F., The use of environmental radionuclides as tracers in soil erosion and sedimentation investigations: recent advances and future developments, *Soil Tillage Res.*, 69, 3, 2003.

57. Walling, D.E. and Quine, T.A., Use of ^{137}Cs as a tracer of erosion and sedimentation: handbook for the application of the ^{137}Cs technique, Report to the UK Overseas Development Administration, Exeter, UK, 1993.

58. Appleby, P.G. and Oldfield, F., Application of lead-210 to sedimentation studies, in *Uranium-Series Disequilibrium: Application to Earth, Marine and Environmental Sciences*, Ivanovich, M. and Harmon, R.S., eds., Clarendon Press, Oxford, 1992.

59. Walling, D.E., Collins, A.L., and Sichingabula, H.M., Using unsupported lead-210 measurements to investigate soil erosion and sediment delivery in a small Zambian catchment, *Geomorphology*, 52, 193, 2003.

60. Wallbrink, P.J. and Murray, A.S., Distribution and variability of [7]Be in soils under different surface cover conditions and its potential for describing soil redistribution processes, *Water Resour. Res.*, 32, 467, 1996.

61. Blake, W.H., Walling, D.E., and He, Q., Fallout beryllium-7 as a tracer in soil erosion investigations, *Appl. Radiat. Isot.*, 51, 599, 1999.

62. Bar'hakhtar, V., Kukhar', V., Los', I., Poyarkov, V., Kolosha, V., Shestopalov, V. (Eds.), Comprehensive risk assessment of the consequences of the Chernobyl accident. Science and Technology. Center in Ukraine/Ukrainian Radiation Training Centre, Kyiv. 1998.

63. Saito, K. and Jacob, P., Gamma ray fields in the air due to sources in the ground, *Radiat. Prot. Dosim.*, 58, 29, 1995.

64. Beck, H.L., De Campo, J., and Cogolak, C., *In situ Ge(Li) and NaI(Tl) Gamma Ray Spectrometry*, USAEC Report HASL-258, U.S. Atomic Energy Agency, New York, 1972.

65. Clouvas, A., Xanthos, S., Antonopoulos-Domis, M., and Silva, J., Monte Carlo calculation of dose rate conversion factors for external exposure to photon emitters in soils, *Health Phys.*, 78, 295, 2000.

66. Ota, Y. and Omura, A., Contrasting styles and rates of tectonic uplift of coral reef terraces in the Ryukyu and Daito Islands, southwestern Japan, *Quatern. Int.*, 15/16, 17, 1992.

6 Radionuclide Transport Processes and Modeling

C. M. Vandecasteele

CONTENTS

6.1   INTRODUCTION

Nuclear electricity production generates large amounts of artificial radionuclides, which may be concentrated through reprocessing into radioactive wastes. The many applications of radioactivity in industry, medicine, and research make use of large quantities of artificial radioisotopes. Finally, some conventional industries (phosphate mills and oil extraction) concentrate naturally occurring radioactive materials (NORMs) in their residues. These activities are responsible for routine and accidental releases of radioactive elements into the environment.

     Radionuclides discharged into the atmosphere as gas, aerosols, or fine particles are transported downwind, dispersed by atmospheric mixing phenomena, and progressively settled by deposition processes. During the passage of the radioactive plume, people are irradiated externally as well as internally by inhalation. After the passage of the cloud, exposure of the population continues via three main pathways: external irradiation from the radionuclides deposited on the ground, inhalation of resuspended contaminated particles, and ingestion of contaminated food products.

When released into surface waters, radionuclides are partly removed from the water phase by adsorption on suspended solids and bottom sediments. As the radioactivity disperses, there is a continuing exchange between the liquid and solid phases. The contaminated sediments deposited on the banks of rivers, lakes, and coastal areas lead to external irradiation of people spending time at these sites. The residual activity in water exposes man internally through the ingestion of drinking water, aquatic food products, and terrestrial food products contaminated by irrigation of vegetation and ingestion of water by livestock.

Radioactivity may also contaminate soil due to lixiviation of waste heaps, shallow land burial, or geological disposal. It migrates slowly with soil water as soluble ions or organic complexes, interacting with the soil compounds in exchange reactions, and contaminates aquifers.

6.2 TRANSPORT IN THE ATMOSPHERE

The atmosphere is the first important path for the dispersion of radioactive pollutants in the environment. Its lower layer, which extends to a height of about 15 km at the equator and 10 km in the polar regions, constitutes the common receptor of routine industrial gaseous discharges and accidental atmospheric releases. This layer, called the troposphere, is a turbulent zone, saturated in water vapor and constantly mixed by winds generated by the heat balance at the Earth's surface.

6.2.1 WINDS

Winds are the driving force for the transport of airborne pollutants. They determine the direction of the plume of pollutants and the speed at which these pollutants are transported downwind. Winds are caused by the interaction of the forces created by the pressure gradients between anticyclones and depressions and the Coriolis forces generated by the Earth's rotation. When equilibrium is reached between these forces, air masses move parallel to the isobars. In the Northern Hemisphere, the flow is clockwise around high pressure areas and counterclockwise around depressions.

Closer to the Earth's surface, however, below 650 m, the shearing forces of contact with the ground modify wind direction and speed. These friction effects can cause the wind to change direction by about 30 degrees (outward around anticyclones and inward around high pressure areas) between altitude (650 m) and the surface. The forces exerted by the roughness of the ground surface due to natural (mountains, hills, valleys, forests) and man-made (buildings and cities) obstacles can change wind trajectories and speed. Variations in wind speed and direction (along the vertical axis) creates turbulence, which increases the dispersion of airborne pollutants.

6.2.2 Atmospheric Stability

Another key parameter influencing the dispersion of airborne contaminants is the stability of the atmosphere, which is determined by the vertical temperature profile of the atmosphere relative to the adiabatic lapse rate, that is, the temperature decrease that a small air parcel undergoes when rising. As pressure decreases with height, rising air masses expand and hence cool down. Considering small air volumes as adiabatic systems (i.e., thermodynamically isolated and not exchanging energy or heat with their environment), the temperature of a rising air bubble decreases at a rate of 9.8°C/km until it becomes water saturated (i.e., when water vapor starts to condense). This rate is known as the dry adiabatic lapse rate. As soon as the air bubble becomes saturated, further rise, and hence cooling, provoke condensation, which causes its temperature to decrease at a reduced rate of 6.5°C/km (termed the saturated or moist adiabatic lapse rate) because the temperature decrease due to expansion is partially compensated for by the recovery of the latent vaporization heat released by condensation of water vapor.

Thus, comparing the actual altitudinal air temperature gradient with the dry or saturated adiabatic lapse rate (Figure 6.1), the atmosphere is

- Neutral if the actual temperature gradient in the atmosphere is equal to the adiabatic lapse rate,
- Stable if its temperature gradient is higher than the adiabatic lapse rate, possibly positive (inversion), and
- Unstable when its temperature gradient is lower than the adiabatic lapse rate.

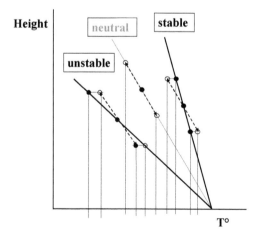

FIGURE 6.1 Illustration of the stability conditions of the atmosphere. The dotted arrows represent the behavior of an adiabatic air parcel.

The vertical temperature profile in the lower troposphere is directly influence by

- The thermal fluxes to (insolation in the day time) and from (infrared radiation during the night) the Earth's surface,
- The heat capacity of the Earth's surface (soil or water),
- The thermal conductivity between the Earth's surface and the lower air layer in contact, and
- The degree of mixing by winds.

Based on experimental observations, Pasquill [1,2] proposed an empirical categorization of the stability of the atmosphere in six classes from A (very unstable) to F (stable), which are based on a few easily observable weather parameters such as wind speed at 10 m and sunshine intensity in the daytime, and wind speed and cloud cover during the night (Table 6.1). Later, a class G was added for very stable atmospheric conditions. The Pasquill stability classification is still used internationally in atmospheric dispersion modeling.

Using more or less comparable approaches, that is, combining synoptic data (wind velocity, solar radiation, solar angle, cloudiness), vertical temperature gradient, horizontal fluctuation of the wind direction, and ground surface roughness, alternative classifications have been proposed by McElroy [3], McElroy and Pooler [4], Klug [5], Bultynck et al. [6], Vogt [7], and Doury [8], which can be more or less correlated (Table 6.2).

The stability of the atmosphere determines the pattern of the plume (Figure 6.2). The "looping" pattern occurs when the atmosphere is unstable, that is, when the temperature gradient of the atmosphere is very negative (superadiabatic). This situation creates whirling air motions that cause the plume to strike the ground repeatedly along its trajectory. Such conditions (very unstable atmosphere) are achieved by strong sunshine and weak winds because they require a warm up of the soil. The "coning" pattern occurs when the atmosphere is neutral or when the gradient is only slightly superadiabatic (weakly unstable). This situation is

---

TABLE 6.1
Stability Classes Related to Meteorological Conditions [1]

Wind Speed at 10 m (m/sec)	In the Daytime; Sunshine			During the Night: Cloudiness	
	Strong	Moderate	Slight	> 3/8	≤ 3/8
<2	A	A–B	B	—	—
2–3	A–B	B	C	E	F
3–5	B	B–C	C	D	E
5–6	C	C–D	D	D	D
>6	C	D	D	D	D

TABLE 6.2
Rough Correspondence of the Stability Classes Between Different Classification Systems

Pasquill [1]	A	B	C	D	E	F	G
McElroy [3] McElroy and Pooler [4]		B_2	B_1	C	D		
Bultynck et al. [6]	E6		E5	E4	E3–E2	E2–E1	E1
Doury [8]	DN					DF	

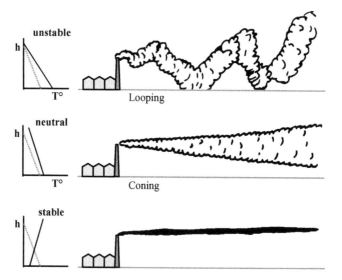

FIGURE 6.2 Typical pollutant dispersion patterns in unstable, neutral, and stable atmospheres. The dotted line on the left graphs represent the air temperature profile as the adiabatic lapse rate.

the one that is the most faithfully represented by the Gaussian model (see Section 6.2.3). The "fanning" pattern occurs in a stable or very stable atmosphere, when the gradient is less negative than the adiabatic lapse rate, or even positive.

6.2.3 THE GAUSSIAN MODEL

The Gaussian model is an empirical model providing an analytical solution to the transport and diffusion equations representing short duration (puffs) or continuous (plumes) releases of atmospheric pollutants. It was developed in the early 1960s by Pasquill [1] and Gifford [9], based on a theoretical description of eddy diffusion in the atmosphere proposed by Sutton [10]. But despite, and also because of its relative simplicity and because it can be run with limited, readily obtainable meteorological information, it is still widely used today.

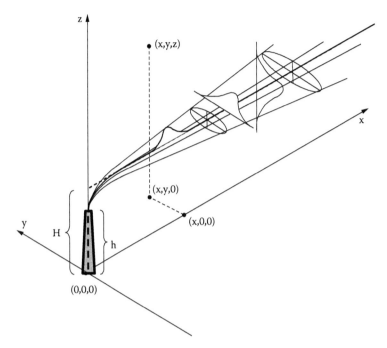

FIGURE 6.3 Coordinate system for dispersion calculations (after Turner [56]).

The Gaussian model is based on the assumption that diffusion of airborne pollutants can be equated to a probabilistic phenomenon, which can be described by a Gaussian equation. In other words, the concentration profiles in the plane perpendicular to the wind axis (plume model) as well as on the wind axis (puff model) adopt Gaussian patterns (Figure 6.3). Therefore the maximum of concentration is centered on the plume axis. The diffusion intensities are expressed by the values taken by the standard deviations, which increase progressively with the distance from the source.

In theory, the model applies only for sites with very simple topography (flat lands, without obstacles or discontinuities) and rather homogeneous meteorological conditions during the release and on the puff or plume travel path. Concentrations observed at some distance from the release point can have extreme fluctuations, depending on variations in wind direction and turbulence, therefore the model provides only average concentrations.

In the case of a puff release, the concentration $(C_{(x,y,z,t)})$ at a given point (x,y,z) and a given time (t) can be estimated by the following mathematical expression:

$$C_{(x,y,z,t)} = \frac{Q}{(2\pi)^{3/2}\,\sigma_x\sigma_y\sigma_z}\exp\left[-\frac{1}{2}\left\{\frac{(x-\bar{u}t)^2}{\sigma_x^2}+\frac{y^2}{\sigma_y^2}+\frac{(z-H)^2}{\sigma_z^2}\right\}\right] \quad (6.1)$$

where

Q = total quantity of pollutants released at the stack (in kg or Bq),

σ_i = standard deviations of the Gaussian distribution, representing the diffusion intensities of the pollutants, along each of the three axes x, y, and z (per m),

$\bar{u}$ = mean wind velocity at the level of the effective release height H (in m/sec),

H = the so-called effective release height; that is, the actual height of the stack incremented by an extra height representing the buoyancy effect (due to initial ejection speed or higher temperature of the gases released at the stack compared to that of the air) (in m).

For a continuous release (plume), the concentration ($C_{(x,y,z)}$) at a given point (x,y,z) is estimated using a similar expression, where the quantity of pollutants released is replaced by the quotient of the mean emission flux Φ (in kg/sec or Bq/sec) divided by the average wind speed $\bar{u}$ (in m/sec). In this case, the diffusion along the y-axis (wind axis), that is, the path of the plume, is neglected because one may suppose that downstream diffusion is compensated for by upstream back-diffusion:

$$C_{(x,y,z)} = \frac{\Phi}{\bar{u}\, 2\pi\, \sigma_y \sigma_z}\exp\left[-\frac{1}{2}\left\{\frac{y^2}{\sigma_y^2}+\frac{(z-H)^2}{\sigma_z^2}\right\}\right]. \tag{6.2}$$

When the puff or the plume strikes the ground, total reflection is assumed (i.e., deposition on the ground is not included at this stage). Mathematically this is achieved by considering a virtual source identical to the actual one, but symmetrical relative to the ground surface (Figure 6.4). The pollutant concentrations in air, beyond the contact point, are the sum of the direct contribution from the source and that resulting from the pollutants reflection on the ground.

The equations become

$$C_{(x,y,z)} = \frac{Q}{(2\pi)^{3/2}\, \sigma_x \sigma_y \sigma_z}\exp\left[-\frac{1}{2}\left\{\frac{(x-\bar{u}t)^2}{\sigma_x^2}+\frac{y^2}{\sigma_y^2}\right\}\right]\times$$
$$\left\{\exp\left[-\frac{1}{2}\frac{(z-H)^2}{\sigma_z^2}\right]+\exp\left[-\frac{1}{2}\frac{(z+H)^2}{\sigma_z^2}\right]\right\} \tag{6.3}$$

for a puff release and

$$C_{(x,y,z)} = \frac{\Phi}{\bar{u}\, 2\pi\, \sigma_y \sigma_z}\exp\left[-\frac{1}{2}\frac{y^2}{\sigma_y^2}\right]\times\left\{\exp\left[-\frac{1}{2}\frac{(z-H)^2}{\sigma_z^2}\right]+\exp\left[-\frac{1}{2}\frac{(z+H)^2}{\sigma_z^2}\right]\right\} \tag{6.4}$$

for a plume release.

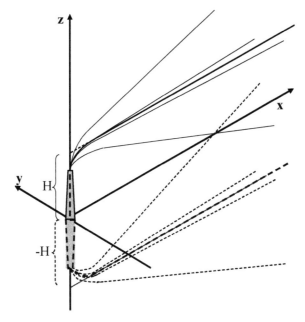

FIGURE 6.4 Schema for coping with the total reflection of the plume on the ground surface.

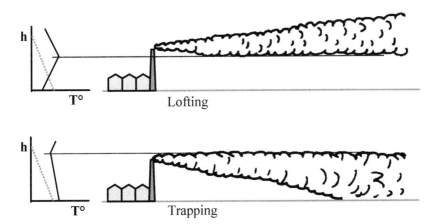

FIGURE 6.5 Example of situations when a temperature inversion is observed below or above the release point.

Similar constructions can be made to cope with temperature inversions (Figure 6.5), through which the penetration of pollutants is not supposed to happen. For example, when the inversion is higher than the effective release, a virtual source of emission must be created at a height corresponding to the height of the inversion plus the difference between the inversion height and the effective release height.

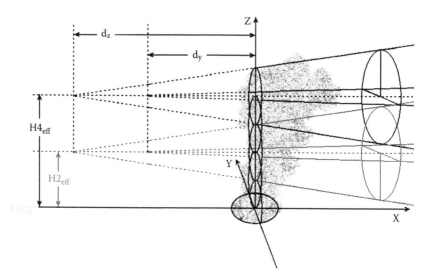

FIGURE 6.6 Gaussian model adapted to cope with the dispersion of radioactivity after the explosion of a radiologic dispersion device (RDD). The picture illustrates the coordinate system for two of the five fractions of the total plume considered by the model. Redrawn from Hotspot 49 [11].

6.2.4 THE GAUSSIAN MODEL APPLIED TO RADIOLOGICAL DISPERSION DEVICES

To cope with recent public and political concerns, the Gaussian model was also adapted (Figure 6.6) to provide a tool to assess the consequences of the dispersion of radioactive material by conventional explosives as a consequence of terrorist actions ("dirty bombs"). Such an application has been developed by the University of California, Lawrence Livermore National Laboratory [11].

Based on the power of the explosion, related to the amount of explosive material expressed in weight equivalent of TNT (in kg), the Hotspot model calculates the height (in meters) of the cloud top ($93 \times w^{0.25}$) and the cloud radius ($r = 0.2 \times$ height of the cloud top). The model then assumes an initial distribution of the dispersed radioactive material between five initial puffs positioned on top of each other at different heights from the ground level up to 0.8 times the cloud top and attributes to each of them a fraction of the total source term (Table 6.3). With each puff are associated two virtual point sources located at a height corresponding to that of the puff and at an upwind distance, d_y and d_z, such that σ_y and σ_z at the vertical of the explosion epicenter ($x = 0$), for the prevalent atmospheric stability class, are equal to one-tenth of the cloud top.

For each individual puff, a Gaussian model calculates the concentrations at any point of coordinates (x,y,z), taking into account possible reflections of the pollutants on the ground or at the level of an inversion. The expected value is the sum of the five individual contributions.

TABLE 6.3
Effective Height and Fraction of the Total Radioactivity Dispersed Associated with the Five Individual Puffs

Puff	Effective Release Height	Fraction of the Total Source Term
4	0.8 × cloud top	20%
3	0.6 × cloud top	35%
2	0.4 × cloud top	25%
1	0.2 × cloud top	16%
0	Ground level	4%

6.2.5 PARAMETERS OF THE GAUSSIAN MODEL

The σ values or diffusion coefficients used by the Gaussian model vary according to the stability of the atmosphere and distance from the source. These values are provided by approximate formulas (see Brenk et al. [12] and Mayall [13]) or abacuses (Figure 6.7). It may reasonably be assumed that the diffusion coefficient along the plume axis, σ_x, is similar to σ_y.

Measuring the wind velocity at the effective release height (H_{eff}) is not necessarily directly feasible. It is possible, however, to estimate it based on measurements at another level (typically at 10 m) according to the following relation:

$$\bar{u}_{H_{eff}} = \bar{u}_{10}\left(\frac{H_{eff}}{10}\right)^m \tag{6.5}$$

where m ranges from 0.03 to 0.64 according to the stability conditions and the type of ground surface (Table 6.4).

6.2.6 IMPORTANT LIMITATIONS OF THE GAUSSIAN MODEL

The application of Gaussian models should, in theory, be limited to environmental conditions compatible with the assumptions that have been used to derive the mathematical expressions, namely,

- Constant wind speed (but no calm), wind direction, and air turbulence along and during the journey of the plume,
- Sufficiently long diffusion times,
- Homogeneous topography and roughness along the plume trajectory, and
- Total reflection of the plume on the ground.

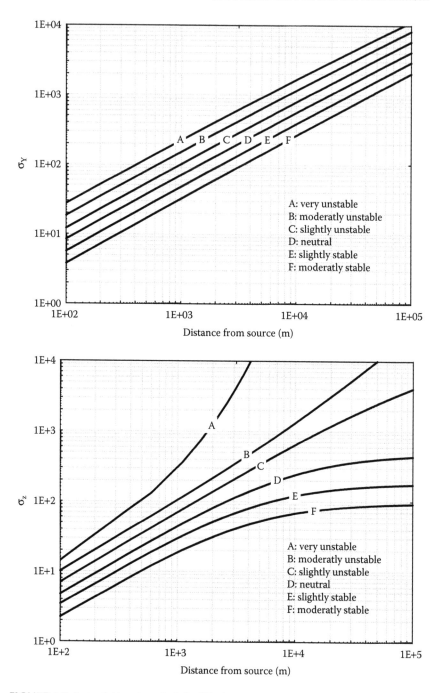

FIGURE 6.7 Lateral $(_y)$ and vertical $(_z)$ diffusion coefficients as a function of the distance from the release point. Redrawn based on Pasquill-Gifford approximated equations for a roughness category 1 [7].

TABLE 6.4
Values of Parameter *m* in Relation with the Type of Ground Surfaces and Pasquill Stability Conditions in the Atmosphere [14]

Type of Ground Surface	Pasquill Stability Class (cf. Table 6.1)					
	A	B	C	D	E	F
Seas and lakes	0.03	0.05	0.06	0.08	0.10	0.12
Agricultural soils	0.10	0.15	0.20	0.25	0.35	0.40
Urban and forest areas	0.16	0.24	0.32	0.40	0.56	0.64

These conditions are rarely completely fulfilled in reality, especially over long distances or long durations. Therefore Gaussian models should only consider short-range travel. There is wide consensus to consider a range from a few hundred meters to a few tens of kilometers as valid, however, in practice, modelers often extend the limit up to 100 km.

The plume occupies a limited space volume, while Gaussian distributions are, by definition, infinite, therefore estimation is limited to situations where the calculated concentration values are greater than or equal to one tenth of the maximal concentration.

6.2.7 Long-Range Dispersion Models

In order to be able to predict plume trajectories over long distances (e.g., the travel of the Chernobyl clouds over Europe), more complex models have been developed that call for a much more complete set of meteorological observations and forecasts from meteorological models (e.g., from the European Centre for Medium Range Weather Forecasting [ECMWF]), including three-dimensional wind fields (Figure 6.8).

Eulerian models are based on equations of air mass motion, radionuclide advection and dispersion, and mass conservation, expressed over a three-dimensional grid, which is fixed with respect to the source origin. Lagrangian models use a mobile grid that follows the travel of the plume. These two model families have their respective advantages and drawbacks.

Eulerian grid models allow full three-dimensional development of pollutant transport, but need more computation time. They are very high-performance tools to cope with atmospheric pollutant chemistry and transformation. They are unable to assess the short-range impact of multiple individual sources, especially when the emission sources do not belong to distinct grid cells. This limitation arises because these models uniformly mix the emissions within the source grid cell, and hence do not properly address the initial growth and dispersion of the pollutants. This drawback might not be crucial in radioactivity dispersion modeling because releases often originate from a single source.

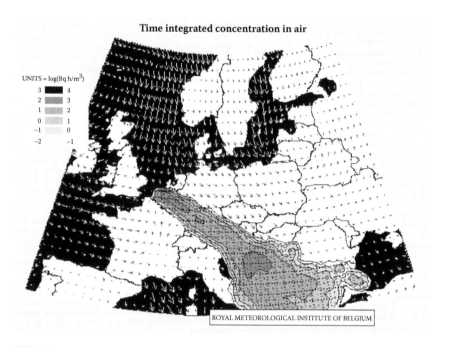

FIGURE 6.8 Example of a long-range plume trajectory. (Courtesy of Dr. L. Van der Auwera, Royal Meteorological Institute, Brussels, Belgium).

Lagrangian plume and puff models are less demanding. Unlike Eulerian models, they do well working with a limited number of different sources and their variation in time. Because they are based on a mobile grid, they are able to trace the plume from individual sources. They cannot treat chemical processes unless they are those that can be approximated by first-order kinetics. When comparisons are made of observed and simulated frequency distributions for fixed receptors, Lagrangian models provide good estimates of maximum concentration values, typically within a factor of two or three of those observed. Many models combine the Lagrangian approach, which follows the history of the release across a region, with the Eulerian approach for the simulation of pollutant dispersion through a three-dimensional grid covering that region.

6.2.8 PLUME DEPLETION

As a first stage, most dispersion models estimate the transport of airborne pollutants from their source without considering the processes that reduce the radioactivity in the air compartment; for example, models consider the total plume reflection on the ground surface and neglect deposition.

6.2.8.1 Radioactive Decay

Radioactive decay must be accounted for when dealing with short-lived radio-isotopes (half-life close to the plume travel duration). The easiest way to perform this correction is by substituting a modified source term in the previously reported equations, that is, replacing Q by $Q = Q \times f_i$, where

$$f_i = e^{(-\lambda_i \times t)} \quad \text{or} \quad f_i = e^{\left(-\lambda_i \times \frac{x}{u}\right)}, \tag{6.6}$$

with λ_i (per sec) being the radioactive decay constant of radionuclide i. Of course, the product of the disintegration might not be a stable isotope, so the source term must also be adapted to take into account the buildup of radioactive daughters.

6.2.8.2 Wet Deposition

Deposition of airborne material onto the ground by the action of precipitation can be assumed to remove pollutants uniformly throughout the entire air column up to the top of the plume with first-order kinetics. As for radioactive decay, a correction factor f_w can be applied to the source term, that is,

$$f_w = e^{(-\alpha_i \times r \times t)} \quad \text{or} \quad f_w = e^{\left(-\alpha_i \times r \times \frac{x}{u}\right)}, \tag{6.7}$$

where

α_i = washout coefficient for a radionuclide i (per mm when t is given in sec),

r = precipitation rate (mm/sec).

Best estimate values of α are 0.58/mm for particulates and 0.40/mm for elemental iodine. The α values are much less than 0.4/mm for organic iodine and insignificant for noble gases [14].

6.2.8.3 Dry Deposition

Airborne contaminants can also be removed from the plume in the absence of precipitation (see Section 6.3.1.1). A correction factor f_D can be similarly applied to the source term:

$$f_D = e^{\left[-\sqrt{\frac{2}{\pi}} \times \frac{v_g}{u} \times \int_0^z e^{\left(-\frac{h^2}{2\sigma_z^2}\right)} \times \frac{\partial z}{\sigma_z}\right]}, \tag{6.8}$$

where v_g is the dry deposition velocity (m/sec).

Best estimate values of v_g are 0.002 m/sec for particulates (less than 4 μm) and 0.04 m/sec for elemental iodine. The α values are much less than 0.0002 m/sec for organic iodine and insignificant for noble gases [14].

6.3 TRANSFER IN TERRESTRIAL FOOD CHAINS

Airborne radionuclides are transported downwind and dispersed by the mixing processes in the atmosphere. They gradually settle on land surfaces as a result of different deposition mechanisms. Plants are contaminated by two main processes: (1) direct deposition on aerial parts of the standing vegetation and (2) indirect contamination by root uptake when radionuclides deposited onto the soil are absorbed by plants along with water and nutrients. In a similar way, radionuclides present in irrigation water reach plants by direct deposition on aerial parts (sprinkling) or via the soil by root absorption. Gaseous radioelements like ^{14}C and ^{3}H (as water vapor or tritiated hydrogen) penetrate the plants through the stomata and are incorporated into organic constituents by photosynthesis and other metabolic processes. Contamination of animals and animal products results from inhalation and ingestion of contaminated soil particles, feed, and water [15]. The most important pathways of radionuclides in agricultural systems are shown in Figure 6.9.

During passage of the radioactive cloud, people are irradiated externally as well as internally by inhalation. Thereafter exposure of the population continues via three main pathways: external irradiation from the radionuclides deposited

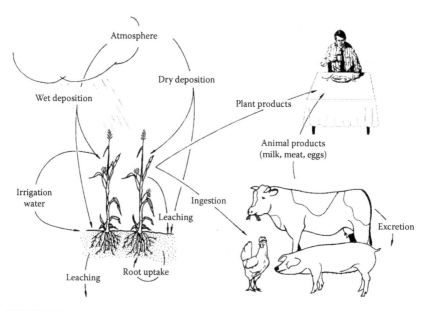

FIGURE 6.9 Main pathways for radionuclides to man in continental agricultural food chains.

on the ground, inhalation of resuspended contaminated particles, and ingestion of contaminated food products.

6.3.1 DIRECT CONTAMINATION OF THE VEGETATION

Direct contamination of the plant aerial parts is the result of two main processes: dry and wet deposition.

6.3.1.1 Dry Deposition

Dry deposition on the surface of plants aerial parts includes diffusion, impaction, or sedimentation of radionuclides as vapor or in association with aerosols or solid particles [16–18]. The interception efficiency of the vegetation depends on several factors.

The physicochemical characteristics of particles. Studies conducted on nuclear weapons test sites have shown that particles with a diameter larger than 45 μm are generally not retained by the vegetation cover but bounce off the leaves and fall to the ground; smaller particles are more easily intercepted by the vegetation [19,20]. For very fine particles (aerosols) or vapor, sedimentation rates are so low that deposition rates are determined by diffusion processes. Chamberlain [21] showed that the deposition of very fine particles is inversely proportional to the thickness of the laminar boundary layer above the leaf surface. The thickness of this layer is perturbed at the edges of plane surfaces where most deposition occurs [22].

The density of the vegetation cover. Chadwick and Chamberlain [23] proposed that the initial interception in grass could be related to the herbage density. Such an interception model based on the vegetation biomass [24] is adequate for plants developing a homogeneous canopy (like pasture grass and cereals in the vegetative growing period) and for which a good correlation exists between biomass and the leaf area index (LAI). However, it cannot properly respond to the situation where the LAI is not a monotonous function of the vegetation biomass, like for cereals from "shooting" onward. In such cases, an interception model based on the LAI gives more reliable predictions [25].

The characteristics of the plants. In grass, most of the particles retained are found on the shoot base below the animal grazing level. Soluble radionuclides accumulated there can subsequently be remobilized and redistributed into plant tissues. The inflorescence of cereals has a shape that favors the interception of fallout particles, which may explain why wheat was found to be the major source of ^{90}Sr from weapons testing fallout in Western diets [26].

The prevailing climatic conditions. Although difficult to account for, the presence of dew on leaf surfaces favors the capture of falling particles.

The initial interception (D_{dry}) of airborne radionuclides by plants due to dry deposition mechanisms (in Bq/m²) can be assessed by

$$D_{dry} = C_{air} \times v_d \times (1 - e^{-\mu LAI}), \tag{6.9}$$

where

C_{air} = time-integrated activity concentration in the air above the plant canopy (in Bq/sec/m³),

v_d = deposition velocity characteristic for the radionuclide, its speciation, and the plant type (in m/sec),

μ = interception coefficient (in kg/m²),

LAI = leaf area index (in m²/kg) characteristic of the plant species and its development stage.

6.3.1.2 Wet Deposition

Wet deposition is the process by which soluble radionuclides dissolved in hydrometeors or bound to aerosol and particles are trapped by water drops (rain, snow, fog, or mist) and deposited on surfaces. Aerosol particles are captured by falling raindrops below the cloud, termed washout, or incorporated in raindrops within the cloud where they can serve as condensation nuclei, termed rainout. The contamination of plants by sprinkling irrigation is similar to wet deposition.

The interception efficiency of the vegetation depends on the size of the droplets and the amount of rainfall, as well as on changes in radionuclide concentrations in the rainwater as a function of the length of the rainfall period. The foliar surfaces are able to retain a certain quantity of water and the excess water is leached to the ground. Moreover, if rain lasts, contamination in the atmosphere is progressively washed out and less-contaminated raindrops reach the plants: the less-contaminated rainfall will also leach part of the already deposited radioactivity down to the soil.

The initial interception (D_{wet}) of airborne radionuclides by plants due to wet deposition processes (in Bq/m²) can be assessed by [27]

$$D_{wet} = \frac{C_{atm}}{t} \times (1 - e^{-\Lambda \times t}) \times \frac{LAI \times k \times S}{r} \times \left(1 - e^{-\frac{\ln 2 \times r \times t}{3 \times S}}\right), \tag{6.10}$$

where

C_{atm} = time-integrated (over the duration of rain) activity concentration in the atmosphere integrated from the ground level up to the height of the clouds (in Bq/sec/m²),

Λ = scavenging coefficient (per sec),

t = duration of the rain (in sec),

LAI = leaf area index (in m²/kg) characteristic of the plant species and its development stage,

S = water storage capacity of the plant surfaces (in mm) characteristic of the plant type (see Müller and Pröhl [27]),

k = radioelement specific factor,

r = rate of rainfall (in mm/sec).

For high biomass density and low rainfall amounts (drizzle), the water retention capacity of the plant biomass might not be exceeded and most of the rainwater will be retained by the vegetation. The expression of the initial interception by wet deposition becomes

$$D_{wet} = \frac{C_{atm}}{t} \times (1 - e^{-\Lambda \times t}). \tag{6.11}$$

Apart from light rain conditions, wet deposition is likely to be much greater than dry deposition for aerosols and a few times greater for elemental iodine [28]. Rains are very efficient at driving airborne pollutants toward the ground.

6.3.1.3 Retention of Radionuclides Deposited on Vegetation

Foliar contamination is reduced by radioactive decay, weathering processes (wind, leaching by rain, fog, dew, mist, or irrigation water), and senescence processes (shedding of cuticular wax, dieback of old leaves). The activity concentration in the plant biomass ($C_{v,t}$, in Bq/m²) at a given time after the deposit is given by

$$C_{v,t} = \frac{Q_{v,0}}{Y_t} \times e^{-((\lambda + \lambda w) \times t)}, \tag{6.12}$$

where

$Q_{v,0}$ = initial contamination in the vegetation biomass (in Bq/m²) resulting from both dry and wet deposition,

Y_t = vegetation biomass (in kg/m²) at the time of measurement,

λ = radioactive decay constant (per sec),

λ_w = weathering coefficient (per sec),

t = time elapsed since the deposit (sec).

The radioactivity in plants is also diluted by plant growth and removal of contaminated parts by harvesting or grazing. The contamination of plants expressed as the activity concentration may also be approximated in early plant development stages by

$$C_{v,t} = \frac{Q_{v,0}}{Y_0} \times e^{-((\lambda + \lambda w + \lambda g) \times t)}, \tag{6.13}$$

where

Y_0 = vegetation biomass (in kg/m²) at the time of the deposit,

λ_g = dilution coefficient due to plant growth (per sec).

Since plant growth depends on the season, λ_g varies with time. For example, in the temperate climate of middle Europe, the growth rate of pasture grass varies from 10 to 2 g/day/m² (dry mass) between May and October, resulting in a half-life on the order of 10 to 50 days [29].

The extent of these processes, excluding physical decay, is estimated by field loss half-life, also called the "environmental" or "ecological" half-life, which is the time needed to reduce the contamination level on vegetation by a factor of two. The combined action of environmental removal processes and physical decay is termed the effective half-life.

Miller and Hoffman [30] reviewed 25 references reporting ecological half-life values for various radionuclides, physicochemical forms of the radionuclides, and plant species. They concluded that ecological half-lives on growing vegetation for iodine vapor and particles were similar (geometric means of 7.2 and 8.8 days, respectively) and, in general, half that for particulate forms of other elements. The ecological half-lives determined on a unit area basis are generally larger than those calculated on a unit mass basis, as the former do not take into account the dilution by biomass growth. Hence seasons that affect the vegetation growth rate play a key role in the field loss parameter on a biomass basis. Hoffman and Baes [31] suggest that the ecological half-lives for pastures are in general half those for cereals.

6.3.2 INDIRECT CONTAMINATION OF VEGETATION

Indirect contamination includes the mechanisms that rule the behavior of radionuclides in the soil and the geosphere, their interaction with soil components, and their uptake by plant roots. These mechanisms depend not only on the element, but also on soil processes and on the physiological properties of the plant roots.

6.3.2.1 Interaction of Radionuclides with Soil

Soils are heterogeneous systems combining three immiscible phases (solid, liquid, and gaseous) in different and changing proportions depending on the humidity level. Each phase is highly complex and variable in composition and physicochemical properties. Soil characteristics and thickness are also highly variable in space. They are often stratified in layers, termed horizons, lying on parent bedrock. The top layer, or topsoil, is rich in organic material, while underlying strata are essentially inorganic. Inorganic compounds are generally categorized on the basis of their size: clay (less than 2 μm), silt (2 to 20 μm), sands (20 to 2000 μm), gravels (2 to 20 mm), and stones (greater than 20 mm).

Soils are dynamic systems; the properties are acquired and modified with time due to the joint actions of natural factors (variations in temperature and humidity, erosion) and farming practices. Radionuclides deposited on the ground or dispersed within the soil are first dissolved in soil water. Dissolving proceeds via kinetics, depending on the speciation of the radioelement: it is quasi-instantaneous for soluble compounds (e.g., CsI), but can be a longer process when radionuclides are included in insoluble matrices (e.g., fuel particles or vitrified wastes), as radionuclides cannot be leached before weathering processes in the soil have altered the matrix [32]. Once in solution, radionuclides can adsorb on the sorption complex by exchange processes; (co-)precipitate as hydroxides, sulfides, carbonates, or insoluble oxides; form complexes with organic molecules; or remain in the water phase in an ionic form [33].

One key property of soil is its ability to adsorb ions and to immobilize them to different extents on the solid phase. Soil colloids (clay minerals and organic matter) contain a high specific density of negative charges acting as cation exchange sites. The ability of a soil to adsorb ions is proportional to the density of exchange sites and is expressed by its cation exchange capacity (CEC, in mEq/kg). Values reported for the CEC range from 0.3 to 1.5 mEq/kg for kaolinite, 1 to 4 mEq/kg for illite, 8 to 15 mEq/kg for montmorillonite, and 30 to 50 mEq/kg for organic compounds.

For most ions, adsorption of ions is reversible and equilibrium tends to be achieved between the concentration in the soil solution and on the sorption complex. This equilibrium is generally expressed as the distribution coefficient K_d (in l/kg), which is the quantity of an element sorbed per unit weight of solids divided by the quantity of the element dissolved per unit volume of water [34]:

$$K_{\mathrm{d}} = \frac{[\ ]_{sol.}}{[\ ]_{liq.}} = \frac{A_{sol.}/M}{A_{liq.}/V}, \tag{6.14}$$

where

$[\ ]_{sol.}$ = activity concentration in the solid phase (in Bq/kg),

$[\ ]_{liq.}$ = activity concentration in the liquid phase (in Bq/l),

$A_{sol.}$ = total radioactivity content in the solid phase (in Bq/kg),

$A_{liq.}$ = total radioactivity content in the liquid phase (in Bq/l),

M = solid phase mass (in kg),

V = liquid phase volume (in l),

or dividing the measured activity in each phase by the total activity in the system,

$$K_{\mathrm{d}} = \frac{f_{sol.}/M}{f_{liq.}/V}, \tag{6.15}$$

where

$f_{sol.}$ = fraction of the activity associated with the solid phase (dimensionless),

$f_{liq.}$ = residual fraction of the activity dissolved in the liquid phase (dimensionless).

Reversibility of adsorption is the rule for most chemical ions, but elements like K^+ and Cs^+ may be trapped and immobilized between the lattices of illite-type clay minerals. The reversibility of this selective binding is very poor and the elements bound at these sites can only be removed by alteration of the crystalline structures due to alternations of drying and rewetting or of freezing and thawing. Hence the modeling of Cs^+ interactions with clays cannot be fairly described by a simple K_d approach and more complex relations must be considered (see, e.g., Hilton and Comans [35]).

Immobilizing ions by fixation onto the soil solid phase or precipitation delays or prevents their leaching with percolation water down to below the rooting zone. However, one should always keep in mind that immobilization might be a transient process. In other words, if the solid phase can be a sink for radioactivity, it may become a source according to changes in concentration gradients between the solid and liquid phases or variations in the soil chemical properties (e.g., variation in pH or oxidoreduction potential $[E_h]$).

Soluble forms of radionuclides move in surface soils, as in geological layers, by diffusion and are carried along by the flow of water. A simple way to describe migration can be derived from the Darcy and Fick laws, taking into account mass conservation:

$$\frac{\partial C_s}{\partial t} + \frac{\partial C_w}{\partial t} = -v_d^* \times \frac{\partial C_w}{\partial x} + D_{app}^* \times \frac{\partial^2 C_w}{\partial x^2}, \tag{6.16}$$

where

C_s = activity concentration in the solid phase (in Bq/kg),

C_w = activity concentration in the solution (Bq/l),

t = time (in sec),

v_d^* = apparent velocity of the radionuclides along the water flow direction (m/sec),

D_{app}^* = apparent diffusion coefficient (m²/sec),

x = travel distance (in m).

The apparent velocity of the radionuclides is related to the Darcy water velocity v_d in the soil pores through the equation

$$v_d^* = \frac{v_d}{\theta + K_d \times \rho}, \tag{6.17}$$

where

θ = soil water content (l/l),

K_d = distribution coefficient (l/kg),

ρ = soil density (kg/l).

6.3.2.2 Root Uptake

Roots absorb their nutrients mainly from the soil solution. The solid phase constitutes a reservoir of nutrients that are made available by the weathering of minerals, humification of dead organic material, and through exchange reactions between the solid and liquid phases. The soil solution is thus continuously depleted of its solutes by root uptake, but it is also continuously replenished from the soil solid phase.

Due to the complexity and temporal and spatial variability of the soil-plant system, the uptake of radionuclides from soil is difficult to quantify. The main physical factors affecting the absorption of nutrients by the roots are

- The chemical properties of ions and ionic interactions, both for adsorption on soil sorption complexes and for root uptake,
- The ionic concentration in the water solution, which depends on the quality and quantity of soil colloids (clay minerals and organic matter) and varies over the course of the growing season according to the weather (e.g., rainfall increasing the soil moisture) and agricultural practices (fertilization, liming, manure),
- The pH and E_h, which affect the solubility of some elements (precipitation and dissolution reaction) and strongly influence K_d values [24].

Because of this complexity and variability, soil-plant transfer is usually quantified empirically by the ratio of the activity concentrations in plants and soil, termed the transfer factor (B_v):

$$B_v = \frac{[\ ]_{plant}}{[\ ]_{soil}},\qquad (6.18)$$

where
$[\ ]_{plant}$ = activity concentration in the plant (in Bq/kg dry or fresh weight),
$[\ ]_{soil}$ = activity concentration in the soil (in Bq/kg dry weight).

By definition, the activity concentration in the soil is averaged over a depth of 10 cm for pasture grass and over 20 cm for other crop species [36]. The activity concentration in plants for human consumption is generally related to their fresh weight, while that in fodders is related to their dry weight.

Immobilizing radionuclides by binding (especially irreversible binding) onto the soil solid phase or precipitation leads to a progressive reduction of their biological availability for root uptake and hence a decrease in the soil-plant transfer factor, which only considers the total activity concentration of the radionuclides in soil, regardless of whether they are bioavailable or not. This is illustrated by the set of transfer data obtained in experimental fields artificially contaminated with $^{134}CsCl$ (Figure 6.10). The calculated transfer factors decrease exponentially

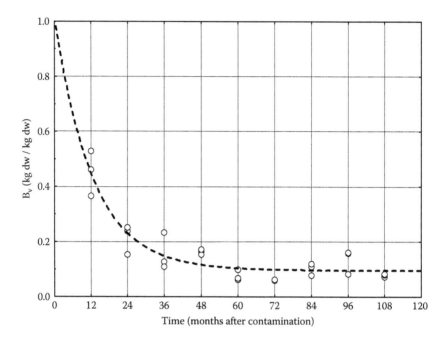

FIGURE 6.10 Changes with time of the transfer factors (B_v) observed in maize leaves.

over 5 years, with a half-life of 8.7 ($\sigma = 1.8$) months, before reaching a constant value corresponding to some 10.4% ($\sigma = 1.4$) of the initial availability.

6.3.2.3 Radionuclide Retention in Soil

The disappearance of radionuclides from the plant root zone can be represented by an exponential decay characterized by an effective removal rate (λ_B, per sec) cumulating the effects of three mechanisms:

$$\lambda_B = \lambda + \lambda_L + \lambda_H, \qquad (6.19)$$

where

λ = radioactive decay constant (per sec),

λ_L = leaching constant accounting for radionuclide migration out of the rooting zone (per sec),

λ_H = removal rate attributable to exportation by harvesting or grazing (per sec).

Losses by leaching (λ_L) can be expressed by the ratio

$$\lambda_L = \frac{v_d^*}{d_s \times \left[1 + \dfrac{\rho}{\theta} \times K_d\right]}, \qquad (6.20)$$

where

v_d^* = apparent velocity of the radionuclides along the water flow direction (in m/sec),

d_s = depth of the rooting zone (in m),

ρ = soil density (in kg/l),

θ = soil water content (dimensionless),

K_d = distribution coefficient (in l/kg).

Removal associated with plant material exportation from the field (λ_H) can be represented by

$$\lambda_H = \frac{B_v \times M_H \times N}{\rho \times d_s},$$ (6.21)

where

B_v = soil-plant transfer factor (dimensionless),

M_H = weight of biomass removed per unit area at each harvest (in kg/m^2),

N = number of harvests per unit of time (per sec),

ρ = soil density (in kg/l),

d_s = depth of the rooting zone (in m).

6.3.2.4 Translocation within Plants

Elements absorbed by plants through the root system (indirect contamination) or through the aerial organs (direct contamination) may be redistributed within plants. After direct contamination, radioactive elements absorbed by nonroot absorption processes are redistributed within the plant depending on their mobility: alkali ions can readily be remobilized, whereas alkaline-earth ions are generally not redistributed from leaves [37]. Movement of ^{90}Sr, ^{144}Ce, and ^{106}Ru into the grain of cereals is minimal if deposition takes place in the early stage of development, while ^{65}Zn, ^{55}Fe, ^{137}Cs, ^{60}Co, and ^{54}Mn are more easily translocated within the plant [38]. Middleton [39] reported that up to 50% of the cesium deposited on potato leaves may be transferred to tubers, while only 0.01% of the strontium deposited onto aerial parts migrates to tubers. Similarly, in wheat plants contaminated before ear emergence, 5% to 10% of the cesium but only 0.1% of the strontium initially retained by the plant is found in the grain at maturity. When absorbed from soil, some elements, characterized by very low mobility in plants (such as zirconium, ruthenium, and plutonium), are retained and accumulated in the roots and exhibit very low translocation to aerial organs; others (such as cesium, strontium, and technetium) are more easily translocated and accumulate preferentially in aerial parts. Consequently the stage of development of the plant at the time of contamination plays a role in determining the contamination level of organs that were not present when the contamination occurred [25].

6.3.3 Transfer to Animals

There are two main routes of pollutant entry in animals: by inhalation of gaseous compounds, aerosols, and particles, and by ingestion of drinking water, food, and soil particles associated with the vegetation grazed by the animal. Ingestion of contaminated soil is generally neglected as a contamination pathway; however, if we consider that grazing animals commonly ingest up to 20% of their dry matter daily intake, this may represent the predominant contamination source for elements that exhibit high K_d values and low soil to plant transfer [40].

6.3.3.1 Contamination by Inhalation

In the case of inhalation, airborne pollutants are transferred from the lungs to organs through the blood. Aerosols and particles penetrate to different extents in the lungs, depending on their size. The largest particles (with diameters of 5 to 30 μm) are deposited in the upper parts of the respiratory system; smaller particles (diameters less than 1 μm) penetrate down to the alveoli. Some of these particles are reexcreted by clearance mechanisms up to the throat and may then pass into the digestive tract. The fate of elements in the lungs depends on their solubility and on their ability to cross the lung barrier. Noble gases, poorly soluble in aqueous media, are not relevant for the contamination of animal organs and products. Iodine, on the other hand, is well absorbed. Radioactive pollutants such as plutonium are more readily absorbed by this route than they are from the level of the gastrointestinal (GI) tract. The contamination of animal products by inhalation is generally insignificant in comparison with ingestion, although actinides might be possible exceptions [41].

6.3.3.2 Contamination by Ingestion

Ingestion of contaminated feed, and water to a lesser extent, represents the most important pathway of contamination in animals. GI absorption of radiopollutants depends on their chemical properties and chemical form, as well as on the animal species and on particular physiological characteristics of the animal [42]. The influence of these parameters is illustrated below.

6.3.3.2.1 Chemical Properties of Radionuclides

Cesium, like other alkali metals, is up to 100% absorbed through the GI tract in monogastric mammals and to a slightly lower extent in ruminants (60 to 80%). GI absorption after oral administration of alkalines varies depending on the element: in general, absorption is highest for calcium, less for strontium (about 20%), and represents only a few percent for radium. Orally dosed plutonium is absorbed to a very small extent (much less than 1%). Increasing dietary concentrations of stable elements with the same or analogous properties (e.g., K^+ vs. Cs^+, Ca^{++} vs. Sr^{++} or Ra^{++}) decrease the absorption flux of corresponding radionuclides by inhibitive competition for the same physiological (absorption, accumulation, excretion) processes.

6.3.3.2.2 Speciation

In monogastric animals, absorption of technetium as pertechnetate is higher than that of technetium bioaccumulated in plant material [43]. In contrast, bioincorporation of plutonium in plants increases its availability for GI uptake [44,45]. Differences in accumulation rates due to the chemical speciation are also noticeable for ingested tritium, depending on whether it is administered as tritiated water or incorporated in various organic molecules, which increase the ^{3}H incorporation [46].

6.3.3.2.3 Species

Food processing in the GI tract may differ markedly between animal species. For example, compared to monogastric mammals, ruminants are characterized by having a four-chambered stomach. The first chamber (rumen) acts as a fermentation vat that receives partially chewed vegetation. Then come three other stomach chambers: the reticulum, the omasum, and finally the abomasum. This last chamber, where elements are subject to enzymatic digestion, has a similar metabolic function as the one-chamber stomach of monogastric animals. The rumen provides an anaerobic, reducing environment ($E_h = -400$ mV) that can modify the chemical form of ingested radionuclides, such as technetium, which administered as TcO_4, is reduced into insoluble forms, resulting in a lower bioavailability [43].

6.3.3.2.4 Physiological Factors

The metabolism of animals also modifies the extent of accumulation of radionuclides in mammals. For example, the transfer of ingested radioactivity to organs is higher in young individuals than in adults. This may be explained by a higher metabolic activity in growing animals than in adults and by a higher permeability of the GI tract in newborns. Animals on an iron-deficient diet have a higher absorption of actinides (uranium, neptunium, americium, and curium) and other nonferrous metals that utilize the same absorption mechanisms as iron [47]. In monogastrics, strontium absorption is enhanced by the presence of lactose in the diet and decreased by oxalates, phytates, and alginates. Diarrhea changes the permeability of the intestine and hence the flux of mineral elements through the intestinal barrier.

6.3.3.3 Distribution in the Animal

Radionuclides absorbed in the GI tract are transported by blood and distributed into the various organs and animal products. The distribution varies according to the physiological status of the animal as well as the nature and chemical form of the pollutant. Radioiodine is known to accumulate in considerable amounts in the thyroid gland. Cesium, like potassium, is distributed in soft tissues. Strontium, radium, plutonium, and rare earth elements are preferentially accumulated in bones. The liver and kidneys, acting as filters for substances penetrating or leaving the body, are preferential storage sites for many pollutants.

Many and complex metabolic steps are involved in the transfer of radionuclides to animals and their products (i.e., meat, milk, and eggs). The transfer to meat, milk, and eggs (F_f, F_m, or F_e, respectively) is usually quantified empirically by the ratio at equilibrium between the activity concentration in the animal product considered and the amount ingested daily in the diet:

$$F_f = \frac{[\;]_{meat}}{Q_{intake}},$$ (6.22)

$$F_m = \frac{[\;]_{milk}}{Q_{intake}},$$ (6.23)

$$F_e = \frac{[\;]_{egg}}{Q_{intake}},$$ (6.24)

where
$[\;]_{meat}$ = activity concentration in meat (in Bq/kg fresh weight),
$[\;]_{milk}$ = activity concentration in milk (in Bq/l),
$[\;]_{egg}$ = activity concentration in egg (in Bq/kg fresh weight),
Q_{intake} = daily radioactivity intake (in Bq/day).

To account for dynamic intakes, biological half-lives must be introduced to cope with the radionuclide buildup in and loss from the organism. ECOSYS-87 [27] calculates the activity in animal products (e.g., in milk) at any time t, even for discontinuous contamination processes, according to the equation

$$[\;]_{milk,t} = F_m \times \sum_{i=1}^{n}\left[a_i \times \int_0^t Q_{intake,\tau} \times \lambda_{b,i} \times e^{\left[-(\lambda_{b,i}+\lambda)(t-\tau)\right]} \times d\tau \right],$$ (6.25)

where
a_i = relative volume of a specific accumulation compartment in the animal, which is characterized by a biological transfer rate, λ_b

(dimensionless), with $\sum_{i=1}^{m} a_i = 1$ in ECOSYS-87,

$Q_{intake,\tau}$ = total radioactivity intake on day τ (in Bq/day),
$\lambda_{b,i}$ = biological transfer rate characteristic of compartment a_i (per sec),
λ = physical decay constant (per sec).

6.3.3.4 Excretion

Unabsorbed radionuclides are rapidly excreted via the feces. The absorbed fraction is progressively eliminated at rates that depend on the turnover rates of analogous/homologous elements or compounds in the body with which the radionuclides are associated. This excretion occurs via urine, feces (endogenous secretion), and animal products (milk and eggs). Retention of radionuclides in the body is generally described as the sum of exponential functions:

$$Q_t = Q_0 \times \sum_{i=1}^{n} a_i \times e^{[-(\lambda_i + \lambda) \times t]}, \qquad (6.26)$$

where

Q_t = total amount of radionuclide in the body at time t (in Bq),
Q_0 = total amount of radionuclide in the body when contamination is stopped, taken as $t = 0$ (in Bq),
a_i = fraction of radionuclides present at $t = 0$ in a specific compartment in the animal (dimensionless), the sum of the number of relative compartments is equal to one,
λ_i = biological elimination half-life characteristic of compartment a_i (per sec),
λ = physical decay constant (per sec).

Each exponential function can be related to a "compartment" (a more or less physically defined reservoir), characterized by two parameters, the initial capacity (a_i) and the half-life (λ_i).

After oral dosing, the first compartment can generally be related to the radioactivity present in the GI tract; other compartments of increasing half-lives represent fractions of radionuclides retained in the body in decreasingly accessible forms and having increasing turnover rates. Excretion rates vary with the chemical properties of the radioelement as well as the physiological characteristics of the target organ. For instance, the half-life of radiocesium is longer in muscles than in organs such as the liver and kidneys, and tritium present in the organism as tritiated water is more readily excreted than organically bound tritium. The long-term retention of ^{65}Zn is attributed to the fraction of the zinc atoms trapped in the matrix or in the crystal lattice of developing bone during the period of intake. Excretion rates also depend on the animal species. Stara et al. [42] reported linear relations between the logarithmic values of the long-term retention of radiocesium and the animal's weight. The explanation can be found in the fact that small animals have increased metabolic rates compared to larger ones.

6.4 TRANSPORT IN AQUATIC SYSTEMS

Nuclear power plants require a large low-temperature sink to transform the heat they produce into electricity. For that reason, they are installed along seashores or on the banks of rivers that maintain a minimum water flow, allowing the evacuation of residual heat while limiting the increase of the river water temperature downstream from the discharge point. Other industries associated with the nuclear fuel cycle (enrichment or reprocessing plants) are also installed in the vicinity of aquatic vectors and take advantage of their large dilution capacity to ensure rapid dispersion of their radioactive effluents (e.g., La Hague on the English Channel, Sellafield on the Irish Sea, Rokkasho Mura on the Pacific Ocean).

Seas and oceans have also been used in the past for radioactive waste disposal [48]: through 1970, the U.S. poured more than 3.7 PBq ("mixed" activities) into the Gulf of Mexico and the Atlantic and Pacific Oceans; western European countries dumped 680 TBq of α emitters and 56 PBq β/γ emitters in the North Atlantic Ocean from 1949 until 1982; the Kara and Barents Seas were used as dumping sites by the former USSR. However, radioactivity released in seas and oceans by waste dumping is far lower than the radioactive contamination due to local and global fallout from weapons tests (42 EBq ^{3}H, 262 PBq ^{90}Sr, and 418 PBq ^{137}Cs estimated for the Pacific Ocean) [49].

Aquatic (freshwater and marine) ecosystems are thus another important pathway for environmental dispersion of radioactive pollutants and potential exposure of populations to artificial radioactivity. Direct exposure can be associated with the consumption of drinking water and foodstuffs (fish, shellfish, algae), but also with entertainment and sport activities (fishing, swimming). Indirect human exposure arises from the use of river water for irrigation and watering of livestock or from the use of algae and sludge as soil amendments.

Radioactivity discharged in aquatic systems is transported by water flows, diluted by diffusion processes, and dispersed by turbulent mixing. Along their path, radionuclides are distributed between the liquid and solid phases, settle with sediments on the bottom, and are incorporated into living organisms. A knowledge of these processes is essential to estimate the transport and behavior of radionuclides in aquatic systems and consequently the radiological dose to populations.

Depending on their structure and characteristics, aquatic systems can be subdivided into four main categories [14]: rivers, lakes and reservoirs, estuaries, and seas and oceans. This subdivision is in some ways arbitrary, as in the real world these categories are interconnected and their physical limits are not always easy to define.

The basic characteristic of rivers is their unidirectional axial flow, from their source to the sea. Lakes and reservoirs are tanklike water bodies, sometimes stratified, having input tributaries and a river output, in which recirculation is possible. Estuaries are defined by their increasing salinity from freshwater to the saltwater of the sea; another property for those that merge into tidal seas is the influence of tides. The upper boundary between river and estuary can be defined as the highest point reached by tidal flow; the lower limit, between estuary and sea, is more difficult to set and is generally deduced from geographical characteristics rather than particular physical properties. Seas and oceans are easily identifiable by their large area, high salinity (35 g/l), and often strong tides.

6.4.1 TRANSPORT AND DISPERSION OF RADIOACTIVITY IN AQUATIC SYSTEMS

Radionuclide transport in surface water systems is driven by three main processes: transport with the water flow, dispersion due to turbulence and diffusion, and interaction with sediments and suspended matter. The large-scale movements of water are responsible for pollutant advection. They are, in essence, determined by gravity, winds, and the Earth's rotation, and temperature and salinity gradients. Depending on the acting forces, the water velocity varies in time and space from strong currents (rivers, tides) to weak ones (ocean circulation, density currents). Modifications of the water flow (breaking waves, friction on the bottom and banks) create turbulence, which disperses pollutants perpendicular to the flow axis. Finally, the fate of radionuclides in aquatic systems depends on interactions (adsorption) with solids present in the water column and physicochemical reactions (e.g., precipitation, complexation) and the transport of particles (sedimentation, solid flow).

Each aquatic ecosystem (stream, river, bay, sea, lake, or ocean) constitutes a unique system with its own mixing properties. Therefore different aquatic dispersion models have been developed to represent the specific transport mechanisms prevalent in each category.

6.4.1.1 Transport in Rivers

A simple way to describe the transport of radionuclides in rivers supposes that mixing and dilution of effluents happen instantaneously after the release and that the transport of pollutants is not affected by any sedimentation phenomenon. In the case of a routine release (continuous and constant in time), the concentration ($[\ ]_{\text{water},\,x}$) in water (in Bq/m³) at a distance x from the discharge point is given by

$$[\ ]_{\text{water},x} = \frac{\Phi_d}{\Phi_r} \times e^{\left(-\lambda \times \frac{x}{v}\right)}, \tag{6.27}$$

where

Φ_d = radionuclide discharge rate (in Bq/sec),
Φ_r = river flow (in m³/sec),
λ = physical decay constant of the considered radionuclide (per sec),
v = mean water velocity between the discharge and the sampling point (in m/sec),
x = distance of the sampling point from the release point (in m).

This model can be adapted further to cope empirically with radionuclide fixation on bottom sediments and sedimentation of radionuclides associated with suspended solids by introducing a removal factor λ_s (per sec). The equation for a routine discharge becomes

$$[\ ]_{\text{water},x} = \frac{\Phi_d}{\Phi_r} \times e^{\left(-(\lambda + \lambda_s) \times \frac{x}{v}\right)}. \tag{6.28}$$

A similar relation can be established for an acute release by modifying the previous equation to account for the volume of water that has passed the discharge point during the very short release time and a relevant diffusion coefficient to account for the pollutant dispersion along the path during transport:

$$[\ ]_{\text{water},x,t} = \frac{Q}{A \times \sqrt{2\pi \times \sigma_L}} \times e^{\left(-\frac{(x-(v \times t))}{\sigma_L^2}\right)} \times e^{\left(-\Lambda_e \times \frac{x}{v}\right)}, \qquad (6.29)$$

where

Q = radionuclide discharge quantity (in Bq),
A = the river cross section (in m^2) at the release point,
σ_L = longitudinal dispersion coefficient (in m^2/sec),
Λ_e = removal coefficient combining physical decay λ and, if needed, sedimentation processes λ_s (per sec).

A generalized expression of river models can be written as a series of equations of mass conservation or pollutants along the river path (i.e., along a one-dimensional axis):

for $i = 1$ to n:

$$\frac{\partial [\ ]_i}{\partial t} + \frac{\partial}{\partial x}\left(v_i \times [\ ]_i\right) = \frac{\partial}{\partial x}\left(D_i \frac{\partial [\ ]_i}{\partial x}\right) + \sum_{j=1}^{m}\left(K_j \times [\ ]_i\right) + \sum_{k=1}^{p} Q_k, \quad (6.30)$$

where

$[\ ]_i$ = activity concentration of the radionuclide in specific river compartments, that is, in water ($[\ ]_w$, in Bq/l) or in sediments ($[\ ]_s$, in Bq/l); a further distinction can be made between bottom sediments and suspended solids and inorganic and organic fractions,
v_i = mean velocity between the discharge and the sampling point of the radionuclide fraction in compartment i (in m/sec),
D_i = apparent dispersion coefficient for the radionuclide fraction associated with compartment i (in m^2/sec),
K_j = rate constants for radioactive decay and any activity concentration-dependent losses and gains (e.g., sorption/desorption and precipitation/dissolution processes) in compartment i (per sec),
Q_k = fluxes of radioactivity per unit of volume for the source terms and sinks (in Bq/sec/l),
x = distance of the sampling point from the release point (in m).

A specific equation must be written to describe the fate of the radionuclide considered in each river compartment. Very often there is no analytical solution to such equations and their resolution appeals to numerical techniques. However, in particular cases when some aspects can be neglected, these equations may be simplified in such a way that an analytical solution becomes possible. The two equations given at the beginning of this section are examples, without and with loss at a constant rate of sedimentation, of such analytical solutions when the longitudinal coordinate system is moving with the flow velocity and no other process but radioactive decay is considered. Other simplified situations are presented and discussed in the National Council on Radiation Protection (NCRP) report 76 [50].

Most sophisticated river models are hydrodynamic models that are based on equations that express the conservation of mass (not only radionuclides, but also water, sediments, etc.) and equilibrium of forces. They are represented by relations between the variation of variables with time and the causes of these variations (external forces, inputs and outputs, internal interactions, transport by water flow). The solutions to these equations are obtained by numerical iteration processes. Hydrodynamic models consist of several submodels, each of them dealing with a particular aspect of the overall problem and producing entry data to the next step [51]:

- A hydrodynamic submodel: based on the river profile (slope, cross section, location of locks and dams, etc.) to calculate hydrodynamic variables like flows, water velocities, and bed shear stress.
- A sediment submodel: to estimate the suspended matter concentrations in the water column, the quantities of sediment deposited on the river bottom, and the movements of these solid phases (downstream transport, sedimentation, and resuspension).
- A radionuclide submodel: which describes the radionuclide activity in water, suspended solids, and sediments.
- A biotic submodel: to include radionuclide transfer in the living compartments of the system.

The structure of hydrodynamic models is based on theoretical concepts and not on characteristics specific to a given site. In this regard they might be considered as general models applicable to any river. However, the input parameters that they use are numerous, very specific for the water body considered, and not easy to obtain. A more detailed description is far beyond the scope of this chapter.

6.4.1.2 Transport in Lakes

Modeling the transport and dispersion of radionuclides in lakes is based on a number of characteristics such as the effective residence time of a soluble radionuclide in the liquid phase, the sedimentation rate of insoluble forms, the input of and dilution by uncontaminated water (including solid particles), and the outputs by water currents [14].

In the case of routine, continuous releases, a dynamic equilibrium is reached when losses from the system are balanced by inputs. For small lakes, such a steady-state equilibrium may be rapidly reached and a simple complete-mixing model can be used to calculate the concentration in the water compartment ($[\ ]_{water}$, in Bq/m³):

$$[\ ]_{water} = \frac{Q}{\Lambda_e * V},\qquad(6.31)$$

where

> Q = radionuclide discharge rate (in Bq/sec),
> V = water volume in the reservoir (in m³),
> Λ_e = effective removal rate constant (per sec).

Λ_e takes into account the physical decay (λ), the losses from the water column (λ_s, e.g., by sedimentation), and the output from the reservoir ($\lambda_r = r/V$) via the outlet with a outflow rate r (in m³/sec).

In large lakes, prompt mixing does not occur and horizontal concentration gradients have to be considered, with higher concentrations close to the discharge area, strongly influenced by the hydrographical conditions at the site. The models used to describe radionuclide transport and dispersion in these lakes are of the same type as those used for the marine environment (see Section 6.4.1.3).

Moreover, in the case of deep lakes, water mixing may be hindered in certain seasons due to thermal stratification phenomena. In spring and summer, surface water, heated by the sun, becomes warmer (thus less dense) than deeper layers. As a result, a thermal gradient appears between the warmed surface layer and the colder bottom water. The gradient intensifies as the season proceeds, limiting the vertical exchanges of water [52]. In such a situation, models divide lakes into two homogeneous layers (the epilimnion at the top and the hypolimnion), separately considered in regard to the tributaries and outlet. In autumn, when strong winds start blowing again, water stratification disappears and the two layers are mixed.

6.4.1.3 Transport in the Marine Environment

The initial dispersion of radionuclides discharged into the marine environment from coastal nuclear installations or from rivers is mainly influenced by the hydrodynamic conditions prevailing at the entrance point, which rule the transport of pollutants by advection and turbulent diffusion. Advection is induced by high amplitude horizontal and vertical movements generated by tidal currents, winds, and density gradients (associated with salinity and temperature gradients), and by differences in water levels between two interconnected basins. Turbulent mixing is caused by friction forces created by winds or shallows (waves). In coastal waters, transport and mixing are essentially driven by tides and winds. In the open ocean, mixing at the surface is principally due to winds and surface currents. In deep waters, radionuclide dispersion is ruled by undertows. Stratification phenomena in open oceans (salinity and temperature gradients) limit the vertical transport and exchange between horizontal layers.

Whereas transport in river systems is considered unidirectional, pollutant movements in oceans must be envisaged in three, or at least two dimensions. Complex hydrodynamic models based on the calculation of the three-dimensional flow field coupled to a radionuclide transport model may be designed to describe the processes involved in the transport and fate of radioactive pollutants. However, a simpler approach in marine radiological assessment, termed the box or compartment model, is commonly used. These models do not consider hydrodynamics and suppose an instantaneous and complete homogenization of the pollutants in each box. Therefore they divide the marine ecosystems into compartments that are as homogeneous as possible, and make a distinction between the so-called local and regional compartments.

The local compartment corresponds to a limited area defined as a single compartment, close to the discharge point, which constitutes the interface between the source and the other (regional) compartments. The local model describes the fate of the radionuclides in this box and allows calculation of the radionuclide content associated with sediments, suspended solids, and water. From there, the contamination levels in the various biological compartments can be estimated. It also allows quantification of the transfer of radioactivity from the "local" zone to contiguous compartments of the regional model. The change in the total (dissolved or associated with suspended solids) radioactivity content in the water compartment of the local model (A_l, in Bq) is given by

$$\frac{\delta A_l}{\delta t} = Q - (\lambda + \lambda_s + \lambda_r) \times A_l = Q - \Lambda_e \times A_l, \qquad (6.32)$$

where
$\quad Q$ = radioactivity discharge rate into the local compartment (in Bq/sec),
$\quad \lambda$ = radioactive decay constant (per sec),
$\quad \lambda_s$ = loss rate due to sedimentation (per sec),
$\quad \lambda_r$ = water renewal rate (per sec),
$\quad \Lambda_e$ = global loss rate (per sec), which is the sum of all particular loss
$\quad\quad$ rates.

The input in the local compartment from the connecting compartments in the regional model is often neglected. The solution of this equation is expressed by

$$A_{l,t} = \frac{Q}{\Lambda_e}(1 - e^{-\Lambda_e \times t}), \qquad (6.33)$$

and the concentration (in Bq/m^3) in the water compartment of the local model is given by

$$[\ ]_{1,t} = \frac{Q}{\Lambda_e * V_l}(1 - e^{-\Lambda_e \times t}) \tag{6.34}$$

where V_1 is the total volume of the compartment (in m³).

When equilibrium is reached ($t \to \infty$), the total activity and radionuclide concentration in the water compartment are given by the relations

$$A_{1,eq} = \frac{Q}{\Lambda_e} \tag{6.35}$$

and

$$[\ ]_{1,eq} = \frac{Q}{\Lambda_e * V_l}. \tag{6.36}$$

The radioactivity (Q_{lr}) leaving the local zone toward the regional compartments depends on the renewal rate in the local compartment, λ_r, and equals

$$Q_{1 \to r} = \lambda_r * A_t = \lambda_r \times \frac{Q}{\Lambda_e}(1 - e^{-\Lambda_e \times t}) \tag{6.37}$$

or, at equilibrium,

$$Q_{1 \to r,eq} = \lambda_r \times \frac{Q}{\Lambda_e}. \tag{6.38}$$

Regional models describe the radiopollutant transport and dispersion toward remote zones from a discharge. To model the movement of a water mass and the radionuclide mass flow, open oceans are subdivided into n different contiguous compartments within which instantaneous mixing is assumed. Changes in the total radionuclide content (A_i, in Bq) in the water compartment in the ith compartment of the system are represented by

$$\frac{\delta A_i}{\delta t} = \sum_{j=i}^{n} (k_{ji} \times A_j - k_i \times A_i) - k_{i0} \times A_i + Q_i, \tag{6.39}$$

where

k_{ij} = transport rate from the ith to the jth compartment (per sec), with $k_{ii} = 0$,

k_{i0} = loss rate within one compartment without transfer into another one (e.g., physical decay, sedimentation) (per sec),

Q_i = discharge rate into the ith compartment (in Bq/sec) (e.g., due to global fallout).

This relation can be written considering radionuclide concentrations (C_i, in Bq/m^3) instead of total quantities (A_i) and flows (R_{ij}, in m^3/sec) instead of transport rates (k_{ij}). The last parameters are interrelated following the relation

$$R_{ij} = k_{ij} \times V_i, \tag{6.40}$$

where V_i is the volume of the ith compartment (in m^3).

The equation then becomes

$$\frac{\delta A_i}{\delta t} = \frac{\delta(C_i \times V_i)}{\delta t} = \sum_{j=i}^{n} (R_{ji} \times C_j - R_i \times C_i) - R_{i0} \times C_i + Q_i. \tag{6.41}$$

6.4.1.4 Transport in Estuaries

Estuaries are complex transition zones between rivers and seas. They present various morphological types which reflect their genesis (e.g., deltas, fjords …) and are characterized by two-way water flow: (1) a one-way freshwater flow and (2) a reversing two-way tidal circulation. The changing pattern of water circulation in the estuary and its morphology define the water mixing patterns between freshwater and seawater. Based on their mixing patterns, estuaries are classified into three categories:

- Poorly mixed: saltwater flows upstream below the downstream freshwater flow, creating a steep vertical salt gradient with practically no horizontal salinity gradient.
- Partially mixed: stronger tidal currents cause mixing between fresh- and saltwater, giving rise to both marked vertical and horizontal gradients.
- Well mixed: strong tidal currents induce enough turbulence to achieve complete mixing between fresh- and saltwater, resulting in the absence of a vertical gradient and leaving only a horizontal salinity gradient increasing toward the open sea.

It should be noted, however, that such a division is not rigid and an individual estuary may evolve in time and space from one pattern to another and back.

The models used to describe the transport of pollutants in estuaries are similar to those designed for rivers, lakes, and oceans: from hydrodynamic models to simple box models, depending on the degree of complexity required to cope with individual processes or the degree of simplification authorized by reasonable assumptions allowed by the specific characteristics of a given estuary. One aspect is worthwhile considering: estuaries tend to be sediment-rich areas within which the reduction of flow velocity favors sedimentation processes and changes in salt concentrations act on the redistribution of radionuclides between water, suspended solids, and sediments.

The radionuclide fraction passing from the liquid to the solid compartment, and vice versa, during transport through the estuarine zone can be estimated from the changes in the characteristic distribution coefficients (K_d; see Section 6.3.2.1) measured in fresh- and saltwater. Some radionuclides are better adsorbed on the solid phase at low salinity and tend to desorb when introduced into brackish and saltwater. Others behave in the opposite way or are unaffected by salinity. Based on their K_d in fresh- and saltwater, the radionuclides can be divided into six classes (Table 6.5).

The distribution of radionuclides belonging to classes A1 and C2 (which are, respectively, strongly or weakly adsorbed on solid particles, regardless of the salt concentration) is not affected by the passage between fresh- and saltwater. Radioelements from classes A2 and B2 (of which the sorption on the solid phase is inversely proportional to the water's salt content) tend to desorb when the solid particles are transferred from a freshwater system to brackish and saltwater. For some of them, up to 30% can be released in saltwater. Finally, radionuclides from classes B1 and C1 (better adsorbed in high-salt medium) tend to adsorb on the solid phase in brackish and saltwater.

TABLE 6.5
Classification of Selected Radionuclides As a Function of Their Adsorption Potential in Fresh- and Saltwater

Radionuclides	Adsorption Class in Freshwater	Adsorption Class in Seawater	Class in Estuary
^{51}Cr			
^{54}Mn			
^{55}Fe, ^{59}Fe			
^{58}Co, ^{60}Co	A	1	
^{106}Ru	High K_d	High K_d	A1
^{239}Np			
^{238}Pu, ^{239}Pu, ^{240}Pu			
^{241}Am			
^{134}Cs, ^{137}Cs	A	2	A2
	High K_d	Low K_d	
^{65}Zn	B	1	B1
^{90}Y, ^{91}Y	Medium K_d	High K_d	
^{14}C	B	2	B2
^{89}Sr, ^{90}Sr	Medium K_d	Low K_d	
^{95}Nb			
^{99}Tc	C	1	C1
^{110m}Ag	Low K_d	High K_d	
^{125}Sb			
^{3}H	C	2	C2
^{129}I, ^{131}I	Low K_d	Low K_d	

6.4.2 PARTITION BETWEEN THE LIQUID AND SOLID PHASES

Aquatic environments consist of an aqueous phase and a solid phase, which is mainly represented by mineral and organic particles present as suspended matter and bottom sediments. Both suspended particles and bottom sediments adsorb radionuclides from the liquid phase; however, the former exhibits a higher relative (per unit weight) sorption capacity than the latter because of its higher content of fine particles and clay. The important role of the solid phase in the transport and behavior of radionuclides in water systems is illustrated by the following two examples:

- Field measurements in the Clinch River near the Oak Ridge (Tennessee) nuclear center show that 90% of the released ^{137}Cs is bound onto suspended solids within 15 km from the discharge point.
- In the Irish Sea, near Sellafield, 95% of the plutonium and 20% of the cesium released by the reprocessing plant are adsorbed and immobilized by the bottom sediment.

Adsorption on the solid phase leads to a decrease in the radiocontaminant concentration in solution and in their bioavailability. Sedimentation of suspended solids can be considered as a decontamination of the system and the bottom sediments as a sink for radioactivity. This immobilization is often temporary, however, since adsorption processes are generally reversible and bottom sediments can be resuspended by the activity of sediment macroflora (bioturbation), tidal regimes, the passage of ships, and dredging.

As for soil particles (see Section 6.3.2.1), suspended particles and sediment materials possess cation binding sites, giving rise to a CEC. The main difference from the situation in soils lies in the volume ratio between the liquid and solid phases (largely in favor of the liquid phase in surface aquatic systems). Radionuclides initially present in the liquid phase as soluble forms tend to adsorb on the solid particles until an equilibrium is reached between both phases. Radionuclides associated with solid particles introduced into uncontaminated or less contaminated water desorb into the liquid phase. The dynamic equilibrium achieved between the two phases can only be maintained if the conditions remain unchanged. Any perturbation of the system (dilution by an uncontaminated tributary, increase of salt concentration in an estuary, introduction of a solid charge by a tributary, industrial activities or sewage) promotes a redistribution of the radioactivity until a new equilibrium is reached (Figure 6.11).

K_ds are estimated by different laboratory and field techniques. In the laboratory, distribution coefficients are obtained after equilibrating a sediment suspension (e.g., 1 g) in a large volume (e.g., 100 ml) of water (distilled water or river or seawater) artificially contaminated with soluble forms of the radionuclide considered. Solid and liquid phases, separated by filtration or centrifugation, are measured for their radioactivity content. *In situ*, suspended solids are separated by continuous centrifugation or filtration, sedimentable particles are collected in special traps through a perforated grid, and bottom sediments are sampled by

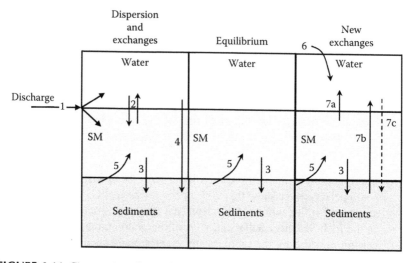

FIGURE 6.11 Changes in radionuclide distribution between the liquid and solid compartments in an aquatic ecosystem. 1. Dispersion. 2. Exchange between the liquid phase and suspended solids. 3. Sedimentation of suspended solids. 4. Exchange between the liquid phase and bottom sediments. 5. Resuspension of bottom sediments. 6. Dilution by an uncontaminated tributary with different physicochemical characteristics. 7. New exchanges to reach a new equilibrium (7a, desorption from suspended matter; 7b, desorption from bottom sediments; 7c, precipitation).

coring or with a grab dredger. Examples of K_d values for different radionuclides and stable elements estimated in sediments from different sites on the Meuse River (Belgium) are given in Table 6.6. One should notice the large variability in the values obtained by different methods.

The radionuclides can be ranked in terms of their sorption affinity on sediments and suspended solids. These sequences give some general trends, but the actual relative position of a radionuclide can be modified depending on its speciation. In marine ecosystems, the following sequence has been established [53]:

^{45}Ca < ^{90}Sr < U, Pu < ^{137}Cs < ^{86}Rb < ^{65}Zn < ^{59}Fe < ^{95}Zr-Nb, ^{54}Mn < ^{106}Ru < ^{147}Pm.

^{144}Ce and ^{60}Co are found somewhere between ^{59}Fe and ^{147}Pm. The position of ^{45}Ca and ^{90}Sr at the low-affinity side suggests a high competition between these radionuclides and their stable isotopes/analogs present in relatively high concentration in seawater. Similar sequences were established for freshwater systems, except that in this case the ^{137}Cs binding affinity is much higher.

6.4.3 CONTAMINATION OF THE BIOCENOSE

The radiocontamination of aquatic organisms is the result of two processes: adsorption of radioactive substances on external surfaces, and uptake and biological incorporation by various absorption mechanisms through external barriers (skin, gills, intestine, etc., in animals; roots, leaves, etc., in higher plants).

TABLE 6.6
In Situ and Laboratory Measured K_ds of Sediments Sampled at Different Sites on the Belgian Section of the Meuse River

Element	Radioactive K_d $\dfrac{Bq/gMs}{Bq/ml}$	Stable K_d $\dfrac{\mu g/gMs}{\mu g/ml}$	Sampling Site on the Meuse River	Conditions
Mn		4.8×10^1	Monsin	*In situ*
	1.9×10^4	1.4×10^1	Hastière	*In situ*
	1.0×10^2		Waulsort	Laboratory
	1.3×10^2		Anseremme	Laboratory
Co	1.3×10^4	8.9×10^2	Monsin	*In situ*
	1.4×10^5	1.3×10^3	Hastière	*In situ* (concerted release)
	2.4×10^3		Waulsor	Laboratory
	3.5×10^3		Anseremme	Laboratory
Sr	7.4×10^2	1.0×10^3	Monsin	*In situ*
	1.7×10^2		Monsin	*In situ*
	1.5×10^2	4.1×10^2	Hastière	*In situ*
Zr	1.3×10^5		Monsin	*In situ*
Cs	5.0×10^3		Monsin	*In situ* (^{134}Cs)
	6.6×10^3		Monsin	*In situ* (^{137}Cs)
	2.8×10^3		Monsin	*In situ* (concerted release)
	3.2×10^3		Ivoz-Val Benoît	*In situ* (concerted release)

The transfer of radionuclides dissolved in the water phase to living organisms (direct contamination for aquatic plants and for animals fed uncontaminated feed under laboratory or fish-farming conditions) is quantified by a concentration factor (CF_{eq}, in l/kg) that expresses the ratio, at equilibrium, of the contamination level in the organisms ($[\ ]_{org.}$, in Bq/kg) to that in water ($[\ ]_{water}$, in Bq/l):

$$CF_{eq} = \frac{[\ ]_{org.}}{[\ ]_{water}}. \qquad (6.42)$$

In aquatic animals, the transfer factor can also be related to the contamination in their feed and expressed by a so-called trophic transfer factor (TTF) as the ratio at equilibrium between the contamination levels in two consecutive trophic levels (in Bq/kg):

$$TTF = \frac{[\ ]_{\text{upper trophic level org.}}}{[\ ]_{\text{lower trophic level org.}}}. \qquad (6.43)$$

In animals, a direct pathway (resulting from direct contamination by substances dissolved in the water phase) can be distinguished from an indirect pathway (due to contaminated food ingestion). The latter pathway is often preponderant in the long term: wild fish caught in the Columbia River downstream from the Hanford nuclear site were about 100 times more contaminated than individuals of the same species from fish-farming, grown in the same water but fed uncontaminated food. However, if the contribution of the direct (water) pathway can be distinguished from that of the indirect (food chain) pathway under laboratory conditions, this partitioning between both pathways is practically impossible in reality. Therefore one generally assumes that the whole system has reached equilibrium and the CF (in l/kg) in aquatic animals can be calculated as the activity concentration ratio in the considered organisms to that of water, regardless of the path of radioactivity.

It is important to note that, depending on the author, concentration levels in an organism or in specific organs are expressed on a dry or a fresh weight basis and that the activity level in water reflects in some cases the soluble fraction (filtered water) and in others the total activity in the water phase, including the activity associated with suspended matter. Part of the variability observed in the literature can be attributed to the difficulty in finding out what is meant by the "activity of water" [48,50].

The accumulation dynamic can be approximated by the relation

$$CF_{\mathrm{t}} = CF_{\mathrm{eq}} \times \left[1 - \sum_{i=1}^{n} \alpha_i \times e^{-\lambda_i \times t} \right] \text{ with } \sum_{i=1}^{n} \alpha_i = 1, \qquad (6.44)$$

where

α_i = fraction corresponding to the ith accumulation compartment (dimensionless),

λ_i = kinetic factor for the ith accumulation compartment (per sec).

As mentioned above, CF values found in the literature can be related to the animal fresh or dry weight, and it is not always clear which fraction of the radionuclides in the water phase is considered. However, even when estimated with the very same method, CF values for a given species can vary over several orders of magnitude. These variations can be explained by differences in the physicochemical characteristics of the water phase (salinity, pH, E_h, stable isotope/analog content, concentration and type of suspended matter) as well as variations in the animal's diet, which depends on the season and the age (size) of the individual.

For instance, large differences in the accumulation of some radionuclides are observed between marine and freshwater organisms (Table 6.7), even if the ranges of values largely overlap. Some radioelements (cesium, rubidium, strontium, tellurium) are more concentrated by freshwater organisms. For example, the mean

TABLE 6.7
Mean Transfer Factors for Marine and Freshwater Fish and Invertebrates [55]

Element	Freshwater		Seawater	
	Fish	Invertebrates	Fish	Invertebrates
H	0.9	0.9	0.9	0.9
Na	100	200	0.07	0.19
Mn	400	900	550	400
Fe	100	3,200	3,000	20,000
Co	50	200	100	1,000
Ni	100	100	100	250
Cu	50	400	670	1,700
Zn	2,000	10,000	2,000	50,000
Rb	2,000	1,000	8.3	17
Sr	30	100	2	20
Y	25	1,000	25	1,000
Zr	3.3	6.7	200	80
Nb	30,000	100	30,000	100
Tc	15	5	10	50
Ru	10	300	3	1,000
Te	400	6,100	10	100
I	15	5	10	50
Cs	2,000	1,000	40	25
La	25	1,000	25	1,000
Ce	1	1,000	10	600

radiocesium concentration factor is about 900 l/kg (range 80 to 4000 l/kg) for freshwater plants and 50 l/kg (range 20 to 240 l/kg) for seaweeds [54]. The corresponding values for radiocobalt are 6800 l/kg in freshwater systems and 550 l/kg in the marine environment. These differences are explained by the salinity and, more precisely, by the stable isotope/analog content. Other radio-elements (iodine, zinc, copper, iron) are more accumulated by most marine organisms than by freshwater organisms.

At the time of the Chernobyl fallout, river fish were only exposed during a very short period of time to a high radiocesium content in the water and their food; they consequently showed lower cesium contamination levels than fish from lakes, where the radioactivity residence time was longer. Moreover, the estimated *in situ* [137]Cs effective half-life of 100 to 200 days for river fish was short compared to the value of several years for species from oligotrophic lakes. It was observed that plankton-eating species were the first to reach their maximum contamination level. Carnivorous species reach their maximum later, but the level achieved is higher than that of plankton eaters. Bottom feeders were the least contaminated compared to plankton eaters and carnivores.

6.5   MODELING THE TRANSFER OF RADIONUCLIDES

The behavior and fate of radioactive pollutants in nature is often difficult to grasp. This is especially true when trying to assess future situations or to reconstruct exposures that occurred in the past. Therefore assessing the impact of environmental releases of radionuclides often calls for modeling to extrapolate beyond the limits of observations and experimentation.

Models are simplified descriptions of systems and may be verbal, mathematical, or physical. Mathematical models are constructed from mathematical equations and appropriate numerical values, or parameters, representing natural processes. Each equation presented in the previous sections to describe a particular process can be considered a mathematical model. The logical combination of these individual models within a branched structure aims to depict, step by step, the path of radioactivity in a given ecosystem and allows us to calculate, from a given discharge, the concentrations in the different compartments of the system. From concentrations in the organisms' tissues, a last dose conversion submodel translates becquerels per kilogram into grays and sieverts.

6.5.1   Model Roles and Uses

Models are mainly used to assess the radiological impact of environmental radioactivity and to predict the doses for man and the environment from various sources. They may consider either NORMs (i.e., uranium and thorium, and their respective descendants, among which are radium and radon) or fission and activation products from nuclear bomb testing, the nuclear fuel cycle, and medical applications. They can be applied to either actual (routine or accidental releases) or hypothetical evaluation of the impact of a possible accident.

The information derived from models lets radiation protection authorities make decisions regarding the issue of a building or operating license for new nuclear installations. Later, it allows them to verify the operating license and, when needed, to revise release permits. In accident situations, dose assessment can direct decision makers regarding evacuation of a population or establishment of a consumption ban for contaminated products. Models must also be able to predict the impact of environmental conditions on the efficiency of countermeasures as well as the expected consequences of the implementation of remedial actions.

Modeling is also used to trace radiopollutants back to the source and to reconstruct the conditions of a past release on the basis of contamination levels measured in environmental bioindicators. Such an approach has been applied in the period since the Chernobyl accident to estimate the composition of the release. Models enable radioecologists to check their understanding of the structure and functioning of ecosystems through comparisons between predictions and observations.

6.5.2   Model Building

Models may be constructed as initially complex models, as replicas of the real world, and discarding nonessential details, or, in contrast, as initially simple models starting with the most essential elements and adding others as needed. Whichever building process is used, model construction is a multistage process that includes a problem definition (scenario), formulation of the conceptual model, development of the mathematical model, estimation of parameter values, calculation of the model output results, and validation of the results by comparison with field measurements.

6.5.2.1 Definition of the Relevant Scenario

The first step in model construction is the definition of the context (characteristics of the release, ecosystem of concern, season, weather conditions) of the release and the identification of the main protagonists (air, water, soil, plant and animal species, general population or critical groups) and the relations between them. This step is generally straightforward, but some elements may be forgotten or ignored, impacting the accuracy of the predictions. For example, contamination through mushroom consumption was generally not considered until measurements carried out after the Chernobyl accident showed this potential critical pathway.

6.5.2.2 Formulation of the Conceptual Model

Once the scenario is thoroughly defined, it has to be translated into a conceptual model. This conceptual model is made up of an ensemble of distinct compartments, interconnected in chains or trees by exchange relations representing individual processes and mechanisms (Figure 6.12). Within the conceptual model, the number of compartments and processes considered depends on the design of a particular scenario, the need for simplification of the real world (e.g., by not considering each individual species), and the feasibility of gathering reliable parameters for the quantification of each individual process.

The conceptual model is necessarily a simplification of reality and its construction relies mainly on the expert judgment and good common sense of its designers. Each compartment is a single entity with typical input, transformation, and output kinetics of a given compound or substance. As such, a compartment is characterized by a parameter representing its apparent or real "volume" and kinetic parameters quantifying the input, transformation, and output fluxes.

These fluxes are most often first-order kinetics (linear response model), that is, the flux of a substance from compartment A to compartment B is directly proportional to its concentration in compartment A, on the whole concentration range. When a transfer process does not respond to a first-order kinetic, it will be referred to a nonlinear response model.

A system is defined as being in (steady state) equilibrium when the inputs strictly compensate the outputs and when the concentration within each compartment remains fairly constant in time. Such a situation is possible for chronic exposure to steady contaminant levels or in the case of elements where absorption and excretion are homeostatically regulated (e.g., K^+ concentration in animal tissues).

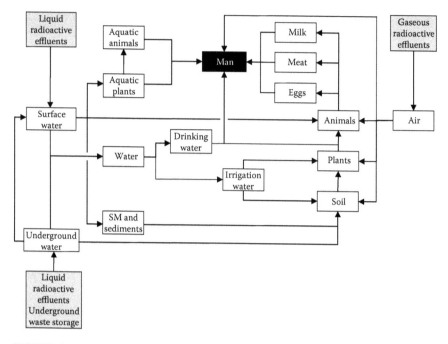

FIGURE 6.12 Conceptual model describing the transfer of liquid and gaseous radioactive effluents to man.

6.5.2.3 Development of the Mathematical Model

While the conceptual model essentially identifies the many processes, paths, compartments, and interactions between compartments needed to describe the scenario, the mathematical model translates the concept into a coherent set of simultaneous equations. It is a tool that generates a quantitative estimation of the processes and interactions the radionuclides undergo within the environment. All mathematical models should be tested and validated.

6.5.2.4 Estimation of Parameter Values

The constants and independent variables of the equations of an environmental transfer model are referred to as the model parameters. These parameters are best estimated from environmental or experimental data obtained under conditions representative of the situation to be addressed. Of course, data gathered for the specific ecosystem considered (site-specific data), when available, provide the most reliable predictions. It is essential to note that even if the scenario and the structure of the model are well defined, improper parameters will never provide satisfactory results.

Model parameters can be subdivided into four categories:

- Those relating to the source term: the time and duration of the release, release kinetics, quantitative and qualitative compositions of the release (spectrum and speciation of the emitted radionuclides).
- Those relating to physical transport and dispersion: wind or current velocity and direction and their variations, rain duration and intensity, atmospheric stability class, water velocity in soil, soil porosity, suspended matter in the water column, K_d.
- Those relating to biological transfers: biological availability of radionuclides for uptake and its variation according to the physicochemical properties of the substrate, soil to plant transfer and translocation toward edible organs as a function of the season, agricultural practices, weathering processes, uptake and accumulation by animals.
- Those relating to human exposure: localization of the habitat, way of life, dietary habits, physiologic and sanitary status of the general population or critical groups.

Considering the complexity and variability of the ecosystems as well as the multiplicity of the situations that can be addressed, it is a real challenge gathering all the experimental data that is needed to estimate the numerous parameters for a given scenario. Often the only alternative is to use average parameters or "best estimates," with questions regarding their representativeness for the conditions addressed.

6.5.2.5 Calculation of Model Predictions

At this stage the calculation is a matter of transforming the equations into a relevant algorithm that can be run on a host computer or PC. However, this step may also generate some errors due to numerical approximations for equation solving and programming bugs.

6.5.3 UNCERTAINTIES AND ERRORS ASSOCIATED WITH MODELING

Several factors may impair the reliability of model predictions. They can be divided into five groups:

- Errors due to an inadequate definition and inappropriate conceptualization of the situation to be addressed and of the scenario.
- Errors associated with an incorrect formulation of the conceptual model.
- Errors in the translation of the conceptual model into the mathematical model.

- Uncertainties inherent in the estimation of parameter values and their statistical distribution or a lack of knowledge relative to the value of parameters relevant for a specific scenario.
- Errors, inaccuracies, and approximations at the level of algorithms and calculations.

Estimating the reliability of model predictions is, *a priori*, extremely difficult because of possible mistakes in the exposition of the problem and the definition of the scenario, since this is essentially based on expert judgment. Likewise, the adequacy of the conceptual model formulation is also a matter of expert judgment and experience, unless there are enough experimental data to allow a thorough validation of the model over a wide range of environmental conditions. In the absence of such datasets, it is impossible to ascertain that no exposure path has been forgotten.

One should also remember that modifications of the assessment question or context may enhance the importance of processes previously neglected as marginal. Errors and uncertainties associated with previously unimportant processes may become significant, even dominate, when the scenario is changed and a model that proved reliable for the initial assessment problem starts to mispredict an even slightly different situation.

6.5.4 MODEL VALIDATION

An obvious model validation method consists of comparing the prediction results with field datasets that are completely independent from the data used to derive the model parameters. If predictions are in agreement with field data, there is a chance that the mathematical formulation is an acceptable representation of the real phenomena. However, the modeler must keep in mind that even concordances may tend to confirm the reliability of his model; a single large discordance may be enough to force the modeler to reconsidering his work or at least to limit the validity range of his model.

In the absence of independent datasets, model intercomparison is another technique that has proved useful to validate hypotheses and computer codes. This method offers no accuracy estimation, however, because of the lack of independent datasets. When discrepancies are evidenced, it is generally difficult to judge which tool provides the best representation of reality. However, this comparison is useful for pointing out obvious mistakes and weaknesses and forces designers to share information and learn about possible alternative approaches. An absence of discrepancy between models is not necessarily proof that the tested models work correctly and are reliable.

6.5.5 MODEL TYPES

Depending on the objectives that have been set and on the particular problem considered, different types of models can be used.

6.5.5.1 Screening Models

By the hypotheses and parameter values that they use, screening models are designed to provide conservative results, that is, they tend to overestimate concentrations and exposure doses compared to reality. These models are designed to provide a quick ranking of potential nuclear plant sites or practices in terms of radiological impact on the population and the environment. They can also identify radionuclides, compartments, and transfer pathways of particular importance.

Screening models must be used with caution, as their inherent simplicity may neglect important processes. It is also essential that all the hypotheses used and parameters chosen for model construction be conservative and remain so for all environmental conditions likely to occur within the screening study.

6.5.5.2 Emergency Models

Emergency models are typically used in radiological crisis management. They have to provide a quick assessment in the case of an accident leading to radioactive discharge. They must enable authorities to rapidly make appropriate decisions in order to protect populations at risk (sheltering, stable iodine intake, evacuation, protection of the food chain). Thus emergency models are simple models. On the basis of limited and easily obtainable information (e.g., wind velocity and direction, atmospheric stability class, release height, river water velocity), they must be able to provide rapid extrapolation regarding the transport, dispersion, and deposition of radionuclides. They deal principally with the short-term consequences and are thus limited to short-term environmental processes such as atmospheric dispersion (external exposure due to radioactive cloud, inhalation, and soil deposition) and dispersion in surface waters (contamination of drinking water). Most do not include food chain contamination or ingestion of contaminated foodstuffs.

6.5.5.3 Generic Models

Generic models attempt to replicate the real world as exactly as possible. They are complex models and designers must balance representing nature in its complexity and all individual transfer mechanisms, while still creating a tool that remains usable. It is irrelevant, not to mention impossible, to explicitly consider a mechanism which, by the end of the day, cannot be characterized in terms of kinetic or thermodynamic constants from observations or experimental evidence (e.g., specifically considering the interactions of radionuclides with each mineral fraction or each clay species in a soil). Therefore generic models, although they take into account all transfer paths, generally neglect the pathways of minor importance and implicitly group within a single step some intermediate paths that cannot be directly characterized by observation or experimentation.

6.5.5.4 Experimental Models

An experimental model can be considered a type of generic model that focuses on a specific process within the transfer chain. Because their scope is limited, they can envisage the processes and mechanisms down to smaller details. Their goal is to check and improve our understanding of particular mechanisms that are experimentally tested.

6.5.5.5 Deterministic and Stochastic Models

A deterministic model is a model in which none of the parameters is represented by a random variable: in other words, all model parameters are represented by single discrete values (e.g., the average of experimentally estimated transfer factors without its associated variability). The results provided by these models are discrete values.

A stochastic or probabilistic model is a model in which at least one parameter is represented by a random variable and its associated distribution function (normal, lognormal, triangular, uniform on a given domain). Therefore, results calculated by these models have a random distribution.

6.5.5.6 Equilibrium and Dynamic Models

Equilibrium models are designed to assess the consequences of routine discharges, rather constant in time, so that all compartments in the receiving ecosystem can reach steady-state equilibrium. Of course, the structure of the ecosystem must also be stable; that is, the relative importance of its compartment and their properties cannot drastically change within a short period of time relative to the time needed to achieve equilibrium. Equilibrium is reached after a period of time, the duration of which is proportional to the transfer velocities between the compartments of the system and the capacities of these compartments. In such a case, transfer parameters from one compartment to another are represented by equilibrium constants (K_d, soil to plant transfer factors [B_v], plant to animal transfer factors [F_m, F_f, F_e]).

Dynamic models are used in nonequilibrium situations, namely to describe and assess accidental releases, variable discharges in time, and situations when the system characteristics change too quickly to allow them to reach equilibrium. In these conditions, model parameters must be represented by transfer fluxes.

6.5.6 Uncertainty Analysis

Even when a model has been duly validated, a certain degree of statistical uncertainty will still remain associated with its predictions. This uncertainty is due to the variability in the available experimental data used to estimate the parameters. Hence the uncertainty associated with a prediction tends to increase with the impossibility to fully grasp a situation in its entirety (e.g., for very long-term predictions or radionuclide transport in deep geological layers). In such cases, the statistical distribution (probability density function) of each random parameter must be reconsidered and possibly corrected by taking into account potential changes in environmental conditions.

An estimation of the uncertainty model predictions can be obtained by different methods, including variance propagation, moment matching, and numerical methods known as Monte Carlo methods (e.g., simple random sampling or Latin hypercube sampling). Monte Carlo methods are widely used in environmental modeling, especially for complex models.

A Monte Carlo uncertainty analysis consists of ranking all random parameters in terms of their weight in the final assessment, and then, for each one within the set selected as the most important ones, to define its statistical distribution within its maximum applicable range. Thereafter, for each selected parameter, a value is generated at random based on the probability density function, taking into account dependencies between factors (e.g., high negative correlation between K_d and B_v) and conditional probabilities. This randomly generated value is introduced in the model together with those obtained in a similar way for the other parameters and the model is run to provide a prediction. This entire process is repeated a large number of times to generate prediction values (Figure 6.13). The distribution of the prediction results are then plotted and analyzed to provide a quantitative estimation of the model confidence (e.g., as a variance or confidence interval).

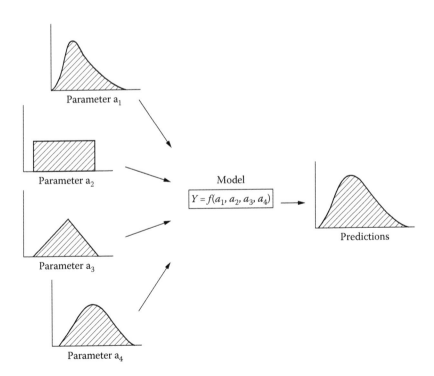

Parameter a_1

Parameter a_2

Model

$Y = f(a_1, a_2, a_3, a_4)$

Predictions

Parameter a_3

Parameter a_4

FIGURE 6.13 Schema of uncertainties propagation through a model.

6.5.7 SENSITIVITY ANALYSIS

A sensitivity analysis models the uncertainty of parameters and identifies those that have the greatest influence on variations in model prediction. It consists of considering each model parameter separately, varying it over a reasonable range, and observing the relative change in model response. In practice, each parameter is increased or decreased by a constant factor (within its uncertainty range) while other parameters remain unchanged. The influence of this perturbation on the prediction is translated as the relative variation of the prediction to that of the modified factor (Figure 6.14). The tested parameter is less sensitive as the variation of the prediction gets close to zero.

Sensitivity analyses enable model designers to identify critical transfer processes and the parameters that contribute most to the variability of model prediction. Hence sensitive parameters must be determined carefully for specific scenarios. Moreover, this analysis also points out the mechanisms most sensitive to the implementation of countermeasures.

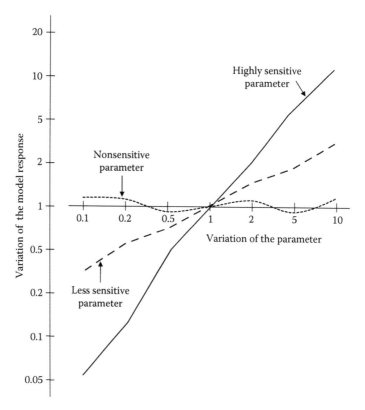

FIGURE 6.14 Example of a sensitivity analysis simulated for model parameters intervening in the model equations as numerator.

REFERENCES

1. Pasquill, F., The estimation of the dispersion of airborne material, *Meteorol. Mag.*, 90, 33, 1961.
2. Pasquill, F., *Atmospheric Diffusion*, Van Nostrand, London, 1962.
3. McElroy, J.L., A comparative study of urban and rural dispersion, *J. Appl. Meteorol.*, 8, 19, 1969.
4. McElroy, J.L. and Pooler, F., *St. Louis Dispersion Study, Vol. II — Analysis*, Publication no. AP-53, National Air Pollution Control Administration, Arlington, Virginia, 1968.
5. Klug, W., Ein Verfahren zur Bestimmung der Ausbreitungsbedigungen aus synoptischen Beobachtungen, *Staub-Reinhalt. Luft*, 29, 143, 1969.
6. Bultynck, H., Mallet, L., Sharma, L.N., and Van der Parren, J., Atmospheric dilution factors and calculation of doses in the environment of SCK•CEN Mol for short and long duration stack discharges, Report BLG-446, SCK•CEN, Mol, Belgium, 1970.
7. Vogt, K.J., Empirical investigations of the diffusion of waste air plumes in the atmosphere, *Nucl. Technol.*, 34, 43, 1977.
8. Doury, A., Une méthode de calcul pratique et générale pour la prévision numérique des pollutions véhiculées par l'atmosphère, Rapport CEA R4280 (Rev. 1), 1976.
9. Gifford, F.A., Use of meteorological observations for estimating atmospheric dispersion, *Nucl. Safety*, 2, 47, 1961.
10. Sutton, O.G., The theoretical distribution of airborne pollution from factory chimneys, *Q. J. R. Meteorol. Soc.*, 73, 426, 1947.
11. University of California, Lawrence Livermore National Laboratory, Hotspot, version 2.06, available at http://www.llnl.gov/nai/technologies/hotspot/, 2005.
12. Brenk, H.D., Fairobent, J.E., and Markee, E.H. Jr., Transport of radionuclides in the atmosphere, in *Radiological Assessment: A Textbook on Environmental Dose Analysis*, Till, J.E. and Meyer, H.R., eds., ORNL-5968, U.S. Department of Commerce, National Technical Information Service, Washington, DC, 1983.
13. Mayall, A., Modelling the dispersion of radionuclides in the atmosphere, in *Modelling Radioactivity in the Environment*, Scott, E.M., ed., Elsevier, Amsterdam, 11, 2003.
14. International Atomic Energy Agency, *Generic Models and Parameters for Assessing the Environmental Transfer of Radionuclides from Routine Releases: Exposure of Critical Groups*, IAEA Safety Series no. 57, STI/PUB/611, International Atomic Energy Agency, Vienna, Austria, 1982.
15. Vandecasteele, C.M., Zeevaert, T., and Kirchmann, R., Factors influencing the transfer of radionuclides in agricultural food chains, in *Anticarcinogenesis and Radiation Protection*, 2nd edition, Nygaard, O.F. and Upton, A.C., eds., Plenum Press, New York, 181, 1991.
16. Chamberlain, A.C., Interception and retention of radioactive aerosols by vegetation, *Health Phys.*, 4, 57, 1970.
17. Chamberlain, A.C., Transport and capture of particles by vegetation, in *Plants and Their Atmospheric Environment, Proceedings of the British Ecology Society Symposium*, Edinburgh, 1979.
18. Simmonds, J.R. and Linsley, G.S., Parameters for modelling the interception and retention of deposits from atmosphere by grain and leafy vegetables, *Health Phys.*, 43, 679, 1982.

19. Russell, R.S., Entry of radioactive material into plants, in *Radioactivity and Human Diet*, Russell, R.S., ed., Pergamon Press, Oxford, 89, 1966.

20. Russell, R.S. and Possingham, J.V., Physical characteristics of fallout and its retention on herbage, in *Progress in Nuclear Energy, Series VI, Biological Sciences 3*, Loutit, J.F. and Russell, R.S., eds., Pergamon Press, Oxford, 2, 1961.

21. Chamberlain, A.C., Aspects of the deposition of radioactive and other gases and particles, *Int. J. Air Pollut.*, 3, 63, 1960.

22. Hungate, F.P., Stewart, J.D., Uhler, R.L., and Cline, J.F., Decontamination of plants exposed to a simulated reactor burn, Report HW-63173, U.S. Atomic Energy Commission, Washington, DC, 1960.

23. Chadwick, R.C. and Chamberlain, A.C., Field loss of radionuclides from grass, *Atmos. Environ.*, 4, 51, 1970.

24. Baes, C.F. III and Sharp, R.D., A proposal for estimation of soil leaching and leaching constants for use in assessment models, *J. Environ. Qual.*, 12, 17, 1983.

25. Vandecasteele, C.M., Baker, S., Förstel, H., Muzinsky, M., Millan, R., Madoz-Escande, C., Tormos, J., Sauras, T., Schulte, E., and Colle, C., Interception, retention and translocation under greenhouse conditions of radiocaesium and radiostrontium from a simulated accidental source, *Sci. Tot. Environ.*, 278, 199, 2001.

26. U.S. Atomic Energy Commission, *Summary of Available Data on the Strontium-90 Content of Foods and of Total Diets in the United States*, Report HASL-90, U.S. Atomic Energy Commission, New York, 1960.

27. Müller, H. and Pröhl, G., ECOSYS-87: a dynamic model for assessing radiological consequences of nuclear accidents, *Health Phys.*, 64, 232, 1993.

28. Higgins, N.A. and Jones, J.A., *Methods for Interpreting Monitoring Data Following an Accident in Wet Conditions*, NRPB-W34, Health Protection Agency, London, 2003.

29. Pröhl, G., Radioactivity in the terrestrial environment, in *Modelling Radioactivity in the Environment*, Scott, E.M., ed., Elsevier, Amsterdam, 87, 2003.

30. Miller, C.W. and Hoffman, F.O., An examination of the environmental half-time for radionuclides deposited on vegetation, *Health Phys.*, 45, 731, 1983.

31. Hoffman, F.O. and Baes, C.F. III, A statistical analysis of selected parameters for predicting food chain transport and internal doses of radionuclides, NUREG CR-1004, Oak Ridge National Laboratory, Oak Ridge, Tennessee, 1979.

32. Konoplev, A.V. and Bulgakov, A.A., Kinetics of radionuclide leaching from fuel particles in the soil around the Chernobyl nuclear power plant, in *Ten Years Terrestrial Radioecological Research Following the Chernobyl Accident, Proceedings of the International Symposium on Radioecology*, Vienna, Austria, April 22–24, 61, 1996.

33. Schulz, R.K., Soil chemistry of radionuclides, *Health Phys.*, 11, 1317, 1965.

34. Sibley, T.H. and Myttenaere, C., *Application of Distribution Coefficients to Radiological Assessment Models*, Elsevier Applied Science, London, 1986.

35. Hilton, J. and Comans, R.N.J., Chemical forms of radionuclides and their quantification in environmental samples, in *Radioecology: Radioactivity and Ecosystems*, Van der Stricht, E. and Kirchmann, R., eds., Fortemps, Liège, 2001.

36. Bell, J.N.B., Minski, M.J., and Grogan, H.A., Plant uptake of radionuclides, *Soil Use Manage.*, 4, 76, 1988.

37. Moorby, J., The foliar uptake and translocation of caesium, *J. Exp. Bot.*, 15, 457, 1964.

38. Aarkrog, A., Radionuclide levels in mature grain related to radiostrontium content and time of direct contamination, *Health Phys.*, 28, 557, 1975.

39. Middleton, L.J., Radioactive strontium and caesium in edible parts of crop plants after foliar contamination, *Int. J. Radiat. Biol.*, 1, 387, 1959.

40. Zach, R. and Mayoh, K.R., Soil ingestion by cattle: a neglected pathway, *Health Phys.*, 46, 426, 1984.

41. Zach, R., Contribution of inhalation by food animals to man's ingestion dose, *Health Phys.*, 49, 737, 1985.

42. Stara, J.F., Nelson, N.S., Della Rosa, R.J., and Bustad, L.K., Comparative metabolism of radionuclides in mammals: a review, *Health Phys.*, 20, 113, 1971.

43. Vandecasteele, C.M., Garten, C.T. Jr., Van Bruwaene, R., Janssens, J., Kirchmann, R. and Myttenaere, C., Chemical speciation of technetium in soil and plants: impact on soil-plant-animal transfer, in *Speciation of Fission and Activation Products in the Environment*, Bulman, R.A. and Cooper, J.R., eds., Elsevier Applied Science, London, 368, 1986.

44. Sullivan, M.F., Actinide absorption from the gastrointestinal tract, in *Actinides in Man and Animals*, Wrenn, M.E., eds., RD Press, Salt Lake City, Utah, 311, 1981.

45. Sullivan, M.F., Garland, T.R., Cataldo, D.A., Wildung, R.E., and Drucker, H., Absorption of plutonium from the gastrointestinal tract of rats and guinea pigs after ingestion of alfalfa containing Pu-238, *Health Phys.*, 38, 215, 1980.

46. Kirchmann, R., Charles, P., Van Bruwaene, R., and Remy, J., Distribution of tritium in the different organs of calves and pigs after ingestion of various tritiated feeds, *Curr. Top. Radiat. Res. Q.*, 12, 291, 1975.

47. Sullivan, M.F. and Rümmler, P.S., Absorption of U-233, Np-237, Pu-238, Am-241 and Cm-244 from the gastrointestinal tracts of rats fed an iron-deficient diet, *Health Phys.*, 54, 311, 1988.

48. Blaylock, B.G., Radionuclide data bases available for bioaccumulation factors for freshwater biota, *Nucl. Safety*, 23, 427, 1982.

49. Eisenbud, M., The status of radioactive waste management: needs for reassessment, *Health Phys.*, 40, 429, 1981.

50. National Council on Radiation Protection, Assessment of radionuclides released to surface waters, in *Radiological Assessment: Predicting the Transport, Bioaccumulation and Uptake by Man of Radionuclides Released to the Environment*, Report no. 76, National Council on Radiation Protection, Bethesda, Maryland, 1984.

51. Smitz, J.S. and Everbecq, E., Modelling of the behaviour of radionuclides in the aquatic ecosystem, in *Proceedings of the Seminar on the Cycling of Long-Lived Radionuclides in the Biosphere: Observations and Models*, vol. I, CEC-Ciemat, 267, 1987.

52. Odum, E.P., *Fundamentals of Ecology*, 3rd edition, W.B. Saunders, Philadelphia, 1971.

53. Duursma, E.K., Chemistry of sediments, in *Annual Report of the International Laboratory on Marine Radioactivity*, Monaco, IAEA Technical Report Series 98, 92, 1969.

54. Eisenbud, M., *Environmental Radioactivity*, 2nd edition, Academic Press, New York, 1973.

55. Nuclear Regulatory Commission, Calculation of annual doses to man from routine releases of reactor effluents for the purpose of evaluating compliance with 10 CFR part 50, appendix I, Regulatory Guide 1.109, Washington, DC, 1977.

56. Turner, D.B., *Workbook of Atmospheric Dispersion Estimates*, Publication no. 995-AP-26, U.S. Department of Health, Education, and Welfare, Washington DC, 1969.

7 Effects of Radioactivity on Plants and Animals

Kathryn A. Higley

CONTENTS

7.1 INTRODUCTION

The literature on the effects of ionizing radiation on plants and animals spans nearly a century. Early studies of radiation effects on drosophila were used to determine that it is a mutagen [1]. The primary intent of these early studies was to better elucidate the nature of radiation interactions to understand their impacts on people. A consequence of the development of nuclear weapons was the developing awareness of the existence and global distribution of radionuclides. Interest grew in understanding where radionuclides went in the environment and helped support numerous studies of radiation effects on species, populations, and ecosystems [2]. While the bulk of the studies have focused on the response of the individual, accidents such as Chernobyl have allowed ecosystem-level investigations to be conducted. Many of these studies are ongoing.

7.2 PHYSICS, CHEMISTRY, AND BIOLOGY OF RADIATION INTERACTIONS

Understanding the effect radiation has on living tissues requires that one first examine the physics and chemistry of the initial interaction. Living cells are

209

composed in large part of water. The remainder consists of organic compounds — lipids, proteins, carbohydrates, and nucleic acids [3]. When ionizing radiation interacts within a cell it rapidly sets in motion a series of events that can lead to chemical and ultimately biological changes. The subsequent damage can be traced to the chemical changes that have come about due to the initial interactions of radiation. The nature and time frame for these events are discussed below. The magnitude of radiation exposure necessary to cause the effects is discussed later in this chapter.

7.2.1 TYPES OF IONIZING RADIATION

There are two types of ionizing radiation: electromagnetic and particulate. X and γ rays are the ionizing electromagnetic radiations. They differ primarily in their origins (atomic vs. nuclear transitions), but are otherwise similar in properties. When X or γ rays are absorbed in matter, energy is deposited — unevenly and in discrete packets. The amount of energy is generally sufficient to break chemical bonds. Hence these radiations are termed "ionizing."

The other type of ionizing radiation is particulate. The most common particulate radiations encountered in environmental settings are α and β particles. α particles are highly energetic helium nuclei lacking orbital electrons. They have a +2 charge when they are initially ejected from the nucleus during decay. β particles are highly energetic electrons that originate in the nucleus and may carry either a −1 or +1 charge.

7.2.2 PHYSICAL AND CHEMICAL ASPECTS OF IONIZING RADIATION INTERACTIONS

Absorption of ionizing radiation energy occurs through indirect and direct mechanisms. Charged particles such as α and β particles have enough kinetic energy to directly dislodge electrons and cause ionization of the atoms and molecules with which they interact. Electromagnetic radiation (X and γ rays) is classified as indirectly ionizing. The radiation must be absorbed in order to transfer its energy to an electron. The end result is virtually the same — the production of an excited or ionized atom.

The result of this interaction is the production of secondary electrons with some kinetic energy (energy of motion). In water, and other low atomic number materials, these secondary electrons have energies on the order of 10 to 70 eV [4]. The life span of these secondary electrons is very brief (approximately 10^{-15} sec) and during that time they transfer their energy to the surrounding environment as they move through it. The initial transfer of energy to water results in the formation of ionized and excited water molecules, most notably H_2O^+ (ionized water) and an electronically excited version of water, H_2O^*. These are accompanied by free electrons that have insufficient energy (less than 7.4 eV) to cause any additional excitation.

Following the initial interaction, the three species that have been created undergo additional changes. The ionized water molecule can interact with an adjacent water molecule to form the following compounds:

$$H_2O^+ + H_2O \rightarrow H_3O^+ + OH.$$

The excited water molecule, H_2O^*, can lose energy in two ways:

$$H_2O^* \rightarrow H_2O^+ + e$$

or

$$H_2O^* \rightarrow H + OH.$$

This process, although not as rapid as the initial ionization event, occurs in the time frame of 10^{-12} sec. The molecule H_2O^+ is an ion radical (it is both electrically charged and contains an unpaired electron). It has a short life span (less than 10^{-10} sec) and decays to form the highly reactive hydroxyl radical ($OH\cdot$), which has a life span of approximately 10^{-5} sec. Once these species have been produced, they go on to react chemically with their environment, based on diffusion-controlled reaction kinetics [4].

7.2.3 DIRECT AND INDIRECT RADIATION INTERACTION

Radiation interactions within cells are typically characterized as direct or indirect in nature. This characterization stems from the historical assessment that DNA is the principal target of concern with regard to radiation damage [3–5]. When radiation interactions occur in the cell, they may do so directly with the atoms of the target or with other atoms or molecules in the vicinity. For α particles, which are considered high linear energy transfer (LET) radiations, direct action is the dominant process by which the critical targets are affected. Sparsely or indirectly ionizing radiations such as β particles and X or γ radiation produce free radicals that can then diffuse and damage the critical target. This mode of delivering radiation damage is called indirect action. It accounts for roughly two-thirds of the damage caused by sparsely ionizing radiations [4].

Although DNA has generally been viewed as the most important target from the perspective of radiation damage, there is a wide range of molecules within the cell that can be adversely affected. These molecules vary in both size and molecular weight, and they too are impacted by the same direct and indirect effects of radiation discussed earlier. Broken chemical bonds, cross-linkages, and conformational changes are the resultant products of radiation interaction within the cell [4,5]. These altered molecules may hinder the molecule's biological function. For example, a change in the orientation of an enzyme or protein (a conformational change) could limit its ability to perform a function in a metabolic pathway. The result could be the interruption or cessation of certain functions [5].

7.2.4 Biological Consequences of Radiation Interaction

The consequences of ionizing radiation interaction can be seen at all levels of biological organization (molecule, cell, organ). However, it is important to note that while events may transpire at the molecular level, impacts do not automatically flow through to the higher levels of organization (individual, population, community, or ecosystem) [6–10].

When DNA is considered the critical target, the impacts of concern are the nature and extent of damage caused by charged particle tracks (or resultant chemical species). Single breaks in a strand of DNA, as well as ruptures in both strands (double-strand breaks), are the immediate products of ionizing radiation interaction within cells. As previously noted, ionization produces highly reactive products that break chemical bonds, including DNA molecules as well as cell membranes. Cell killing, mutation, and carcinogenesis are the longer-term consequences of these events. However, to complicate matters, many living cells have systems in place to repair damage to the DNA [11].

There are several characteristics of radiation that are important in determining the extent of the biological response. These include

- Type and energy of radiation (e.g., α, β, or γ). As noted previously, these can be densely ionizing radiations (i.e., α) that directly impact critical targets, or sparsely ionizing radiations (X or γ rays, or β particles), which have an indirect effect as their principle mode of radiation damage. These radiations are not the same with respect to their effectiveness in causing biological damage [12]. An absorbed dose of α particles, for example, can cause more biological damage than an equal absorbed dose of photons. In translating absorbed dose to a measure of biological effect, radiation "weighting" factors have been developed for humans. They have been assigned a value of 1 for photons and electrons and 20 for α particles. However, they account for the potential to cause cancer, a stochastic effect, and do not address deterministic effects. Data on deterministic radiation effects for α particles have been reviewed and evaluated by the International Commission on Radiological Protection (ICRP) [13] and appear to lie in the range of about 5 to 10 [12]. A weighting factor of one is typically used for electrons and photons, even for deterministic effects.
- Spatial distribution of delivered energy, both micro- and macroscopic. At the macroscopic scale, the physical unit that describes energy deposition is the absorbed dose (in Gy or rads). It is defined as the average energy absorbed in a target tissue or organ divided by its mass. However, this average value does not depict the enormous variability in energy deposition that occurs at the microscopic (e.g., cellular and molecular) level due to the stochastic nature of energy deposition events.

- Total dose (energy per mass) delivered. With moderate to high doses of sparsely ionizing radiation (greater than 100 mGy), cells and tissues receive a nearly uniform exposure [14]. However, for substantially lower doses (approximately 1 mGy) more than a third of the cells remain undamaged [11]. The number of cells struck by an ionizing event depends significantly on the radiation energy as well as the type of radiation (i.e., α, β, or γ).
- Rate at which the dose is delivered. It is well known that dose response can be modified by changing the duration of exposure [5]. The biological effects from low-LET radiation are smaller when low dose rates are used than for higher ones (0.5 to 1.0 Gy/min). Fractionation also can reduce the impact. High-LET radiations, because of the direct nature of the damage they inflict, do not show the same degree of dose-rate response.

Radiobiological studies have shown that, in general, cells most sensitive to the effects of ionizing radiation are those that are undifferentiated, well oxygenated, are highly metabolically active, and rapidly reproduce. In mammalian cells, the most sensitive are spermatogonia and erythroblasts, epidermal stem cells, and gastrointestinal stem cells [3,4,15,16]. The least sensitive are the highly differentiated and mitotically inactive nerve cells and muscle fibers. Interestingly, oocytes and lymphocytes are also very sensitive, although they are resting cells and consequently do not match the criteria noted earlier. The reasons for their sensitivity are unclear.

There are also several areas of radiobiological research that are challenging our fundamental understanding of radiation damage at the cellular level (where DNA has historically been viewed as the principal target of concern). Three of these areas are

- Genomic instability. Also known as genetic and chromosomal instability, it refers to genetic change occurring serially and spontaneously in cell populations as they replicate. The concept of genomic instability is that radiation can induce a genome-wide process of instability in cells. This instability is transmitted over many generations of cell replication, leading to an enhanced frequency of genetic changes occurring among the progeny of the original irradiated cell [17]. The phenomenon has been observed with cell systems *in vivo* and *in vitro* and for low- as well as high-LET radiation [18]. These effects have been noted not only in cells that have been hit by ionizing radiations, but by adjacent, unirradiated cells (see the section below on bystander effects). While genomic instability is generally accepted, there are many unanswered questions concerning the mechanisms, in particular how it is initiated and how it is maintained over many generations of cell replication [17,18].

- Bystander effects. The conventional model of radiation-induced damage requires damage of DNA either from direct interactions of radiation or from free radicals created nearby. Recent studies have demonstrated damage (such as altered gene expression) occurring in cells not directly exposed to radiation [18,19]. This is known as the bystander effect. There is evidence that this damage may be a consequence of intercellular signaling, production of cytokines, or free radical generation. It is also thought that these effects are related to inflammatory-type responses. The significance of the bystander effect as it relates to organisms and environmental consequences of radiation exposure is not yet known [17,18].

- Adaptive response. The technical literature contains an increasing number of studies that show that adaptive protection responses occur in living cells after single as well as protracted exposures to X or γ radiation at low doses [20]. This has been observed both *in vivo* and *in vitro* and has been documented across a wide range of organisms from bacteria and viruses to plants and animals. Two types of protection are identified. One prevents and repairs DNA damage, the other removes damaged cells. The adaptive response mechanism is not immediate, but develops, presumably in response to physiologic stress. It manifests within hours and may persist weeks to months. However, there are no strong data supporting adaptive response following exposures to high-LET radiation [5].

By convention, the delivery of radiation dose has been categorized as acute (short term) or chronic (protracted). The resultant impacts of exposure are further apportioned into deterministic or stochastic effects. There is some confusion in the application of the terminology, as well as imprecision in describing both. In general, large radiation doses (the definition of large depends upon the organism) delivered within a short period of time (an acute dose) leads to short-term, acute (deterministic) effects. The expression of acute effects does not preclude the later occurrence of stochastic impacts (stochastic meaning an effect for which the probability of occurrence, rather than the severity, is a function of dose without a threshold). The most notable stochastic effects are cancer and genetic effects.

Impairment of reproductive capability is one example of a deterministic effect [21]. A more severe one is death. Many effects, such as skin reddening or sterility, only appear when a threshold dose has been exceeded. There are also confounding factors (noted earlier) such as total dose, dose rate, fractionation, and partial body irradiation that can alter an organism's response.

Protracted (chronic), lower-dose radiation exposures that do not exceed the threshold for deterministic effects can still lead to increased probability for stochastic impacts. The definition of chronic depends on the life span and metabolism of the receptor, but it is generally on the order of days to weeks (or longer). Chronic irradiation effects data are generally given in terms of the daily dose (e.g., mGy/day) rather than the total dose (e.g., Gy).

7.3 EFFECTS OF RADIOACTIVITY ON INDIVIDUAL PLANTS AND ANIMALS

When radiation effects at the level of the organism are examined, it becomes apparent that radiosensitivity generally increases with increasing organism complexity [2,21,22]. The generally accepted hierarchy of radiosensitivity to acute radiation doses has mammals, including man, among the most radiosensitive, and primitive organisms (bacteria, protozoa, viruses) among the most resistant [2].

Extrapolations and generalizations of effects must be made with caution. Even within similar species, radiosensitivity can vary by more than an order of magnitude [21]. During the course of their life span, individuals may also exhibit a range of radiosensitivities, based on a number of factors, including age, health, and genetic predisposition. In general, the young are more radiosensitive than adults (which can be attributed to cell proliferation being higher). However, considering the wide range of organisms (plants, animals, viruses, bacteria) found in the environment, the United Nations Scientific Committee on the Effects of Atomic Radiation (UNSCEAR) [21] noted that the data do not allow one to "reliably predict the potential radiation effects in the wide variety of organisms likely to be present in a contaminated area."

The difficulty in providing clear-cut evaluations of the effect of radioactivity on plants and animals is that much of the available radiation effects data are based on short-duration (e.g., seconds to hours), high-dose exposures, which are expressed in terms of the total dose rather than a dose rate. These data, unaltered, do little to help address the issue of radiation exposures at low dose rates and in chronic conditions.

In a sweeping study, Rose [16] conducted an extensive, critical review of the published literature to summarize and categorize the levels at which radiation-induced changes were detected in organisms following both acute and chronic exposures. Three broad categories of impact were examined: death, behavioral or developmental, and teratogenic or genetic. This review encompassed more than 600 citations and included data from all five kingdoms: protista, animalia, monera, fungi, and plantae. Viruses were also examined.

The bulk of the work examined by Rose was conducted with animals and plants and utilizing X or γ radiation. It is interesting to note that considering the large dataset, only a few species were represented; the majority were mammalian. Most also focused on acute, high-dose exposures in laboratory.

Past approaches to addressing the absence of chronic exposure data have been to use the acute effects data to estimate which effects are expected from chronic exposures. This approach is very conservative because, as noted earlier, a much larger total dose can be tolerated if it is received gradually rather than all at once [16]. Repair and compensation mechanisms that can be used at low dose rates are overwhelmed if the dose is received rapidly. One example cited by Rose [16] is an acute:chronic ratio of 10 or more observed for the most sensitive stages of fish development, growth reduction in plants, and damage to somatic organs in mammals.

As part of the EPIC project (Environmental Protection from Ionizing Contaminants), a database of approximately 1600 records spanning 440 publications on dose-effects relationships for wildlife in northern temperate climate zones was recently published [23]. This database is built on records from Russian/FSU experimental field studies and addresses what had previously been a large gap in knowledge on low to moderate dose rate effects. As a consequence, much more information is now being made available on the effects of chronic radiation in animals. The data are still being reviewed, but some of the results are noted here.

In an article examining radiation protection criteria for northern wildlife, Sazykina [23] proposed that five potentially measurable parameters be considered when assessing the potential impacts of radiation exposure in the environment. Three of these categories were similar to those identified by Rose [16]. These five were

- Cytogenetic effects. Radiation interaction in tissue can leave indications at the cellular and subcellular level. One example of a molecular endpoint is reciprocal chromosome aberrations [25]. The advantage of examining this molecular marker is that the abundance of such aberrations can be related to cell killing, mutation and carcinogenesis, and also reproductive successes (for germ cells). The problem is that there are insufficient data at the present time to relate the chromosome aberrations to individual and population-level effects.
- Radiation hormesis. Similar to the mechanism of adaptive response, radiation hormesis is considered to be the consequence of stimulation of the immune system from low-level irradiation. While results have been observed, the data are inconsistent, and at this time do not appear to be useful as a measure of assessing impacts of dose.
- Morbidity. In the context of Sazykina [23], morbidity as a parameter referred to the appearance of illness and the general deterioration of specific aspects of an organism such as suppression of the immune system, changes in blood/lymph systems, and an overall decline in health.
- Reproductive effects. Reproductive organs are known to be sensitive to radiation exposure. Sazykina [23] included damage to both the reproductive organs of adults as well as its eggs and embryos. In its literature review of radiation effects on biota, the International Atomic Energy Agency (IAEA) [22] suggested that reproduction was an important endpoint for assessing the effects of radiation on plants and animals, within the context of developing guidelines for radiation protection. Cataloging the doses necessary to cause sterility is important because for some organisms a dose which may cause complete sterility may result in only minor changes within the organism [23]. And while sterilization may not directly impact the organism's life span, it may indirectly effect the population in which it lives [7]. While tissues and organs within an organism vary in their radiosensitivity,

reproductive processes and the early stages of development are seen as the most radiosensitive due to the ongoing activities of cell division and differentiation.

- Mortality and life shortening. The classic measure of radiation impact has been to measure mortality. Within confined experimental settings, determination of mortality and comparison of the life span of control as compared to exposed animals is relatively straightforward. In the natural environment, confounding factors may make the analysis more complicated [7,14,23–26].

While obscuring some of the finer points, it is possible to combine the work of Rose [16] and the summary of Sazykina [23] and an earlier summary of Brechignac [15] to develop an overall assessment of radiation exposure on organisms. These will be examined using the five-kingdom convention of Rose [16] and incorporating the effects analyses of Sazykina [23]. Rose noted that within individual kingdoms there was a wide range of sensitivity to radiation. Sometimes the response appeared beneficial rather than harmful at low radiation exposures.

- Animalia. The bulk of the literature on radiosensitivity is for mammals, and they have been observed to be the most radiosensitive, with lethal doses, of 6 to 10 Gy for small mammals and 1.5 to 2 5 Gy for the largest wild and domestic animals [15]. The lowest dose rate observed to cause death was in the range of 3 to 6 Gy/yr for several species of rodents [16].

  Protraction of the lethal dose such that it is delivered over the life span of the organism substantially decreased its impact. UNSCEAR [27] noted that if a mouse was given the lifetime equivalent of its lethal dose, 7 Gy, the mean reduction of the life span was estimated to be 5% from cancer induction. In summarizing the literature on radiation effects for animals, Brechignac [15] noted that while there was a variation between species, if dose rates were less than 4 Gy/yr the mortality rate of the corresponding population would not be seriously affected.

  The lowest chronic exposure to produce a detectable change in behavior or development was about 10^2 Gy/yr (detected in planarium worms and mud snails) [16]. For acute exposures, a dose of only 10^{-6} Gy could be visually detected in cockroaches.

  Reproductive capacity is more sensitive to the effects of radiation than life expectancy [2,15,16,26–29]. The lowest chronic exposure to produce a reliable teratogenic or genetic change (reduced birth mass and increased brain mass of laboratory rats irradiated as fetuses) was 3×10^{-3} Gy/yr. Acute exposures of 10^{-2} Gy to pregnant rats impaired the reflexes of their offspring. The lowest lethal dose rate was 3.6 Gy/yr and was found for several species of American rodents. The lowest dose rate found for detectable teratogenic or genetic effects was 3×10^{-3}

Gy/yr. This dose rate reduced the birth mass and increased the brain mass of laboratory rats irradiated as fetuses toward the end of the intrauterine life. The lowest single dose to cause a teratogenic effect was 10^{-2} Gy, which impaired reflexes in the offspring of irradiated pregnant rats [15,16].

It is important to note that while mammals have comprised the bulk of studies, work has been done on birds, reptiles, aquatic organisms, and invertebrates. The radiosensitivity of birds is similar to those of small mammals. Studies on reptiles, while appearing to show them as less radiosensitive, are being reexamined because of differences in physiology that may not have been appropriately accounted for [15]. Invertebrates, while less sensitive, still exhibit age-specific radiosensitivity, with gametogenesis, egg development, and their young being most sensitive.

In the aquatic environment, fish are the most sensitive. Doses of 10 to 25 Gy to ocean species are lethal, although embryos are substantially more sensitive (e.g., 0.16 Gy for salmon) [15,26]. Embryo development in fish and the process of gametogenesis appear to be the most radiosensitive stages of all aquatic organisms tested [22].

- Plantae. It has been noted that the plant kingdom contains the most radiosensitive species. The lowest acute dose, 0.8 Gy, killed a small proportion of young Douglas fir trees (*Pseudotsuga douglasii*). Yet a different species, eastern white pine (*Pinus strobus*), required doses of 2.7 Gy [16]. In his review of the literature, Brechignac [15] observed that literature values of lethal radiation doses are between 10 and 1000 Gy for plants. As has been reported several times, larger plants appear more radiosensitive than small ones. The order of radiosensitivity, from greatest to least, is conifers to deciduous trees, thicket species, herbaceous plants, lichens, and mushrooms.

The review by Rose [16] indicated that dose rates on the order of 6 Gy/yr were found to kill red pine (*Pinus resinosa*), but a 50% reduction in dose rate had no observable effect on pitch pine (*Pinus rigida*). Nonlethal effects on plants have also been observed, as well as variable sensitivity in plant structures. Nonlethal effects observed include inhibition of growth and seed production, delay in bud opening, increased leaf dormancy, and greater susceptibility to infestation [15]. Examples of ranges of sensitivity include seeds (very insensitive) and apical meristems (most sensitive). The data of others [15,26] is in general agreement with that of Rose [16], and dose rates of approximately 4 Gy/yr will produce only minor effects on sensitive plants and have minimal impacts on the large majority of plants in natural communities.

The literature has provided limited data on the radiosensitivity of other organisms. The data provided below are summarized from Rose [16].

- Protista. A dose of 100 Gy was lethal to diatoms (*Nitschi closterium*). An acute dose of 10^6 Gy temporarily slowed the rate of growth of slime mold.
- Fungi. Doses in excess of 600 Gy have failed to kill yeasts and molds (e.g., *Penicillium camemberti*). Species of lichens were predicted to be unaffected by dose rates up to 1800 Gy/yr.
- Viruses. Doses in excess of 440 Gy are required to inactive viruses.
- Monera. Doses in excess of 80 Gy are survived by blue-green algae (*Oscillatoria limosa*); bacteria (*Bacillus cereus*) survived doses of 2000 Gy. Studies on algae colonizing a reactor primary coolant estimated dose rates of 870 Gy/yr.

7.4 ECOLOGICAL CONSEQUENCES OF RADIATION EXPOSURE

While studies in laboratory settings can provide insights into the radiation responses of individual organisms, it can be difficult to extrapolate these data to a contaminated environment where entities of concern are exposed populations, communities, or ecosystems rather than individual members of species. Unfortunately studies of radiation effects at the level of populations, communities, and ecosystems have been limited. The few that have been done were *in situ* irradiation experiments from enclosures of natural systems to follow the dynamics of animal populations or in areas subjected to increased levels from accidental or intentional radioactive contamination [10,15,16]. Most of these studies lack sufficient rigor to support strong statements as to effect [15]. One extraordinary example is found at Chernobyl. Although severe impacts to biota occurred as a consequence of the reactor accident, a net ecological improvement has been measured. This is attributed to the removal of a more radiosensitive species (humans) from the environment [7,26].

In an effort to understand radiation effects on a broad scope, Polikarpov [10] developed a conceptual model that sought to address the issue of chronic exposure, across all levels of organization. He related specific ranges of dose rates with resultant impacts using a model that spanned 12 orders of magnitude from less than 10^{-5} to greater than 10^6 Gy/yr. This model contained five zones of exposure which summarized radiation effects on cells/organisms, populations, and biotic communities [10,28]. The lowest, zone 1 (less than 1×10^{-5} to 4×10^{-5} Gy/yr), was identified as the zone of biological uncertainty. The dose rate for this zone was below the natural background rate from cosmic radiation. The second, zone 2 (4×10^{-5} to 5×10^{-3} Gy/yr), was labeled the natural background, or the zone of well-being. Zone 3 (5×10^{-2} to 5×10^{-3} Gy/yr) was classified as a region where masking of the physiological effects of radiation exposure occurs, as the dose rates can overlap with those of natural background. In zone 4 (4×10^0 to 5×10^{-2} Gy/yr), there are effects on individuals, but these are masked by the interactions with the population and community. Finally, in zone 5 (4×10^0 to greater than 3×10^3 Gy/yr), the consequences are catastrophic to ecosystems because the damage to the underlying populations and communities is severe. Polikarpov also provided examples of environments that delivered dose rates corresponding to these zones. The zones proposed by Polikarpov appear to be supported by the current and past literature on radiological effects [10,15,16,23,28]. A comparison of the model of Polikarpov [10] with data from Rose [16] and Sazykina [23] is provided in Table 7.1.

It is relatively straightforward to identify ranges of exposure and potential effects. The difficulty arises in trying to measure them, either in the field or in a laboratory setting, and then interpret them with regard to an organism's radiosensitivity. The radiation field generated by a source is rarely uniform — either spatially or temporally. This makes an accurate determination of dose problematic. Several individuals are working on molecular probes in an effort to address this problem [7,25,29,30]. The utility of such tools is obvious, but their ability to link microscale measurements to ecosystem level impacts has not yet been demonstrated [7,25,29–31].

Also, until recently there were only a limited number of studies published in the Western literature that examined the responses of plant and animal populations to radiation exposure in their natural environments [15,23]. Instead, the bulk of the research has emphasized individual over population responses. Because of the ease and immediacy of information retrieval, mortality rather than reproduction was assessed. Similarly, acute rather than chronic doses were given. Due to technical considerations surrounding the delivery of doses, external γ irradiation rather than internal contamination studies were favored. All of these factors have contributed to an incomplete understanding of the consequences of low-level radiation exposure in natural settings [11,25,27,32].

In the last 15 years, acute and chronic radiation effects data have been reviewed by several organizations [16,21,22,33]. Based on their reviews, the National Council on Radiation Protection and Measurements (NCRP) [33] identified an expected safe level of exposure of approximately 4 Gy/yr (10 mGy/day) for populations of aquatic animals. Shortly thereafter the IAEA [22] identified an expected safe level of exposure of approximately 4 Gy/yr (10 mGy/day) for populations of terrestrial plants and an expected safe level of exposure of approximately 0.4 Gy/yr (1 mGy/day) for populations of terrestrial animals. At the time, these levels of exposure were selected based on the understanding that the population would be adequately protected if the dose rate to the maximally exposed individual did not exceed that level of exposure [22,33]. The radiological data suggest that approximately 0.4 Gy/yr represents a threshold for effects, however, the data are sparse for nonmammals, particularly with respect to ecosystem level effects.

It is also important to note that the previously proposed safe levels of exposure have largely been derived from observed dose-response relationships for deterministic effects. This has led to some concern that stochastic radiation effects, which might be important in the protection of biota, are not being adequately considered [7,34]. Information on stochastic effects in biota was considered in the 1996 UNSCEAR report on the effects of radiation on the environment [21], which concluded that as long as the dose was kept below the expected safe levels

TABLE 7.1
A Comparison of Dose-Effects Relationships Found in the Literature

Dose Rate, Gy/yr	Polikarpov [10]	Rose [16]	Sazykina [23]
$<1 \times 10^5$	Uncertainty		Natural background
4×10^5	Well-being		
4×10^4			
3×10^3		Teratogenic effects (Animalia)	
4×10^3	Physiologic masking		No data
5×10^3			
1×10^2		Developmental (Animalia)	
2×10^2		Behavioral (Animalia)	
4×10^2	Ecological masking		Minor cytogenetic effects, stimulation of vertebrate species
5×10^2			
2×10^1		Teratogenic (Plantae)	Threshold for minor effects on morbidity in vertebrates
4×10^1			
7×10^1			Threshold for reproductive effects on vertebrates
2×10^0			Threshold for life shortening of vertebrates, threshold for invertebrates and plants
3×10^0		Lethality (Animalia)	
4×10^0	Obvious effects		Life shortening of vertebrates; damage to conifers
6×10^0		Lethality (Plantae)	
4×10^1			Acute radiation sickness of vertebrates, death of conifers, damage to invertebrate young
4×10^2			
8.7×10^2		Lethality (Monera)	Acute radiation sickness of vertebrates, increased mortality of invertebrate young; damage to deciduous plants
3×10^3		Lethality (Fungi)	
5.3×10^3		Teratogenic (Monera)	

of exposure based on reproductive effects, stochastic effects should not be significant at a population level.

The available stochastic effects data are difficult to interpret in regard to harm to an individual organism [21,22,33,34]. The expected safe levels of exposure were based on the dose–response relationships for reproductive effects, rather than all effects that might be important for the viability of any given individual organism (e.g., early mortality). Thus the levels of exposure expected to protect the viability of natural populations may not be protective for individual members of a species. The implication was, however, that although a few individuals could be damaged, the population would remain viable [21,22,33].

7.5 CONCLUSION

Research on radiation effects on living systems spans more than half a century. It is well known that a range of more than four orders of magnitude exists in radiosensitivity among taxonomic groups, largely from differences in cellular and molecular characteristics [2,3,10,15,16,27,35]. Consequently discussions of radiation effects on plants and animals must take place within the context of the circumstances of exposure. As with humans, plants and animals can exhibit acute and chronic responses to ionizing radiation. Effects which can be documented at the cellular level may not transfer to observable impacts at the organism or ecosystem level. Studies on acute exposure of individuals may provide only limited insight into effects at the ecosystem level from chronic exposures. Current research is under way to try and link the data produced by molecular probes to impacts on organisms and populations. There are sufficient new data to help fill in many of the gaps in knowledge on the effects of chronic exposures [15,16,23,24]. While remaining in general agreement with past research, some differences have been found that can be attributed to environmental conditions of exposure [23].

Finally, at a very broad level, the preponderance of data suggest that the lowest dose rate at which deterministic effects of chronic irradiation would be expected from low-LET radiation are in the range of 0.4 to 1 Gy/yr. The lowest dose at which effects of acute irradiation might be observed is 0.01 Gy. It is important to note, however, that the complexity of the environment is such that adverse impacts might not be observed at considerably higher doses and dose rates.

REFERENCES

1 Muller, H.J., Artificial transmutation of the gene, *Science*, 66, 84, 1927.
2. Whicker, F.W. and Schultz, V., *Radioecology: Nuclear Energy and the Environment*, CRC Press, Boca Raton, FL, 1982.

3. Hall, E.J., *Radiobiology for the Radiologist*, 4th edition, J.B. Lippincott, Philadelphia, 1994.
4. Turner, J.E., *Atoms, Radiation, and Radiation Protection*, 2nd edition, Wiley-Interscience, New York, 1995.
5. Streffer, C., Bolt, H., Follesdal, D., Hall, P., Hengstler, J.G., Jakob, P., Oughton, D., Prieß, K., Rehbinder, E., and Swaton, E., *Low Dose Exposures in the Environment, Dose-Effect Relations and Risk Evaluation*, Springer, New York, 2004.
6. Florou, H., Tsytsugina, V., Polikarpov, G.G, Trabidou, G., Gorbenko, V., and Chaloulou, C.H., Field observations of the effects of protracted low levels of ionizing radiation on natural aquatic population by using a cytogenetic tool, *J Environ. Radioactiv.*, 75, 267, 2004.
7. Hinton, T.G., Bedford, J.S., Congdon, J.C., and Whicker, F.W., Effects of radiation on the environment: a need to question old paradigms and enhance collaboration among radiation biologists and radiation ecologists, *Radiat. Res.*, 162, 332, 2004.
8. Jackson, D., Copplestone, D., Stone, D.M., and Smith, G.M., Terrestrial invertebrate population studies in the Chernobyl exclusion zone, Ukraine, *Radioprotection*, 40, S857, 2005.
9. Hingston, J.L., Wood, M.D., Copplestone, D., and Zinger, I., Impact of chronic low-level ionising radiation exposure on terrestrial invertebrates, *Radioprotection*, 40, S145, 2005.
10. Polikarpov G.G., Conceptual model of responses of organisms, populations and ecosystems to all possible dose rates of ionising radiation in the environment, *Radiat. Protect. Dosim.*, 75, 181, 1998.
11. United Nations Scientific Committee on the Effects of Atomic Radiation, *Scientific Committee on the Effects of Atomic Radiation, Report to the General Assembly, with 10 Scientific Annexes*. United Nations, New York, 2000.
12. Kocher, D.C. and Trabalka, J.R., On the application of a radiation weighting factor for alpha particles in protection of non-human biota, *Health Phys.*, 79, 407, 2000.
13. International Commission on Radiological Protection, *RBE for Deterministic Effects*, Publication 58, Pergamon Press, Oxford, 1989.
14. International Commission on Radiation Units and Measurements, *Microdosimetry*, Report 36, International Commission on Radiation Units and Measurements, Bethesda, MD, 1993.
15. Brechignac, F., Impact of radioactivity on the environment: problems, state of current knowledge and approaches for identification of radioprotection criteria, *Radioprotection*, 36, 511, 2001.
16. Rose, K.S.B., Lower limits of radiosensitivity in organisms, excluding man, *J. Environ. Radioactiv.*, 15, 113, 1992.
17. Little, J.B., Radiation-induced genomic instability, *J. Radiat. Biol.*, 74, 663, 1998.
18. Little, J.B., Radiation carcinogenesis, *Carcinogenesis*, 21, 397, 2000.
19. Lorimore, S.A., Coates, P.J., and Wright, E.G., Radiation-induced genomic instability and bystander effects: inter-related nontargeted effects of exposure to ionizing radiation, *Oncogene*, 22, 7058, 2003.
20. Feinendegen, L.E., Evidence for beneficial low level radiation effects and radiation hormesis, UKRC 2004 debate, *Br. J. Radiol.*, 78, 3, 2005.
21. United Nations Scientific Committee on the Effects of Atomic Radiation, *Effects of Radiation on the Environment*, Report to the General Assembly, United Nations, New York, 1996.

22. International Atomic Energy Agency, *Effects of Ionizing Radiation on Plants and Animals at Levels Implied by Current Radiation Protection Standards*, Technical Report Series no. 332, International Atomic Energy Agency, Vienna, 1992.

23. Sazykina, T.G., A system of dose-effects relationships for the northern wildlife: radiation protection criteria, *Radioprotection*, 40, S889, 2005.

24. Copplestone, D., Howard, B.J., and Brechignac, F., The ecological relevance of current approaches for environmental protection from exposure to ionising radiation, *J. Environ. Radioactiv.*, 74, 31, 2004.

25. Hinton, T.G, Coughlin, D.P., Yi, Y., and Marsh, L.C., Low dose rate irradiation facility: initial study on chronic exposures to medaka, *J. Environ. Radioactiv.*, 74, 43, 2004.

26. Baker, R.J., The Chernobyl nuclear disaster and subsequent creation of a wildlife preserve, *Environ. Toxicol. Chem.*, 19, 1231, 2000.

27. United Nations Scientific Committee on the Effects of Atomic Radiation, *Ionizing Radiation: Sources and Biological Effects, Report to the General Assembly with annexes*, United Nations, New York, 1982.

28. Kuz'menko, M.I. and Polikarpov, G.G., Radioecology of natural waters at the turn of the millennia, *Hydrobiol. J.*, 38, 13, 2002,

29. Ulsh, B.A., Miller, S.M., Mallory, F.F., Mitchel, R.E.J., Morrison, D.P., and Boreham, D.R., Cytogenetic dose-response and adaptive response in cells of ungulate species exposed to ionizing radiation, *J. Environ. Radioactiv.*, 74, 73, 2004.

30. Wickliffe, J.K., Chesser, R.K., Rodgers, B.E., and Baker, R.J., Assessing the genotoxicity of chronic environmental irradiation by using mitochondrial DNA heteroplasmy in the bank vole (*Clethrionomys glareolus*) at Chernobyl, Ukraine, *Environ. Toxicol. Chem.*, 21,1249, 2002.

31. Suter, G.W. II, Efroymson, R.A., Sample, B.E., and Jones, D.S., *Ecological Risk Assessment for Contaminated Sites*, Lewis, Boca Raton, FL, 2000.

32. Smith, J.T., The case against protecting the environment from ionising radiation, *Radioprotection*, 40, S967, 2005.

33. National Council on Radiation Protection and Measurements, *Effects of Ionizing Radiation on Aquatic Organisms*, Report no. 109, National Council on Radiation Protection and Measurements, Bethesda, MD, 1991.

34. International Commission on Radiological Protection, *A Framework for Assessing the Impact of Ionizing Radiation on Non-Human Species*, Publication 91, Pergamon Press, Oxford, 2003.

35. Woodwell, G.M., Effects of ionizing radiation on terrestrial ecosystems, *Science*, 138, 572, 1962.

8 Radionuclides in Foodstuffs and Food Raw Material

Pascal Froidevaux, Tony Dell, and Paul Tossell

CONTENTS

8.1 INTRODUCTION

Everybody needs to eat food to survive and develop. Food can become contaminated with a wide range of pollutants including radioactivity.

The goal of this chapter is to show the importance of monitoring food for levels of radioactivity. We will look at the important sources of radioactivity, both natural and anthropogenic, and relevant transfer pathways through the food chain, identifying the combinations of food groups and radionuclides of most interest.

In order to assess the impact of food contamination exposure on the population, we will develop the concept of radioactivity monitoring programs for food, including important driving forces such as developing international safety and trade legislation, and public reassurance. We show that data generated can be used for both retrospective and prospective dose assessments, and the effect that food processing methods may have on these doses. In addition to what might be regarded as routine programs, we will look at examples of special investigations, such as postaccident monitoring of food.

8.2 SOURCES OF RADIOACTIVITY

Radioactivity has two different origins in the environment. Some radionuclides are naturally present in soil, rocks, underground water, oceans, and the atmosphere. Their mobility and potential transfer to the food chain are directly linked to parameters such as their chemical form, redox conditions of the environment, alteration of minerals and hydrogeological conditions. Chemistry within the rhizosphere is critical in the transfer of radioactivity from soils to plants [1,2]. Air mass exchange within the atmosphere is also a key parameter for radionuclides produced by cosmic rays in the atmosphere. For technologically enhanced naturally occurring radioactive materials (TENORMs), both soil mineralogy and human parameters (e.g., fertilizers, petroleum or mining industries) are of importance when considering the transfer of radioactivity to the food chain.

The distribution of anthropogenic radionuclides in the environment is less associated with the mineralogy of soils, and depends mostly on the presence of authorized or accidental releases from the nuclear power industry, military facilities, and nuclear weapons tests.

While naturally occurring radionuclide distribution can be seen as approximately homogeneously distributed on Earth, with the exception of ore deposits, anthropogenic radionuclides have been distributed along plumes of contamination. In that case, sources of contamination are of the utmost importance as far as transfer of radionuclides to the food chain is concerned. For instance, Bundt et al. [3] show that ^{137}Cs from the Chernobyl accident has been enriched in flow paths present in soils due to heavy rain and water runoff during the deposition. Consequently enrichment of radionuclides during wet deposition in a part of the soil where roots are present in higher density led to higher activity in plants than with dry deposition. When looking at the presence of radioactivity in food, emphasis should be placed on the sources of radionuclides or dispersion in the environment.

8.2.1 NATURAL SOURCES

Our planet and its atmosphere contain many different naturally occurring radioactive materials (NORMs). Most cosmogenic radionuclides are produced from spallation of atoms in the atmosphere due to bombardment by cosmic rays. Of all the radionuclides produced in the atmosphere, only ^{14}C, ^{3}H, and to a lesser extent ^{7}Be are of any significance in foodstuffs, these three radionuclides being easily transferred to the food chain. The residence time of a radionuclide produced by cosmic rays in the atmosphere is about 1 year before gravitational settling and precipitation processes deposit it on the ground. Due to its short half-life (53 days), ^{7}Be is only observed in grass and leaves following direct deposition (e.g., leafy vegetables). In Switzerland, ^{7}Be activity in grass ranges from 50 to 400 Bq/kg dry weight, with higher activities measured in alpine grass than in lowland grass. ^{14}C (5500 yr) is rapidly oxidized to ^{14}CO, then to ^{14}CO$_2$, and incorporated to all living beings, first as a result of photosynthesis. ^{14}C reference activity in all living organisms is close to 0.23 Bq/g carbon. As a result of the introduction of large amounts of fossil carbon in the atmosphere from burning fuel and oil, the ratio of ^{14}C to nonradioactive carbon (^{12}C) has been reduced starting from the second part of the 19th century [4]. The detonation of hundreds of nuclear weapons during the 1960s led to a sharp increase in the atmospheric ^{14}C inventory, roughly doubling the previous ratio to 0.5 Bq/g carbon. Since the signing of the Nuclear Test Ban Treaty, which stopped the testing of nuclear bombs in the atmosphere, a regular decrease in ^{14}C activity has been observed, with a "half-life" of about 13.5 yr. At the present time, and without the input of ^{14}C associated with nuclear power plant operations, the ^{14}C activity ratio has returned to pretesting levels [5]. However, ^{14}C is also a by-product of nuclear energy production. Where atmospheric releases from the nuclear power industry occur, an increase in the ^{14}C/^{12}C ratio in vegetation has been locally observed [6].

^{40}K is present in all soils as an isotope of stable potassium and is transferred, as an alkaline cation, to the food chain. Soils of Switzerland contain ^{40}K activities from 250 to 1000 Bq/kg dry weight, while activities in grass range from 400 to 1300 Bq/kg dry weight. Milk contains high levels of potassium (up to 1.4 g/l) and [40]K activity is close to 45 Bq/l [7]. The activity of wheat cultivated in lowland Switzerland is 116 ± 10 Bq/kg. Thus high activities of [40]K found in food lead to a body activity due to [40]K of 4.4 kBq for the reference man (70 kg), and is mainly located in muscles [8]. Accordingly [40]K represents the largest contributor to internal exposure to radioactivity by ingestion of food.

Soils contain three series of naturally occurring heavy radionuclides. The [232]Th series and the [238]U series are of most importance, the [235]U series being less important because of the low natural [235]U content of uranium ores (0.72%) and its long half-life (7.04 × 10[8] yr). Virtually all soils contain uranium and thorium. Typical [238]U activity is close to 30 Bq/kg [9]. Soil to plant transfer factors for uranium and thorium are very low, so root uptake is not the main pathway of uranium and thorium in the food chain, even if their progeny can find their way to food in larger quantities [10]. In an investigation of the phytoremediation of uranium contaminated sites, Ebbs [11] suggested that some plants preferentially accumulate uranium, but to no more than 3.5 μg/plant (12 Bq/plant). In Switzerland, the range of values for uranium in grass is 0.25 to 14 Bq/kg dry weight [7]. Cows inadvertently eat soil while grazing and grass can be contaminated by soil particles. However, the authors showed that milk (less than 5 mBq/l) and cheese (less than 30 mBq/kg) contain very low levels of [238]U. Analysis of the [234]U/[238]U ratio suggests that the contamination of milk and cheese by uranium originates from the water that the cows drink, not the grass they eat. It was assumed that uranium dissolved in water is more readily available for absorption through the gastrointestinal tract than uranium contained in grass, either as the result of root uptake or by adherent soil particles. Nevertheless, source-dependent bioavailability is an important factor in determining the radioactivity contamination of ruminant-derived food products [12].

Technologically enhanced naturally occurring radioactive materials are produced through various industrial operations and these may lead to discharges to the environment. One of the major contributions of radiological exposure to man from TENORMs is mining and mill tailings, where enhanced concentrations of NORMs are observed [13]. Thus enhanced accumulation of uranium in forage or in drinking water could lead to enhanced uranium in milk and beef [14]. In the European Commission MARINA II Study Part II, Betti et al. [15] suggested that, in the 1980s, the radiation dose rates to marine biota in the region around a phosphate plant on the northwest coast of England were as high as those near the Sellafield reprocessing plant due to its own discharges. It was estimated that since 1981, the total discharges from the phosphate industry of the α emitters [226]Ra and [210]Po to the North Sea and the English Channel amounted to 65 TBq. Since the 1990s, discharges from the phosphate industry have decreased, being replaced by discharges from the oil and gas industry, mostly as releases of contaminated water by offshore platforms.

As a member of the [238]U series, [226]Ra is associated with uranium deposition, but, as a member of the alkaline earth group, its behavior is similar to that of calcium. Thus [226]Ra can be transferred to food by similar mechanisms to calcium. [226]Ra has been used throughout the 20th century. Its radiotoxicity was established in 1924, when dentist Theodore Blum noted the prevalence of "radium-jaw" disease among radium dial painters [16]. ^{226}Ra used in industrial products may still be a source of environmental contamination (e.g., contaminated buildings, waste disposal). The petroleum industry is a major source of ^{226}Ra dispersal to the environment [17]. In the geological process of oil formation, ^{226}Ra, being slightly soluble, accumulates on the liquid phases of subsurface water formation. When brought to the surface, some ^{226}Ra precipitates with barium sulfates and carbonates, yielding concentrated levels of radium in scales and sludges. Smith et al. [17] calculated that disposal of radioactive petroleum waste in municipal solid waste landfills would result in exposure to the public of a small fraction of the recommended 1 mSv/yr.

8.2.2 Anthropogenic Sources

Since the discovery of nuclear fission, a large number of anthropogenic radionuclides have been produced. Some of them are produced due to fission of nuclei, like ^{137}Cs, ^{131}I, or ^{90}Sr, while others are produced by activation of uranium fuel (e.g., plutonium isotopes) or reactor components (e.g., ^{60}Co) by neutrons. The release of anthropogenic radionuclides in the environment follows different pathways, all having their importance in the way radioactivity finds its way to the food chain. The production of electricity from nuclear power plant is responsible for the introduction of anthropogenic radioactivity into the environment through authorized discharges, accidental discharges such as the Chernobyl accident, and to a lesser extent unauthorized discharges. The production and testing of nuclear weapons is responsible for both localized contamination, due to onsite incidents, and global dispersion of radioactivity from fallout. Fallout from weapons tests occurred for several months following each atmospheric test as wet and dry deposition. For instance, rainfall and snowfall deposition rates are higher in mountainous areas, and deposition of ^{137}Cs, ^{90}Sr, and $^{239/240}$Pu is always higher in mountainous areas than in lowland areas [7,18,19]. A significant relationship has been observed between ^{137}Cs deposition and rainfall rates [20–22].

The transfer of radioactivity to food has been observed as a consequence of some of the previously discussed sources. Nuclear weapons tests released large quantities of plutonium, ^{90}Sr, and ^{137}Cs throughout the Northern Hemisphere, with maximum levels found around 40°N to 50°N latitude [23]. In Switzerland, particular attention has been paid to the highly radiotoxic ^{90}Sr since the beginning of the nuclear era [24]. As milk and dairy products constitute an important part of the diet of the Swiss population, it was recognized that ^{90}Sr, an alkaline earth cation, follows the same metabolic pathways as calcium, and represents the main contributor to the internal dose by fission products. Since the beginning of the 1950s, milk samples, milk teeth, and vertebrae have been collected yearly for ^{90}Sr determination. The results presented in Figure 8.1 show a large increase in ^{90}Sr activity in milk samples during the 1960s, corresponding to nuclear testing in the atmosphere. The ^{90}Sr activity profile in milk teeth matches that of milk, illustrating that ^{90}Sr present in the environment has been transferred to the food

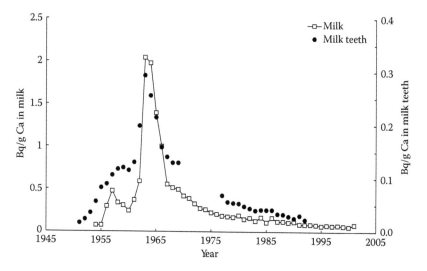

FIGURE 8.1 Average ^{90}Sr activity (in Bq/g of calcium) in milk and milk teeth from 1950 to 2000 in Switzerland. Activity in milk teeth is reported to the year of birth.

chain, then to milk teeth through breast-feeding. Since the signing of the Limited Nuclear Test Ban Treaty in 1963, ^{90}Sr activity has decreased exponentially, with an apparent biological half-life of about 12 years in milk and 10 years in milk teeth.

After the Chernobyl accident, it was observed that the ^{90}Sr activity of milk and dairy products in Switzerland doubled from 0.1 to 0.2 Bq/l during the first months after the accident [25]. Unexpectedly, ^{90}Sr activity in Swiss milk returned to its pre-Chernobyl level after just a few months. Rapid migration of Chernobyl-derived ^{90}Sr in the deepest parts of the soil profile was observed, indicating that the chemical form of the Chernobyl radiostrontium was more mobile than radiostrontium from nuclear weapons test fallout [26].

^{137}Cs in the environment results from two main deposition pathways. Fallout from nuclear weapons tests spread large quantities of radiocesium. The average deposition in the Northern Hemisphere ranges between 2000 and 5000 Bq/m^2 (reference date 2000), with greater activities found in highlands than in lowlands. The Chernobyl accident approximately doubled the deposition of radiocesium in large parts of western Europe. Levels as high as 85 kBq/m^2 were recorded in Sweden, while the Tessin region in Switzerland and Bavaria in Germany received up to 45 kBq/m^2 [27]. Furthermore, reconcentration phenomena as a result of soil particle runoff during heavy rainfall episodes yielded hot spots with very high activity [18,28]. The ^{137}Cs contamination of food following the Chernobyl accident was very dependent on meteorological conditions during the passage of the contaminated cloud.

Following a release of radioactivity in the environment, it is very important to determine the bioavailability of the most radiologically significant radionuclides.

For instance, it has been demonstrated that the availability of the initial deposit of Chernobyl fallout for transfer to grazing animals was considerably less than the value for radiocesium incorporated into grassy herbage via root uptake. Beresford et al. [12] reviewed the source-dependent bioavailability in determining absorption from the ruminant gastrointestinal tract for the most significant radionuclides (^{137}Cs, ^{90}Sr, and ^{131}I). The review showed that absorption of radioiodine through the gastrointestinal tract is complete whatever the source. ^{90}Sr absorption is very dependent on the calcium requirement of the animal, but not on the source, while radiocesium absorption is very source dependent. Plutonium's absorption coefficient is very low (1.21×10^4) compared to ^{137}Cs (0.2 to 0.8), but might be source dependent. However, Froidevaux et al. [7] were unable to detect plutonium isotopes in cheese produced in western Europe (less than 0.3 mBq/kg), showing that absorption of plutonium from ingested soil (maximum activity of 3 Bq/kg) through the gastrointestinal tract is very low and does not represent a significant contribution to internal exposure.

Directly after a gaseous radioactive contamination incident (e.g., the Chernobyl accident), contamination of foodstuffs is essentially the result of vegetation interception of the deposition (i.e., direct surface contamination). The combined effect of the radioactive decay (for short half-life radionuclides), weathering effects, dilution due to biomass growth, and transfer into nonedible or unused parts of the plant, and increasing fixation of radionuclides in soil account for an apparent "half-life" of the radioactivity that is usually less than 1 year. From the first to the second year after deposition, a significant decrease in the activity concentration in all foodstuffs is observed due to the change from direct contamination to contamination caused by root uptake [29]. This change in the mechanism of food contamination accounts for a long-term exposure and apparent "half-life" that increases to about 6 years. For Chernobyl ^{137}Cs, this long-term increase in apparent half-life is even longer in some specific environments such as Scandinavian lakes, where fish contamination by ^{137}Cs still represents a significant exposure to the population [30]. A similar situation is observed in the Cumbrian region of the U.K., where sheep meat with activity levels greater than 2000 Bq/kg were still observed in 2000 [31]. It is worth noting that contamination of milk by Chernobyl-derived ^{137}Cs reached the same peak value (about 8 kBq/kg) observed in 1964 following nuclear weapons testing fallout in Germany. Afterwards the decrease is very similar in both cases [29].

The presence of anthropogenic actinides in the environment is essentially due to the nuclear weapons testing fallout during the 1960s and 1970s, and locally to nuclear facilities. Average plutonium deposition in the Swiss lowland is about 75 Bq/m^2, but deposition as high as 300 Bq/m^2 has been observed in the Jura Mountains [3,7]. ^{241}Am deposition is 0.4 times that of $^{239/240}$Pu, indicating that fallout from nuclear weapons tests is the origin of the contamination. Because of the very low soil to plant transfer factors (less than 10^{-4}), fallout plutonium and americium are not significant contributors to internal exposure by ingestion of terrestrial foods.

8.3 PATHWAYS OF TRANSFER TO FOOD

Discharge routes for radioactive waste from a nuclear site can be liquid, gaseous, and solid (as shown in Figure 8.2). Solid disposals are usually of little relevance to the food chain in the short term and thus are not considered further here. This leads to two broad categories of pathways for the movement of radionuclides into and around the food chain: aquatic and terrestrial. The aquatic pathway covers potential contamination of oceans, rivers, and lakes due to liquid discharges. The terrestrial pathway deals with potential contamination of land predominately due to gaseous discharges to the atmosphere.

The aquatic pathways affect water systems both locally and at great distances. An input of radioactive material into a river can contaminate fish and shellfish directly, but that river will also drain into an ocean, where currents can carry the contamination to a wide area. These currents are slow but important pathways for areas such as the Arctic [32]. At a local level, radioactive waste discharges can have an immediate affect on the food chain. For instance, fish can incorporate ^{3}H in the form of ^{3}H$_2$O into their tissue very rapidly (with a turnover time in the order of a few minutes to a few hours) and reach concentrations near that of the surrounding water [33]. Thus if discharges increase, it is likely that the activity level in fish will increase as well.

Direct deposition of some radionuclides, such as ^{210}Po and ^{210}Pb, can have a significant impact on the level of these radionuclides from gaseous sources [34]. Leafy green vegetables can be directly contaminated in this manner.

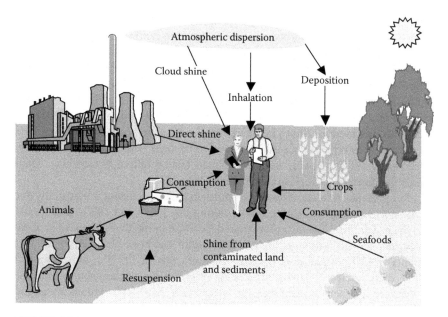

FIGURE 8.2 Potential radioactivity and radiation exposure pathways from a nuclear site.

Gases, such as $^{14}CO_2$, can become incorporated into plant tissue at the primary level of production. At the heterotrophic level, either farm animals eat the plants and then people eat the animals, or people eat the plants directly.

Terrestrial samples can also receive contamination from liquid discharges via the sea to land pathway. Sea spray can result in airborne contamination and tide-washed pastures can be contaminated directly from the waters, albeit to a lower level than from actual gaseous releases [35]. Irrigation of crops or livestock drinking river water are also ways that liquid discharges can enter the terrestrial food chain. Other pathways are investigated because of specific circumstances, such as pigeons near the Sellafield, U.K., site (discussed in Section 8.5.2).

8.3.1 FOOD GROUPS AND RADIONUCLIDES OF INTEREST

8.3.1.1 Milk

For terrestrial radiological monitoring programs, cow's milk is often the predominant sample taken because it is readily available, consumed by a large number of people, consumed by children in relatively large quantities, and is a good indicator of radionuclides present in the environment. In the U.S., the Environmental Protection Agency (EPA) runs the Environmental Radiation Ambient Monitoring System program, which covers air, drinking water, precipitation, and milk [36]. Quarterly samples of milk from 42 locations (66 in 1988) are analyzed by γ spectrometry, looking for fission products such as ^{131}I, ^{140}Ba, and ^{137}Cs. On a less frequent schedule, samples are analyzed for ^{90}Sr.

As part of the requirements under Article 35 of the Euratom Treaty, the European Union (EU) recommends that member states analyze ^{137}Cs and ^{90}Sr in milk from large milk processing sites [37]. Figure 8.3 shows "maximum average" levels of ^{90}Sr and ^{137}Cs in dairies sampled throughout England between 1996 and 2003. The maximum average value is the mean concentration at the farm or dairy with the highest individual result. For most foods, the maximum concentration can be selected for a dose assessment, as there is the possibility of storage of that food following harvesting, which could coincide with a peak level of activity in the food. Milk is generally not stored for long periods, so maximum averages may be used on the basis that the farm or milk production site where the highest value is found can supply milk to a consumer who consumes it in large quantities (a "high-rate" consumer).

^{14}C is a naturally occurring radionuclide, so some will be present in all milk samples. The U.K. uses a carbon content of 7% in milk, a background activity value of 250 Bq ^{14}C/kg total carbon, and a subsequent background level of 18 Bq/l ^{14}C for milk samples [38]. Average levels in milk samples taken from up to 17 farms per year around the nuclear reprocessing site at Sellafield, U.K., since 1991 have been shown to slightly exceed the background on a few occasions over this period.

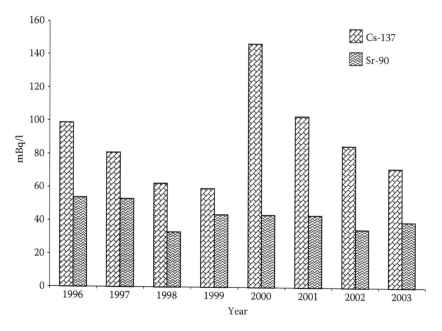

FIGURE 8.3 Annual "maximum average" ^{137}Cs and ^{90}Sr levels in milk from English dairies (1996 to 2003).

8.3.1.2 Total Diet Samples

In addition to data from milk sample analysis, the EU requires that member states report measurements for a list of recommended radionuclides in mixed diet samples to derive doses from general food consumption [37]. In the U.K., the Food Standard Agency's Total Diet Study (TDS) is used to analyze for a range of both radioactive and nonradioactive contaminants in the general diet. The TDS samples used for radionuclide analysis were comprised of all the food groups (except beverages) in proportion of their significance in the diet. The amounts of each of the food groups eaten are derived from studies of consumption, such as the National Food Survey [39]. The use of TDS samples allows a more representative exposure estimate than analyzing all food types from an area, as people rarely obtain all their food from a local source [40].

Figure 8.4 shows the highest levels of ^{210}Pb and ^{210}Po in the U.K. TDS samples for 1995 to 2003 and the doses calculated from both naturally occurring and anthropogenic radionuclides. The figure shows that natural radionuclides dominate the dose, with only a fraction (no more than 13%) coming from artificial radionuclides. In 2003, ^{210}Po dominated, accounting for 50% of the total dose, with ^{210}Pb accounting for another 25% [38].

The U.S. Food and Drug Administration (FDA) has monitored levels of radionuclides in their TDS samples since 1961 [41]. Their approach has been to use a "mixed basket" and analyze individual parts of the diet separately instead

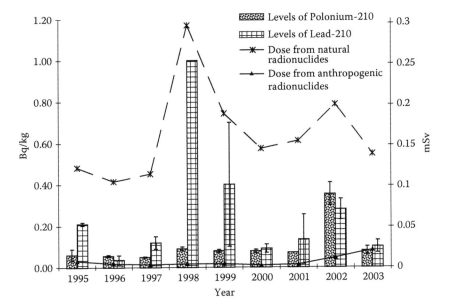

FIGURE 8.4 Levels of ^{210}Pb and ^{210}Po in English TDS samples and average doses to U.K. consumers from natural and anthropogenic radionuclides in TDS samples (1995 to 2003).

of in a representative diet. ^{226}Ra, ^{232}Th, ^{241}Am, ^{140}Ba, ^{134}Cs, ^{60}Co, ^{131}I, ^{140}La, ^{103}Ru, and ^{106}Ru were below reporting levels in all samples, while ^{137}Cs, ^{90}Sr, and ^{40}K were detectable in some of the food types. The highest level of ^{90}Sr was found in mixed nuts, at 1.9 Bq/kg. A study of the individual food groups that make up the U.K. TDS found ^{90}Sr at 0.8 Bq/kg for nuts [42].

Syria introduced a National Food Monitoring Program in 1996 to look at natural radionuclides in the Syrian diet. The study found that for infant food, ^{210}Po and ^{210}Pb were relatively low in most samples [43], while ^{40}K was relatively high in most samples consisting of wheat. ^{40}K is under homeostatic control in the body, so there is little variation in doses to adults. Even so, the Syrian study found that ^{40}K was the main contributor at the first 6-month stage due to high consumption rates of milk.

8.3.1.3 Naturally Occurring Radionuclides

Naturally occurring radionuclides in foodstuffs are known to vary in direct relationship to levels in soil and also according to direct deposition. A study by the U.K.'s National Radiological Protection Board (NRPB) looked at variability in the levels of naturally occurring radionuclides between areas of differing environmental background [34]. The radionuclides of interest were ^{210}Pb, ^{210}Po, ^{226}Ra, ^{234,238}U, and ^{230,232}Th. Foods were grown at organic farms (one in an area of typical U.K. levels and one in an area with elevated levels) to avoid interference from artificial phosphate-based fertilizers. At both sites, the contribution from isotopes of uranium and thorium to the dose from a given foodstuff was small. For ^{226}Ra, doses from vegetable crops at the test site were generally much greater than those at the control site, a consequence of the higher activity concentrations in the soil and, in some cases, a higher soil to plant transfer factor. Levels of ^{210}Po and ^{210}Pb, particularly in leafy green vegetables, were most associated with direct deposition, as discussed previously. The study suggested that ^{210}Po and ^{210}Pb in offal could be a significant contributor to dose.

A further study by the NRPB also looked at naturally occurring radionuclides, but this time in so-called free or wild foods [44]. Habit surveys were conducted to identify those people who collected the most "free foods." In total, 400 people were identified and between them they collected 54 different types of free food. Blackberries were by far the most common species collected, although various types of mushrooms and nuts were also popular.

8.3.1.4 Free Foods

Around the typical location in 2000, an individual who consumed free foods at average rates would receive an annual dose of about 29 μSv compared with the dose estimate for the TDS of 140 μSv [45]. The corresponding value for a high-rate consumer was 84 μSv, with the majority contribution (more than 95%) for all foodstuffs measured was from ^{210}Po and ^{210}Pb. The foodstuffs of importance were field mushrooms and elderflowers. For the samples from the elevated area, more than 98% of the dose from consumption of free foods measured was from ^{210}Po and ^{210}Pb. An average consumer of these free foods would receive an annual dose of about 156 μSv compared with a high-rate consumer receiving up to 273 μSv. Boletus mushrooms (*Suillus luteus*) were the highest contributors to dose, although nettles and horse mushrooms were also important. Honey was chosen as a foodstuff of interest because it is derived from upland heather and for which there was previous evidence of elevated activity concentrations of ^{137}Cs from the Chernobyl accident. However, activity concentrations of the radionuclides measured in this U.K. study were among the lowest found. The FDA TDS study reported that all samples except honey were below the detection limit for ^{137}Cs. Honey was found to contain 6.7 Bq/kg [41].

The NRPB also looked at radionuclide levels in free foods from around the following four nuclear sites in the U.K.: the Atomic Weapons Establishment at Aldermaston, the radiopharmaceutical plant in Cardiff, Hinkley Point nuclear power station, and Sizewell nuclear power station [46]. A total of 802 people were found to collect free foods. Between them they collected about 85 different types of free food: 86% collected blackberries, 34% collected some type of mushroom, 18% collected sloes, 15% collected chestnuts, 15% collected cobnuts or hazelnuts, 9% collected elderberries, 6% collected elderflowers, 5% collected crab apples, 5% collected rabbits, and other foods were collected by 4% or less. The radionuclides analyzed were selected on the basis of the discharge data for each individual site together with likely radiological importance. In all cases, even assuming a high rate of consumption, no dose estimate exceeded 6 μSv/yr, well below the annual dose limit of 1000 μSv/yr. These values are also significantly lower than the dose of natural radionuclides from the consumption of the free foods discussed above. A similar project conducted earlier around the Sellafield site also found the collection of free foods to be a relatively common practice [47]. In a household survey of 181 individuals (from 72 households), 129 collected blackberries. High-rate consumers were estimated to receive a dose of up to 32.2 μSv/yr, mainly from honey and hedgerow fruits. Two samples of honey were reported — one from Bootle Fell, an area 20 km south of the Sellafield site, the other from Wellington, much closer to the site. The honey from Bootle Fell had the highest concentration of ^{137}Cs, at 254 ± 1 Bq/kg (giving a dose of 23 μSv/yr), compared to 20.5 ± 0.37 Bq/kg for the Wellington sample. It is suggested that the high ^{137}Cs result was due to deposition from the Chernobyl accident. The next highest dose estimate, 25.1 μSv/yr, was for an individual eating 134 kg/yr of venison from upland areas. ^{137}Cs dominated the dose, with 23.7 μSv/yr coming from the venison alone. The level of ^{137}Cs in venison was 13 Bq/kg, but the report suggested that this was due to Chernobyl deposition, as venison from nearer the Sellafield site and at a lower level had previously been noted to be much lower at 2.6 Bq/kg. These values are comparable to levels in other animals, but the consumption rates are lower, so subsequently doses are lower. ^{137}Cs levels in goose were reported as 3.84 ± 0.03 Bq/kg, rabbit at 12.5 ± 0.33 Bq/kg, mallard duck at 3.55 ± 0.14 Bq/kg, and pheasant at 4.52 ± 0.14 Bq/kg.

8.3.1.5 Freshwater Foods

The terrestrial environment also includes foods that are grown in freshwater, such as rice plants. Rice, which is a staple food crop for most of the world's population, was reported in December 2004 to have an estimated global paddy production of 611 million tons [48]. Rice is grown under flooded conditions primarily because the water provides a nonchemical control of weeds, as plant growth involves chemical reactions that require oxygen. Flooded fields have less oxygen available for plant roots than dry or aerated soils. Rice leaves and stems have internal air spaces, like a series of small tunnels, through which air is collected and passed down to the root cells. This is a route by which radioactive gases can pass into the plant. They may also pass into the plant by root transfer. Muramatsu et al. [49] found that soil types influenced the uptake and desorption of radioiodine into the edible part of the rice plant. Another study found that virtually no radioiodine deposited onto the leaves and stalks of rice plants was translocated to the edible portion [50].

The water lily (*Nympaea* sp.) is another plant that grows in freshwater. Accumulation of radionuclides can occur as a result of uptake from the water column and uptake into roots and rhizomes from the sediment in which the plant is rooted, with the possibility of subsequent translocation into the plant [51]. Along with freshwater mussels (*Velesunio angasi*), which have been noted to have very high flesh concentrations of ^{226}Ra, these foods are a potential pathway for transfer of TENORM radionuclides into the food chain of aboriginal people (discussed below).

A study of the levels of radionuclides in food in Hong Kong found about a third of rice samples had levels of ^{210}Pb up to 0.5 Bq/kg. The majority of samples had levels of ^{137}Cs up to 0.59 Bq/kg. ^{40}K was detectable in all samples in the range 0.1 to 17 Bq/kg, but a previous study by the Royal Observatory of Hong Kong found levels up to 38 Bq/kg. ^{238}U, ^{226}Ra, ^{228}Ra, and ^{60}Co were not detected in any sample.

In addition to the TDS concept of exposure estimates, another form is the analysis of duplicate diets. A study by Iyengar et al. [52] looked at the daily dietary intake of ^{232}Th and ^{238}U in adults living in a number of Asian countries. The study covered Bangladesh, China, India, Japan, Pakistan, the Philippines, Republic of Korea, and Vietnam. Together these countries represent more than half the population of the world and many of their diets are dominated by rice. The study found the median daily intake of ^{232}Th ranged between 0.6 and 14.4 mBq, the lowest being the Philippines and the highest being Bangladesh. Daily intakes of ^{238}U ranged from 6.7 mBq for India up to 62.5 mBq for China.

8.3.1.6 TENORM Radionuclides

As discussed in Section 8.2.1, TENORMs are an important source of contamination for some pathways. In Australia, there has been interest in levels of natural series radionuclides in foods because of the uranium mining occurring there. A study by Martin and Ryan [51] looked at levels in traditional aboriginal foods in northern Australia. The aboriginal people eat both commercial foods brought into the area and also flora and fauna from the local environment, so-called bush foods. One study suggests that 40% of the total calorific intake and 81% of the protein in the aboriginal diet comes from bush foods [53]. A total of 170 species of flora and fauna were observed and it was noted that a single species will generally have several edible parts (e.g., various organs of an animal). Buffalo, pigs, and magpie geese are animals known to be eaten by the aborigines. Analysis of these animals has shown that naturally occurring radionuclides are found in higher concentrations in kidney and liver than other parts of the animal, particularly for ^{210}Po.

Other countries where uranium mining has taken place have also undertaken studies of the transfer of TENORM radionuclides into the food chain. In northern Saskatchewan, Canada, the lichen-caribou-human food chain has been studied [54]. Lichens accumulate atmospheric radionuclides more efficiently than other vegetation because of their lack of roots, large surface area, and longevity. Lichens are the main winter forage for caribou, which in turn are the main food source for many northern Canadians. It was found that levels of ^{210}Po generally increase as one moves north or east across the Canadian Arctic. The Beverly herd in central Canada has levels of 15 Bq/kg, but those in the northeast have been found with up to 40 Bq/kg. The partitioning of radionuclides in animals was studied and

^{226}Ra was found to be highest in the bone (72 Bq/kg), but was in the range 0.23 to 1.7 Bq/kg in other tissues. The report added that ^{226}Ra levels in caribou were similar to other native animals such as prairie rodents. ^{210}Po was found at greater than 400 Bq/kg in bone, fur, and feces, but as low as 1 Bq/kg in muscle. ^{137}Cs was highest in kidney (557 Bq/kg), but was 232 Bq/kg in liver and 370 Bq/kg in muscle. Assuming an intake of 100 g/day of caribou meat, ^{210}Po, followed by ^{137}Cs, contributed most of the dose of 0.85 mSv/yr. Additional consumption of 1 liver and 10 kidneys per year doubles the dose to 1.7 mSv/yr.

8.3.1.7 Fish and Shellfish

As discussed in Section 8.2.1, TENORMs can be a major factor in the activity levels found in seafood. High-rate fish and shellfish consumers near Sellafield received about 66% of their dose from natural radionuclide elevated by TEN-ORMs [38]. The dose from the consumption of fish and shellfish from both natural and artificial radionuclides for 2003 was 0.62 mSv/yr. Thus the fish and shellfish pathway of the human food chain is very important.

Consumption habits for aquatic samples can vary significantly between groups around different nuclear sites. For instance, consumption of fish and shellfish around Dungeness Nuclear Power Station (NPS) in southern England is about 59 kg/yr of fish, 17 kg/yr of crustaceans, and 15 kg/yr of mollusks. This can be compared to the Wylfa NPS in north Wales, where a consumption habit survey found 94 kg/yr of fish, 23 kg/yr of crustaceans, but only 1.8 kg/yr of mollusks. Consumption habits can also be detailed enough to denote species. For instance, at another Welsh NPS — Trawsfynydd — consumption was noted as 1.8 kg/yr of brown trout, 22 kg/yr of rainbow trout, and 0.9 kg/yr of perch. Where samples are being analyzed for a dose assessment, it is very important to get the correct species, as the feeding habits of fish can affect their levels of radionuclides. A study of four lakes in Finland found predatory species such as pike, perch, and burbot had higher radiocesium levels than whitefish and vendace [32]. The predatory species showed an increase in ^{137}Cs levels for a couple years after the Chernobyl accident due to the accumulation up the trophic level.

8.3.1.8 Indicator Materials

Sometimes it is more appropriate to collect indicator materials, such as seawater, tidal grasses, sediments, and seaweeds in order to ensure the aquatic pathway is adequately monitored. These materials can concentrate particular radionuclides. Some radionuclide levels in fish can be estimated by analyzing samples of seawater. Seawater surveys can also support international studies such as the Oslo and Paris Commission (OSPAR) [55].

An indicator material such as seaweed is a cost-effective means of determining levels of activity in the environment. In addition, seaweeds are sometimes used as fertilizers and soil conditioners [38]. Although seaweed harvesting in the Sellafield area was found to be rare, several plots of land fertilized with seaweed were identified and investigated [56]. Samples of soil were analyzed for a range of radionuclides by γ ray spectrometry and for ^{99}Tc. The soil and compost data show enhanced levels of ^{99}Tc and small amounts of other radionuclides, as would be expected from the activity initially present in the seaweed. Various vegetables that had been grown in the soils from these plots were sampled. The ^{99}Tc concentrations in vegetables ranged from 3 to 270 Bq/kg in the edible parts.

Table 8.1 provides a summary of activity levels found globally in foodstuffs.

8.4 MONITORING RADIOACTIVITY IN THE FOOD CHAIN

8.4.1 WHO/WHAT DRIVES LEGISLATION?

The aim of this section is to give the reader a broad overview of some of the key organizations worldwide that both directly and indirectly shape legislation in the area of radioactivity in food. Countries throughout the world have generally based legislation on recommendations set out by international bodies that have a wealth of expertise in the field of radioactivity, and some of those of importance will now be briefly discussed.

The International Commission on Radiological Protection (ICRP) is an independent registered charity established to advance the science of radiological protection. It does this by providing recommendations and guidance on all aspects of protection against ionizing radiation. Many of the reports of this organization have been used to develop dose-limiting legislation throughout the world.

There are several key parts of the United Nations (UN) that warrant a mention. The UN Scientific Committee on Atomic Radiation (UNSCEAR) was set up in 1955 to assess and report levels and effects of human exposure to ionizing radiation. The reports produced by UNSCEAR over many years review exposures from nuclear power production, nuclear weapons tests, natural radiation sources, exposures from medical radiation (diagnosis and treatment), and occupational exposure to radiation. The Food and Agriculture Organization of the UN, whose broad aim is to "defeat hunger," also plays a key role in determining guidelines for food safety standards. This is particularly so in the joint approach with the World Health Organization (WHO) and the development of the Codex Alimentarius. The Codex has the aim of "protecting the health of consumers, ensuring fair trade practices in the food trade, and promoting coordination of all food standards work undertaken by international governmental and nongovernmental organizations."

The International Atomic Energy Agency (IAEA) has an important role to play in protecting consumers from potential radiation hazards associated with food. Its broad remit includes nonproliferation of nuclear technology, as well as ensuring that in countries already using nuclear technologies, best practices are followed to reduce the risk of accidents. One of its major themes is to cover emergency preparedness and response to potential radiological incidents. The agency is also well placed to share vital information with affected countries at all stages of a major nuclear accident.

TABLE 8.1
Radionuclide Levels for a Variety of Food Samples from Around the World

Food Type	Location	Median	Minimum Value	Maximum Value	Ref.
		^{14}C			
Milk (Bq/l)	U.K.	18	4	33	
		^{90}Sr			
Water (Bq/l)	Switzerland	$<5 \times 10^{-3}$			
Milk (Bq/l)	Swiss lowland	0.053	0.018	0.103	
	Swiss Alps	0.37	0.08	0.77	
Cheese (Bq/kg)	Western Europe lowlands	0.49	0.29	0.68	7
	Western Europe uplands	3.28	0.77	6.27	7
Wheat (Bq/kg)	Swiss lowlands	0.37	0.11	0.85	
Potatoes (Bq/kg dw, unpeeled)	Swiss lowlands	0.37	0.12	0.81	
Salad (Bq/kg dw)	Swiss lowlands	6.2	4.6	9.7	
Herbage (cow food) (Bq/kg dw)	Swiss lowlands	3.8	0.5	11	
	Swiss Jura Mountains	6.9	3	14	
	Swiss Alps	12.3	9	38	
	Swiss South Alps (Tessin)	16	14	50	
	Maritime Alps (France)	88	47	156	
Milk (Bq/l)	U.K.	0.066	0.029	0.293	
		^{40}K			
Milk (Bq/l)	Switzerland	43	34	48	
Cheese (Bq/kg)	Western Europe	17	15	21	7
Wheat (Bq/kg)	Swiss lowlands	105	91	121	
Herbage (cow food) (Bq/kg dw)	Switzerland	750	400	1300	
Cereal products	Syria		56	382	43
Vegetables	Syria		29	3680	43
Marine mammals (Bq/kg ww)	Entire world		56	127	99
		^{137}Cs			
Milk (Bq/l)	Maritimes Alps (France)	3.3	1.3	6.2	
	Swiss lowlands	<1			
	Swiss Alps and Tessin		0.3	25	
Cheese (Bq/kg)	Maritimes Alps (France)	4.3	2	6.0	
	Western Europe lowlands	<0.2			7
Wheat (Bq/kg)	Swiss lowlands	<0.4			

(continued)

TABLE 8.1 (continued)
Radionuclide Levels for a Variety of Food Samples from Around the World

Food Type	Location	Median	Minimum Value	Maximum Value	Ref.
Mushrooms (Boletus edulis)	Switzerland	120	3	2000	
Mushrooms (Xerocomus badius)	Switzerland	20	3	470	
Mushrooms (Rozites caperata)	Switzerland	460	195	680	
Mushrooms (basidiomycetes, Bq/kg dw)	Taiwan		<1	7.5	100
Mushrooms (all sorts, Bq/kg dw)	Czech Republic	30	1.7	116	101
Wild pig (Bq/kg)	Swiss South Alps (Tessin)	55	13	293	
Marine mammals (Bq/kg ww)	Entire world		nd	66	99
Fish (Bq/kg)	NE Atlantic	2.4			102
	Mediterranean Sea	1.0			102
Fish (Bq/kg ww)	Cuba	0.1			103
Shellfish (Bq/kg ww)	Cuba	0.1			103
Mollusks (Bq/kg ww)	Cuba	0.9			103
Onions (Bq/kg fw)	Egypt	0.7	nd	1	104
Tomatoes	Egypt	0.32	nd	1.0	104
Green peas	Egypt	1.7	0.6	4.0	104
^{226}Ra					
Groundwater (mBq/l)	Swiss Alps (southeast)	15	6	50	
Mineral water (mBq/l)	Swiss Alps (southeast)	25	12	100	
Mineral water (mBq/l)	Northern Italy	41	2	200	105
Mineral water (mBq/l)	Taiwan	3.5	nd	12	106
Rice (Bq/kg fw)	Taiwan	0.08			106
Milk (Bq/kg)	Taiwan	0.03			106
Fish (Bq/kg fw)	Taiwan	0.04			106
Fish and shellfish (Bq/kg fw)	West Irish Sea		0.03	9.6	15
Brazil nuts (Bq/kg)	Brazil	50			96
^{238}U					
Groundwater (mBq/l)	Swiss Alps (southeast)	20	5	200	
Mineral water (mBq/l)	Swiss Alps (southeast)	20	5	200	
Mineral water (mBq/l)	Northern Italy	28	4	120	105
Cheese (mBq/kg)	Western Europe	12	1.7	27	7
Fish and shellfish (Bq/kg fw)	West Irish Sea	0.45	0.009	1.7	15

TABLE 8.1 (continued)
Radionuclide Levels for a Variety of Food Samples from Around the World

Food Type	Location	Median	Minimum Value	Maximum Value	Ref.
		^{210}Po			
Fish (Bq/kg)	NE Atlantic	2.4			102
	Mediterranean Sea	2.4			102
Shellfish (Bq/kg ww)	NE Atlantic	15			102
	Mediterranean Sea	15			102
Fish and shellfish (Bq/kg ww)	West Irish Sea	21	1	53	15
Fish (Bq/kg ww)	Cuba	19.5	5	89	103
Crustaceans (Bq/kg ww)	Cuba	100	50	125	103
Mollusks (Bq/kg ww)	Cuba	25	21	33	103
Tea (Bq/kg)	Syria	14	6	39	107
Cereals (Bq/kg dw)	Syria		0.8	2.6	43
Vegetables	Syria		0.2	8.3	43
Fish (Bq/kg)	U.K. waters	0.82	0.18	4.4	38
Crustaceans (Bq/kg)	U.K. waters	9.1	1.1	35	38
Crabs (Bq/kg)	U.K. waters	19	4.1	35	38
Lobsters (Bq/kg)	U.K. waters	5.3	1.9	10	38
Mollusks (Bq/kg)	U.K. waters	17	1.2	69	38
Winkles (Bq/kg)	U.K. waters	13	6.1	25	38
Mussels (Bq/kg)	U.K. waters	42	19	69	38
Cockles (Bq/kg)	U.K. waters	18	11	36	38
Whelks (Bq/kg)	U.K. waters	6.5	1.2	11	38
Limpets (Bq/kg)	U.K. waters	8.4	5.9	15	38
		^{210}Pb			
Fish (Bq/kg)	U.K. waters	0.042	0.003	0.55	38
Crustaceans (Bq/kg)	U.K. waters	0.025	0.013	2.4	38
Crabs (Bq/kg)	U.K. waters	0.24	0.043	0.76	38
Lobsters (Bq/kg)	U.K. waters	0.080	0.02	0.79	38
Mollusks (Bq/kg)	U.K. waters	1.2	0.18	6.8	38
Winkles (Bq/kg)	U.K. waters	1.5	0.69	2.6	38
Mussels (Bq/kg)	U.K. waters	1.6	0.68	6.8	38
Cockles (Bq/kg)	U.K. waters	0.94	0.59	1.3	38
Whelks (Bq/kg)	U.K. waters	0.39	0.18	0.61	38
Limpets (Bq/kg)	U.K. waters	1.5	0.68	4.9	38

Note: dw, dry weight; fw, fresh weight; nd, no data; ww, wet weight.

The Nuclear Energy Agency of the Organization on Economic Cooperation and Development is an organization whose aims are broadly "to help create sound national and international legal regimes required for the peaceful uses of nuclear energy, including international trade in nuclear materials and equipment, to address issues of liability and compensation for nuclear damage, and to serve as a centre for nuclear law information and education." This organization has, since 1968, produced a widely distributed publication entitled "Nuclear Law Bulletin," that provides the reader with a great deal of useful information relating to nuclear law throughout the world.

The EU plays a key role in determining the legal framework for member states. Indeed Article 35 of the Euratom Treaty, clearly requires that member states "establish the necessary facilities to carry out continuous monitoring of the level of radioactivity," which includes soil, air, water, and foodstuffs.

At the national level there are often organizations that are set up to give informed opinion to governments prior to legislation being drawn up. A prime example in the U.K. is the NRPB, which has the role of advancing knowledge connected with the protection of mankind from ionizing radiation and providing advice in the field of radiological protection. In general, legislation is drafted with the philosophy that the safety of the most vulnerable section of society is considered a priority and the view is then taken that the levels set will protect this group and other less vulnerable groups too.

8.4.2 INTERVENTION-LEVEL GUIDELINES

These are derived from the primary legislation within national boundaries, but the effects of international trade are such that the approach in recent years has been to attempt to harmonize intervention levels. Often the barriers to complete harmonization across international borders are constrained by the fact that the national law of a country takes precedence over other "foreign" legislation. At the time of the Chernobyl accident, there was a large and varied range of "intervention levels" set by different countries, which undoubtedly caused confusion. There is currently a new set of guideline proposals for radionuclides in food for use in international trade (see Section 8.6).

8.4.3 EFFECTS OF PROCESSING

Consideration should always be given to the effects of food processing on the concentrations of radionuclides. Indeed, some food products may be converted into other nonfood items, for example, the use of some edible herbs such as chamomile and lemon balm in pharmaceutical products [57].

Jackson and Edwards [58] demonstrated the effects of domestic food preparation on radionuclide concentrations. It was demonstrated that the outer layer of vegetable peel contained elevated levels of strontium, plutonium, and americium relative to the flesh, with up to one third of americium being removed by peeling potatoes. However, while peeling potatoes and discarding the skin could be recommended in "accident" situations, normal dietary habits often include eating the skin of the potato, and this must be accounted for in any subsequent dose assessment.

Often the cooking of foods will have an effect on the concentrations of radionuclides. Water-soluble ones will often concentrate in the liquid if food is boiled. If this liquid is discarded, then potential radiological doses may be reduced, but often the water is subsequently used as a stock to produce other edible products such as soup or gravy. It has been reported by Travnikova et al. [59] that preboiling fish contaminated with radiocesium prior to cooking can reduce the levels ingested by up to 50%.

Milk that is contaminated with radiocesium and strontium can be processed into cheese, with much of the ^{137}Cs activity staying in the whey (the liquid fraction) and not being present in the final cheese product. The effect can also be useful at eliminating short-half-life radionuclides such as ^{131}I. In this case, the product is stored for a long period prior to human consumption and the radionuclide harmlessly decays during the storage period.

8.4.4 RECOMMENDATIONS FOR FOOD MONITORING PROGRAMS

The main aim of any monitoring scheme must be to ensure that any radioactivity present in food does not compromise food safety. The program is often set up to identify inputs from authorized and unauthorized discharges of radioactive material into the environment as well as sources of natural radioactivity. The program should cover terrestrial and aquatic food sources. The types of locations around which foods are monitored are likely to include

- Nuclear fuel cycle sites including nuclear power plants.
- Nuclear weapons testing and manufacturing facilities.
- Hospitals, where a wide range of radionuclides can be used for medical diagnosis and treatment.
- Research laboratories.
- Industrial facilities (e.g., phosphate processing, where the by-products can contain enhanced levels of naturally occurring radionuclides such as ^{210}Pb/^{210}Po).
- Locations that are remote from sites known to use radionuclides (like those above) — such data are useful background and to identify potential inputs that were not anticipated.

It is important that the publication time for data that is generated is not delayed for an unreasonable length of time. The public will not gain reassurance from routine monitoring data that is not up to date. Figure 8.5 gives an overview of the most important components of a comprehensive monitoring program. Further expansion of some of the themes identified is provided in Section 8.4.4.1 to Section 8.4.4.6. When designing these monitoring programs, consideration should be given to the food groups and radionuclides summarized in Table 8.2, which have been included in monitoring programs throughout the world.

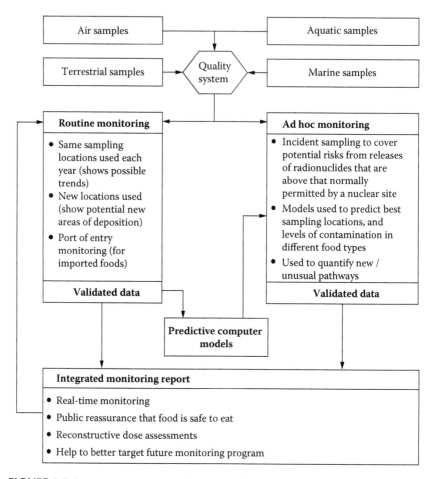

FIGURE 8.5 Important components of a comprehensive monitoring program.

8.4.4.1 Provide Real-Time Monitoring Data to Detect the Presence of Radionuclides

This can be effective in identifying potential exposure at an early stage, often before significant incorporation into the food chain. A good example of this is the Radioactive Incident Monitoring Network (RIMNET), set up and operated by the U.K. Department of Environment, Food, and Rural Affairs. This currently comprises of about 90 dose meters that measure γ radiation. The dose meters are spread throughout the United Kingdom and data are sent automatically to a central computer every hour. The data are then checked to identify any possible increase in radiation that may be attributed to a nuclear accident. Automated systems such as RIMNET play a vital role in monitoring air for γ-emitting radionuclides and run continuously, giving 24-hour-a-day coverage.

TABLE 8.2
Radionuclides and Food Groups Often of Interest in Routine Radiological Monitoring Programs

Food Group	Natural	Artificial
Beverages	^{226}Ra, ^{238}U	^{90}Sr, ^{131}I, ^{137}Cs
Cereals	^{40}K	^{90}Sr, ^{131}I, ^{137}Cs
Fish and shellfish	^{210}Pb, ^{210}Po	^{99}Tc, ^{137}Cs, Pu, Am
Fruit	^{14}C	^{35}S
Game food and venison	^{210}Po	^{137}Cs
Honey	^{14}C	^{137}Cs
Meat and offal	^{210}Po	^{90}Sr, ^{137}Cs, Pu, Am
Milk and dairy products	^{14}C, ^{40}K	^{90}Sr, ^{131}I, ^{137}Cs
Vegetables	^{40}K	^{90}Sr, ^{131}I, ^{137}Cs

8.4.4.2 Provide Public Reassurance That the Food Being Consumed Is Safe to Eat

The sampling scheme needs to be comprehensive to ensure that any relevant pathways are not overlooked. The monitoring programs typically look at foodstuffs from the terrestrial and aquatic environments. It is essential to undertake surveys of consumers' eating habits that can identify food types that may provide a significant dose to high-rate consumers. Byrom et al. [60] used data from three national representative dietary surveys of the U.K. to derive mean, median, and 97.5 percentile consumption rates. It may be that the most at-risk food types are from a small range of imported products, and these should be targeted as part of reassurance monitoring.

8.4.4.3 Produce Reconstructive Dose Assessments

These can provide valuable data to be input into models that are designed to predict potential "at-risk" members of the population:

- To target critical groups, that is, those that may have a high consumption rate of particular food groups, for example, young infants who consume a large volume of milk in their diet.
- To look at the dose for groups identified through consumer habit surveys.
- To review data obtained and, if appropriate, reduce the limits for discharges of radioactivity from nuclear sites that are licensed or authorized to discharge radioactivity.

8.4.4.4   Aid in the Estimation of Prospective Dose Assessments

This aspect of monitoring programs is often overlooked, and yet it is important in determining discharge authorizations (both new and revised) for nuclear installations. Nuclear sites throughout the world generally require prior authorization, often after extensive public consultation, by industry regulators. Information generated in routine monitoring programs is invaluable in determining the effect on the environment and food of proposed emissions and routes and levels of radionuclides in those emissions.

8.4.4.5   Emergency Response

It is essential that a component of a routine monitoring system should be set up to act as a contingency should there be an unusual release of activity, including a major nuclear disaster or potential terrorist attack (e.g., use of a dirty bomb). Such contingency plans are often set up to ensure effective communication between many organizations, in the first instance nationally, but also internationally. They may include plans for evacuation of the population, sheltering, iodine prophylaxis, and restrictions on the consumption of at-risk food supplies. Guidance for emergency planning in the United Kingdom has been produced by the NRPB [61].

Equipment used to monitor food includes mobile detection systems, especially those capable of making γ measurements. Such equipment has become increasingly sophisticated in the last few years and includes portable germanium-based γ spectrometers that are electrically cooled rather than relying on a potentially cumbersome liquid nitrogen supply. Measurements of samples *in situ* can be useful in selecting areas of contamination to allow better targeting of samples for laboratory analysis. Good emergency plans also have provisions for mobile laboratories that can be transported close to the site (though not so close as to contaminate the lab or personnel), and will have a range of α and β detectors, as well as fume cupboards to allow a limited amount of chemical separation to be carried out on the samples. It is very important that contingency plans be tested on a regular basis and refinements made as necessary to ensure the plans are fully effective.

8.4.5   Quality Assurance

It is vital that any data that are produced in a monitoring program are obtained in a way that enhances both scientific and public trust. Independently verified accreditation such as that provided under ISO 17025 is internationally recognized as an appropriate standard for laboratories carrying out analytical measurements. Other relevant certifications include ISO 9001:2000, which covers a broad range of company activities. The public is often distrustful of data published in the scientific literature, and the publication of results to an independently verifiable standard should enhance the acceptability of data.

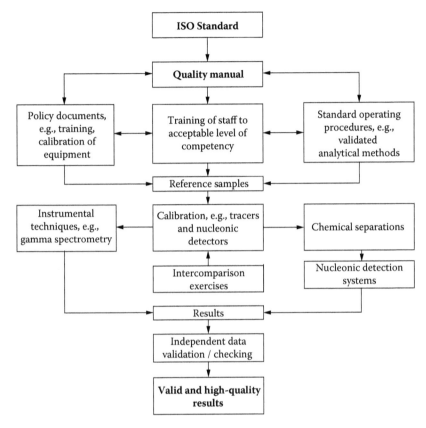

FIGURE 8.6 An overview of a typical quality assurance system and its key components.

Laboratories that have accreditation for carrying out radiochemical analysis of foods will have a well-documented quality system underpinned by a quality manual. A guide to an approach to accreditation was published by Dell and Lally [62], and then a review 10 years after gaining accreditation was written, outlining the benefits of accreditation [63]. It is essential that laboratory staff be appropriately trained to carry out any analytical work prior to analyzing routine samples. Figure 8.6 gives an overview of a typical quality system and its key components. Some points in the overview warrant further explanation at this stage.

The quality manual (QM) is how an individual laboratory puts the quality standard into practice and can be very specific to an individual organization. The QM lays out the laboratories approach to quality and sets the scene for how key policy documents and standard operating procedures are produced and managed. The quality of any laboratory carrying out food monitoring is very much affected by the staff working within it and training, and its documentation is an essential part of an effective quality system.

Any calibration sources, radionuclide tracer solutions used as part of the radiochemical separation methods, or γ spectrometry systems should be traceable to a recognized national or international standard, as measurements with inaccurate standards has a serious detrimental effect on the quality of data produced.

While it is common practice for laboratories carrying out radiochemical analysis of samples to have some form of accreditation or certification, often the same standards are not applied during the data manipulation phases of producing reports. It is essential that any data that are to be published should go through a rigorous review stage.

8.5 INTRODUCTION TO SPECIAL SITUATIONS

National authorities and nuclear operators who conduct radiological monitoring of foodstuffs have defined routine programs that state the frequency and location of sampling, and the range and frequency of analysis of radionuclides. These programs are primarily aimed at providing reassurance to regulatory bodies and the public that discharges from the routine operation of nuclear sites do not result in undue contamination of any local foods and that the exposure dose to people living near the site in question are below limits and constraints.

On occasion, such as an unusual event at a nuclear site or through raised public interest in a particular food or radionuclide, there may be the need for extra sampling, extra analysis, or reprioritization of sample analyses from a routine program. Competent authorities in each country set their own policy on which level of the International Nuclear Event Scale turns the monitoring from reassurance toward a sampling strategy aimed at defining areas requiring possible restriction of the movement or sale of foods due to contamination. After what may be called the acute phase of an emergency, the monitoring becomes more akin to a routine program, and this work may go on for many years or even decades. Other "special situations" include monitoring specific foods or radionuclides because of the unique nature of the pathway of interest or the circumstances of the potential contamination.

8.5.1 Chernobyl

The accident at Chernobyl on April 26, 1986, can be regarded as one of the most significant accidents involving a civil nuclear reactor. The aftereffects of the reactor fire have been felt widely throughout the Northern Hemisphere, with many parts of Europe suffering contamination of land and consequent transfer to the food chain [64]. The deposition consisted of a variety of radionuclides, including ^{110m}Ag, ^{144}Ce, ^{134}Cs, ^{137}Cs, ^{89}Sr, ^{90}Sr, ^{132}Te, ^{239}Pu, ^{103}Ru, ^{106}Ru, and ^{131}I. While the short-half-life radionuclides no longer present a problem, radionuclides with longer physical half-lives, such as ^{137}Cs, persist in food products after nearly 20 years, even several thousands of kilometers from the Chernobyl reactor. This following information demonstrates the geographical spread of contamination, as well as the range of food products that were affected.

Levels of contamination in Byelorussia and the Ukraine were, unsurprisingly, among the highest found. De Ruig and van der Struijs [65] showed that certain food types, including mushrooms, had contamination with radiocesium in excess of 100 kBq/kg, and ^{90}Sr in excess of 1.5 kBq/kg. A study of a drainless peat lake in the contaminated region showed levels of ^{137}Cs in pike fish in excess of 23 kBq/kg and crayfish in excess of 4 kBq/kg. These were based on a survey carried out 10 years after the accident, showing the persistence of cesium in this type of ecological environment. They estimated that this was the main ingestion pathway for the local population, typically accounting for 40% to 50% of the dose. They also reported the continued feeding of Prussian blue to dairy cattle, which reduced the ^{137}Cs levels in milk to about 15% of that if the animals were not fed Prussian blue. This demonstrates that relatively simple countermeasures can be effective in reducing mans' exposure to contamination via dairy products.

In Italy, levels of contamination were particularly high in the northeast, such as in the Friuli Venezia Giulia region. Giovani et al. [66] showed that, as in many other nations, the contamination of mushrooms was a real problem. It is interesting to note that between 1986 and 2001, the average ^{137}Cs activity from eight survey sites used by the authors has remained relatively constant at 20 kBq/kg dry weight. Generally, marine species in the Ligurian Sea, near the northeast Italian coast, show much lower levels of activity. Gallelli et al. [67] showed very low concentrations of cesium in marine species, reflecting the dilution of contaminants in the open ocean. It was shown that the contamination in mollusk species was higher than that of fish and shellfish, and the common octopus (*Octopus vulgaris*) can be used as a good indicator of radioactive contamination in the ocean.

In Greece, Assikamakpoulos et al. [68] showed levels of ^{131}I in sheep milk were in excess of 18 kBq/kg. It should be noted that throughout the literature, levels of ^{131}I were consistently higher in sheep than cattle, which may be due to the feeding habits of sheep, which tend to have a higher soil intake when grazing.

In Finland, in 1986, Rantavaara et al. [69] identified levels of radiocesium as high as 10.5 kBq/kg in several species of waterfowl.

In Germany, Bunzl and Kracke [70] identified levels of ^{131}I in honey in excess of 14 kBq/kg and ^{103}Ru at 0.7 kBq/kg. Prohl et al. [71] showed that 29% of ^{137}Cs from contaminated barley was transferred through to beer via the fermentation process. This was identified as an important pathway of cesium to man, where average consumption of beer in Germany for adults has been estimated at 150 l/yr.

Scandinavian countries were greatly affected by deposition from Chernobyl. Ahman and Ahman [72] reported ^{137}Cs as high as 80 kBq/kg in reindeer meat in 1986, and later demonstrated a marked seasonal variation in the concentration linked with the migration of the animals between their summer range in the mountains and their winter range spent nearer the Baltic Sea. Rosen et al. [73] indicated an effective ecological half-life for cesium of 3.4 years in lambs, with average concentrations decreasing from 1.1 kBq/kg in 1990. It should be understood that the ecological half-life often varies from region to region due to the underlying soil type. Ahman et al. [74] showed effective half-lives in two different regions of 11.0 and 7.1 years.

In the U.K. in 1986, concentrations of ^{131}I in cow's milk analyzed by the Central Veterinary Laboratory were found at up to 0.4 kBq/l, and radiocesium in ovine muscle was found at up to 4.2 kBq/kg in ovine meat from Cumbria and north Wales [75]. The consequences of the accident have lingered for many years, especially in upland areas of north Wales, Cumbria, and southern Scotland. In 2004 it was reported to the Scottish and U.K. Parliaments that 359 farms in Wales covering an area of 53,000 ha, 9 farms in Cumbria, and 18 farms in Scotland were still under animal movement restrictions as a result of deposition of ^{137}Cs from Chernobyl. Fisk and Sanderson [76] carried out a study of radiocesium concentrations in heather honey in Scotland between 1993 and 1995 and showed concentrations up to 0.7 kBq/kg. Problems within the U.K. are particularly persistent where the soil type is peat based and where there is an absence of clay particles to bind the cesium to make it unavailable for uptake by plants, and thence from plants to animal.

8.5.2 SELLAFIELD AND THE CUMBRIAN COAST

In October 1957, the core of the no. 1 pile of the U.K. Windscale plant at Sellafield overheated and caught fire, releasing radioiodine into the atmosphere. The NRPB estimated that the fire caused the release of 740 TBq of ^{131}I and 22 TBq of ^{137}Cs, as well as a wide range of other radionuclides [61]. The principal dose exposure pathway immediately after the fire was from the consumption of milk contaminated with ^{131}I. A ban on milk was put in place for about 200 mi^2 around Windscale. The NRPB also estimated that the fire resulted in the release of about 8.8 TBq of ^{210}Po into the atmosphere [61].

A full review ("habit survey") of seafood consumption rates at Sellafield was undertaken in 1998. The review revealed that a single family was consuming material caught as bycatch by the local fishing industry. The bycatch products included uncommon species that were not normally eaten, such as sea mice (a marine worm [*Aphrodite aculeata*]), sea urchins (*Echinoidea*), brittle stars (*Ophiuroidea*), common shore crabs (*Carcinus maenas*), and hermit crabs (*Eupagurus* sp.). Some of these species were consumed directly after cooking, other material was used in soups [77]. A consumption of 8.3 kg/yr of sea mice was found and the dose calculation suggested that a dose of up to 0.33 mSv could potentially be received by the consumption of these by-products. This was mostly due to the relatively high concentration of actinides, including 7.6 Bq/kg ^{238}Pu, 37 Bq/kg $^{239+240}$Pu, and 110 Bq/kg ^{241}Am. By comparison, the next highest activity levels found that year were from a winkle sample from St. Bees, just south of the Sellafield site, with 3.9 Bq/kg of ^{238}Pu, 19 Bq/kg $^{239+240}$Pu, and 34 Bq/kg of ^{241}Am. Only 4.5 kg/yr of winkles were estimated to be consumed, which together with the activity levels gives a significantly lower dose than for bycatches. This started a further investigation of the possible consumption of uncommon foods, including those caught near other sites around the U.K. [78]. By 2002 the family had moved out of the area and the habit survey for that year and subsequent years did not

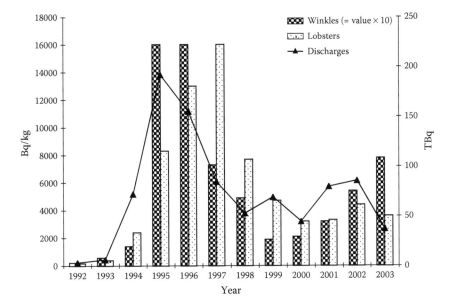

FIGURE 8.7 ^{99}Tc activity levels in lobsters and winkles around Sellafield and annual site discharges of [99]Tc (1992 to 2003).

find any other consumption of uncommon seafood or bycatches, but the exposure pathway will remain under review.

The Sellafield site has been reducing discharges of most radionuclides for many years now. An exception to this is [99]Tc. Figure 8.7 shows the discharges of ^{99}Tc from Sellafield and the corresponding levels in winkles (multiplied by a factor of 10) and lobsters near Sellafield since 1992. It can be seen that the levels in winkles closely match the discharge profile, while lobsters appear to have a lag of about 2 years. In 2003, discharges of ^{99}Tc were estimated to have added 0.030 mSv to the dose of Sellafield seafood consumers, accounting for about 15% of the dose. Figure 8.8 shows the relationship between ^{99}Tc discharges since 1992 and the corresponding percentage of dose to members of the local fishing community from consumption of fish and shellfish.

[99]Tc from Sellafield can be detected in the Irish Sea, in Scottish waters, the North Sea [38], and as far away as the Arctic [32]. Analysis of seaweed from Hillesøy, on the northern coast of Norway, showed a steep increase of ^{99}Tc in seaweed in the late spring and early summer of 1997. It has been suggested that this was due to the rapid increase in discharges from Sellafield in the spring of 1994 [32].

Another unusual exposure pathway at Sellafield that required special investigation was the contamination of feral pigeons. On February 6, 1998, the U.K. Ministry of Agriculture, Fisheries, and Food (MAFF) was informed that feral pigeons were found to be contaminated in the village of Seascale, close to the

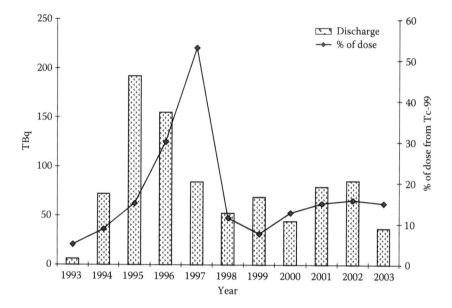

FIGURE 8.8 Annual ^{99}Tc discharges from Sellafield and the percentage of the aquatic pathway dose due to ^{99}Tc (1993 to 2003).

Sellafield site. These birds were part of a group of about 700 birds that were being fed at a pigeon sanctuary in the village. Around 150 of the birds had been humanely killed in order to reduce the number of birds at the sanctuary, and some of these were sent for monitoring.

The site operator's initial measurements gave a dose rate of around 1.4 mSv/h, but it was not clear whether this was all from surface contamination of the birds or internal contamination as well. The MAFF investigated the level of internal contamination in the birds. Results showed that there was significant internal contamination of up to 110 kBq/kg. More than 50 kBq/kg ^{137}Cs was found in one sample of pigeon breast meat, about 40 times the community food intervention level (CFIL) for ^{137}Cs in meat, which is 1250 Bq/kg. The CFILs are maximum permitted levels of radionuclides in foodstuffs that would apply in the event of a nuclear accident or emergency, and therefore do not actually apply in this case, but are a good measure for comparison.

Results from the site operator supplied to the MAFF indicated that for birds with the highest radionuclide concentrations, only six birds need to be consumed to achieve a dose of 1 mSv. However, the MAFF found no evidence of anyone consuming feral pigeons or the meat entering the human food chain. Nevertheless, as a precaution, the MAFF issued advice on February 14, 1998, not to handle, slaughter, or consume pigeons within a 10-mile radius of the Sellafield site [79].

Although no pathway for consumption of feral pigeons was found, for reassurance purposes, local wood pigeons have been regularly monitored since 1999 and have been found to have little or no contamination. Since 1998, the site

TABLE 8.3
Levels of ^{90}Sr and ^{137}Cs in Pigeon Meat
from Around the Sellafield Site

| | Year | Activity Levels in Meat (Bq/kg) | | Reference |
		^{137}Cs	^{90}Sr	
Feral pigeon	1998	50,388	520	77
Wood pigeon	1999	4.5*	0.06	88
Wood pigeon	2001	1.5*	0.02	89
Wood pigeon	2003	1.0*	0.03	38

* Total cesium.

operator has implemented remediation and dose reduction procedures at the site and also substantially reduced the feral pigeon population. Table 8.3 shows the levels of ^{90}Sr and ^{137}Cs in feral and wood pigeon meat since 1998.

8.5.3 TECHA RIVER

The Mayak Production Association site, situated between Ekaterinburg and Cheliabinsk, was the site of the first production reactor complex built in Russia for the production of weapons-grade plutonium. A number of natural lakes and ponds have been used as reservoirs for the management of radioactive effluents. The construction of dams along the Techa River system considerably reduced direct radioactive discharges to the river compared to discharges made between 1949 and 1956. It is believed that 100 PBq of radioactive material was discharged to the reservoirs during that period, causing severe contamination along the entire length of the Techa River [80]. Meanwhile, 7500 people evacuated from 20 settlements along the Techa River received radiation doses ranging from 35 mSv to 1.7 Sv [81]. Maximum contamination occurred along the riverbanks, at an height of about 1 m above the normal water level. Reported contamination ranged from hundreds of kilobecquerels per square meter to hundreds of megabecquerels per square meter for ^{137}Cs [82] and hundreds of kilobecquerels per square meter for ^{90}Sr (2002 reference date) [83], with good correlation between ^{90}Sr and ^{137}Cs [84]. Grass activity levels ranged from 100 Bq/kg to 8 kBq/kg for ^{137}Cs and 450 Bq/kg to 8.4 kBq/kg dry weight for ^{90}Sr. ^{90}Sr soil activity in villages near the Techa River is at least an order of magnitude higher than expected from global fallout due to weapons tests [83].

The effects of such soil contamination by ^{137}Cs and ^{90}Sr on local foodstuffs, mainly produced in private gardens, reveal large variations, possibly as a result of some inhabitants watering their gardens with Techa River water or fertilizing it with river silt. For instance, ^{90}Sr activity levels in potatoes ranged from 0.1 to 7.0 Bq/kg fresh weight and spring onion ranged from 0.2 to 93 Bq/kg fresh weight. The range is even larger for ^{137}Cs, with milk activity levels from 0.1 to 174 Bq/kg fresh weight and from 0.1 to 34 Bq/kg fresh weight for ^{90}Sr. Results are consistent with the likelihood that some cows have access to the contaminated floodplain, leading to very different milk activities than for herds grazing on land further from the river banks.

Using the average contamination density in nearby villages, excluding the contaminated floodplain, Shutov et al. [83] calculated the aggregated transfer parameter (T_{ag}) (see Section 8.5.6) for ^{90}Sr in milk of 4.0×10^5 m^2/kg, compared with a value of 7.2×10^5 m^2/kg in Switzerland in 2003. The authors calculated the maximum activity of milk in all herds grazing on the contaminated floodplain as 60 Bq/l for ^{137}Cs and 30 Bq/l for ^{90}Sr. Meanwhile, there was no statistically significant change in ^{137}Cs and ^{90}Sr activity in cow milk produced in villages close to the Techa River over the sampling period (1992 to 1998). This may indicate an equilibrium state, which will lead eventually to a decrease in milk activity only with the physical half-life of both radionuclides. It was recognized recently that the registry of Mayak workers and the general population are as valuable as the data on survivors of the Hiroshima and Nagasaki bombs for the assessment of long-term, low-level, internal dose risk [85].

8.5.4 CARDIFF, WALES

GE Healthcare currently operates a plant in Cardiff, Wales, that produces radio-isotopes for medical use. Since 1982 the site has been authorized to release ^{3}H as liquid waste into the local sewage system, where it is mixed with sewage wastes and is subsequently discharged into the Severn estuary at a place called Orchard Ledges.

Most U.K. nuclear sites discharge ^{3}H in the form of ^{3}H$_2$O, which is rapidly diluted and dispersed with prevailing currents when released into the marine environment. The Cardiff site releases ^{3}H in this form, but also as organically bound tritium (OBT). The exact chemical composition of the organic component of the effluent is unknown, as it contains many reaction intermediates and by-products as well as the final radiolabeled compound. It is estimated that up to 30% of the ^{3}H discharged into the sewage system through May 1998 consisted of OBT [86].

Organisms incorporate ^{3}H into their tissues in the form of ^{3}H$_2$O very rapidly and reach concentrations approaching that of the external medium. Incorporation of ^{3}H in the form of OBT into cells occurs at a much slower rate than free water and typically reaches a concentration about half that of the external medium. The dose coefficient for ^{3}H as OBT is up to 2.5 times that of ^{3}H$_2$O [87]. Taking these factors together suggests that analyzing ^{3}H levels in seawater would give a reliable indicator of total ^{3}H in fish and shellfish samples, which was what the MAFF did until 1997.

In 1997, four samples of flounder were found to contain a mean of 19 kBq/kg total ^{3}H, while the seawater only contained a mean of 53 Bq/l [88]. This pattern of results was repeated in 1998 and in subsequent years (see Figure 8.9) and was

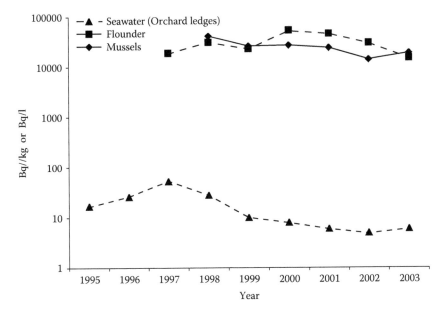

FIGURE 8.9 Total ^{3}H activity levels in mussels, flounders, and seawater from Cardiff Bay (1995 to 2003).

TABLE 8.4
Mean ^{3}H Concentrations in Flounder and
Mussels from Around Cardiff (1997 to 2003)
[38,45,77,88–91]

	Bq/kg (Wet) in Flounder		Bq/kg (Wet) in Mussels	
Year	Total ^{3}H	OBT	Total ^{3}H	OBT
1997	19,000	N/A	N/A	N/A
1998	31,000	N/A	41,000	N/A
1999	23,000	16,000	26,000	20,000
2000	54,000	51,000	27,000	24,000
2001	46,000	NA	24,000	25,000
2002	30,000	27,000	14,000	12,000
2003	15,000	14,000	19,000	19,000

Note: NA, not available.

also seen in mussels, with 41 kBq/kg found in 1998. Further analysis of ^{3}H showed that OBT accounted for about 70 to 100% of the total ^{3}H in flounders and mussels, as shown in Table 8.4.

Other species of fish and shellfish have shown similar activity levels of ^{3}H, with high fractions of OBT [38,45,77,89–91]. Annual averages for total ^{3}H in sole since 1998 have been in the range of 3.7 to 43 kBq/kg, and the annual average for cod since 1999 has ranged from 2 to 33 kBq/kg. In 2000, a wide variety of species were caught and analyzed for total ^{3}H: chubb (10 kBq/kg), barbel (30 kBq/kg), grayling (17 kBq/kg), roach (15 kBq/kg), and eel (30 kBq/kg). In 1998, lugworms were found to contain 16 kBq/kg, and in 2000, green crabs had concentrations of 59 kBq/kg, shrimp 40 kBq/kg, and whelks 74 kBq/kg.

Following the initial findings in 1997, the Environment Agency required the site to reduce its ^{3}H discharges. Prior to 1997, annual discharges of total ^{3}H ranged from 397 to 609 TBq. In May 1998, certain tritiated methanolic wastes and ^{3}H$_2$O were withheld from the discharge, resulting in a reduction in total ^{3}H discharged. However, the proportion of the OBT increased to around 80% [92]. Since then the annual discharges have steadily decreased, to 30 TBq in 2003. As can be seen from Figure 8.9 and Table 8.4, even after the reduction in discharges, levels of ^{3}H in fish and shellfish have remained very high in comparison to the levels in seawater. This implies that either there is a biological sink or the source still remains.

Warwick et al. [92] suggested short-term temporal variations (observed by sampling sediments monthly over a 2 year period) were due to weather or were tide related. Spatial variability shows an approximate symmetrical decline with distance from the effluent pipe carrying the ^{3}H discharges, based on measurements from multiple sediment sampling sites along the coast on either side of the discharge point. ^{3}H activities up to a maximum of 0.83 Bq/g have been found near the discharge point, declining to less than 0.2 Bq/g further away.

Relatively low concentrations have been found in the herbivorous winkle (*Littorina littorea*), with 4 kBq/kg observed in 1998 [77], and the pelagic sprat (*Spratus spratus*) compared with other benthic organisms (e.g., green crabs and lugworms) and demersal fish (e.g., flounder and sole) [33]. Demersal fish species live on or near the bottom of the sea, while pelagic fish live in the water column. McCubbin et al. [33] suggested that the variation between fish was most likely a result of differences in environmental behavior rather than age.

Since lower benthos species, such as burrowing worms, were found to contain high levels of ^{3}H, it has been suggested that the sediment plays an important role in the transfer of ^{3}H to the food chain [33]. This is in agreement with the work of Warwick et al. [92], who found that ^{3}H was mostly associated with the fine-grained mud/silt fraction and was not water extractable, with a low extraction efficiency of less than 10%. They also found freeze drying had little effect on the levels in sediment, suggesting a strong association for the ^{3}H with the sediment. Sediment cores also suggest a correlation with discharge records, although McCubbin et al. [33] noted that the cores did not reflect the decline in recent discharge levels, which they attributed to the mixture of organic material.

Wildfowl were analyzed for levels of ^{3}H in 1999 to see if ^{3}H was moving through the trophic levels. Shelducks contained up to 61 kBq/kg (mean 24 kBq/kg) of total ^{3}H, with 42 kBq/kg being OBT. These levels can be compared with levels of ^{3}H in ducks from Sellafield. In 1998, ducks from near Sellafield contained less than 3 Bq/kg of total ^{3}H, even though the site discharged 2310 TBq of ^{3}H in 1998, while Cardiff discharged only 105 TBq in 1999.

All the data for OBT levels suggest a bioaccumulation process due to incorporation of the radiolabeled biologically active compounds discharged from the Cardiff site. Investigations were undertaken to see if gaseous discharges of ^{3}H where affecting the terrestrial food chain in the same manner as the aquatic.

In 1999, grass samples were taken from tide-washed pastures on both the Welsh and English sides of the Bristol Channel. Levels of ^{3}H on the English side ranged from less than the limit of detection (LoD) up to 10 Bq/kg total ^{3}H (8 Bq/kg of OBT), while those along the Welsh coast on either side of the Cardiff discharge point ranged from 170 to 320 Bq/kg, with OBT in the range of 73 to 210 Bq/kg. Grass samples taken inland nearer the site had concentrations up to 2000 Bq/kg [89].

In 2000, a wide variety of terrestrial samples were taken from around the Cardiff site and analyzed for total ^{3}H and OBT [45]. Levels of total ^{3}H were significantly lower than in aquatic samples. The highest level found was 630 Bq/kg total ^{3}H (230 Bq/kg of OBT) for cabbage, and it was noted that concentrations for most samples decreased with distance from the site [93]. OBT rarely accounted for more than 50% of the total ^{3}H, often being less than 25%. Where the OBT accounted for more than 50% of the total, the actual levels reported were very low (almost at the LoD) and the uncertainty on the measurement was such that ratios between OBT and ^{3}H$_2$O were potentially subject to large variations. These results suggested that the bioaccumulation processes noted in aquatic samples due to liquid ^{3}H discharges were not repeated for terrestrial samples exposed to gaseous ^{3}H discharges.

Reductions in ^{3}H levels in milk were also noted. Figure 8.10 compares the annual maximum average ^{3}H levels in milk for farms up to 3.5 km from the site with farms more than 3.5 km from the site. Farms more than 3.5 km from the site consistently had levels at or around the LoD. Figure 8.10 also shows the annual discharges of gaseous ^{3}H since 1997. The reduction in ^{3}H levels at farms within 3.5 km of the site closely matches the reduction in gaseous discharges over the period since 1997.

In April 2002, a new sewage treatment plant was commissioned. This sewage plant takes the radioactive liquid waste from the Cardiff site and treats it in an activated sludge treatment plant, resulting in a high-quality effluent being discharged into the estuary. It is hoped that this will further reduce the discharges of ^{3}H into the Severn estuary.

8.5.5 Brazil Nuts

Brazil nuts are seeds of the tree *Bertholletia excelsa*, found in many parts of the Amazon River valley, on clay and argillous sandstone, a formation of low NORM content. As early as 1933, it was shown that Brazil nuts accumulated unusual amounts of barium [94]. Turner et al. [95] measured NORM activity in Brazil nuts as high as 300 Bq/kg. Later, Penna-Franca [96] measured ^{226}Ra and ^{228}Ra

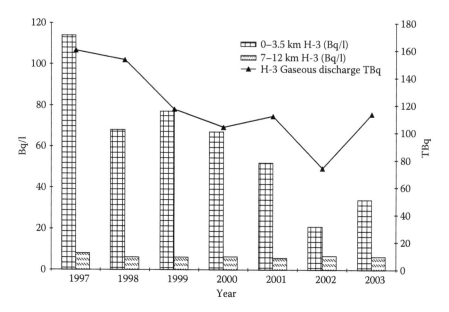

FIGURE 8.10 The effect of gaseous (soluble) ³H discharge from Cardiff on the concentration of ³H in milk (1997 to 2003).

in Brazil nuts and found both isotope activities to be around 50 Bq/kg. It was shown that *Bertholletia excelsa* possess an enormous radicular system that is able to absorb a large amounts of nutrients from the soil. Unlike the vast majority of plants, *Bertholletia excelsa* discriminates against calcium in favor of barium, with barium and radium preferentially absorbed in all parts of the tree, especially in the fruits and nuts [10].

In Switzerland, ^{90}Sr activity for imported Brazil nuts was measured and was found to range from 11 to 15 Bq/kg. The ^{90}Sr/calcium ratio was 50 ± 5 Bq ^{90}Sr/g of calcium, a value far greater than those routinely determined for other food products in Switzerland. For comparison, grass samples have an average ratio less than unity (range 0.2 to 0.9). It amounts to 0.22 ± 0.02 Bq ^{90}Sr/g of calcium in wheat and 0.07 ± 0.02 Bq ^{90}Sr/g of calcium in apples.

The aggregated transfer parameter (T_{ag}) is calculated by using the following relation:

$$T_{ag} = \frac{^{90}Sr \ activity \ concentration \ in \ food \ \left[\dfrac{Bq}{kg}\right]}{^{90}Sr \ activity \ deposited \ in \ soil \ \left[\dfrac{Bq}{m^2}\right]}.$$

Table 8.5 shows the T_{ag} for some foodstuff samples analyzed in 2003 in Switzerland, taking an average deposition of 700 Bq/m² for the Swiss lowland

TABLE 8.5
^{90}Sr Aggregated Transfer Factors (T_{ag}) for Some Food
Samples Determined in Switzerland in 2003

Food Product	Average ^{90}Sr Activity (Bq/kg)	T_{ag}
Grass	4.4	7.1×10^{-3}
Milk	0.05	7.2×10^{-5}
Wheat	0.3	4.3×10^{-4}
Apples	0.08	1.1×10^{-4}
Potatoes	0.7	1.0×10^{-3}
Brazil nuts	12	5.0×10^{-2}

[7]. Added to this table is the T_{ag} for Brazil nuts, taking an average deposition for the Brazil Amazonian zone (0°–15°S latitude) of 250 Bq/m^2 [97]. Results show that the T_{ag} for Brazil nuts is almost 50 times higher than that of potatoes, which can be directly contaminated by ^{90}Sr translocation from soil to potatoes. Taking into account only cereals or fruits with no contact with soil (e.g., wheat or apples), the increase in T_{ag} for Brazil nuts is more than 400 times.

Brazil nuts have by far the greatest ^{90}Sr aggregated transfer factor known at the present time. Brazil nut trees or related species with similar behavior regarding calcium may be very useful for bioremediation of sites highly contaminated by ^{90}Sr or radium.

8.6 FUTURE ISSUES

The Codex Alimentarius Commission (CAC) has been tasked with producing a set of guidelines for levels of radioactivity in food for use in international trade. The proposals have been published for the first stage of consultation [98]. The suggested levels (shown in Table 8.6) are designed to protect public health and harmonize international trade. The radionuclides included are deemed to be those of greatest importance in terms of uptake into the food chain. The activity of each radionuclide within a group is to be summed and the total compared with

TABLE 8.6
Draft Guideline Levels (in Bq/kg) for Radionuclides in Food [98]

Radionuclides in Food	Draft Guideline Level (Bq/kg)
^{238}Pu, ^{239}Pu, ^{240}Pu, ^{241}Am	1
^{90}Sr, ^{106}Ru, ^{129}I, ^{131}I, ^{235}U	100
^{35}S, ^{60}Co, ^{89}Sr, ^{103}Ru, ^{134}Cs, ^{137}Cs, ^{144}Ce, ^{192}Ir	1000
^{3}H*, ^{14}C, ^{99}Tc	10,000

* Represents organically bound tritium.

the guideline level. At the time of writing, worldwide consultation is ongoing, with individual countries assessing the impact on their food industries. It may be that the suggested guideline levels will have to be modified in light of the response from international consultation. Once again, this reflects the importance of gathering appropriate monitoring data. Assuming that these proposals are accepted, countries will need to review their monitoring programs to demonstrate compliance.

REFERENCES

1. Lu, N., Kung, K.S., Mason, C.F.V., Triay, I.R., Cotter, C.R., Pappas, A.J., and Pappas, M.E.G., Removal of plutonium-239 and americium-241 from Rocky Flats soil by leaching, *Environ. Sci. Technol.*, 32, 370, 1998.
2. Perrier, T., Martin-Garin, A., and Morello, M., Remobilisation of [241]Am in a calcareous soil under simplified rhizospheric conditions, studied by column experiments, *J. Environ. Radiactiv.*, 79, 205, 2004.
3. Bundt, M., Albrecht, A., Froidevaux, P., Blaser, P., and Flühler, H., Impact of preferential flow on radionuclides distribution in soil, *Environ. Sci. Technol.*, 34, 3895, 2000.
4. Suess, H.E., Radiocarbon concentration in modern wood, *Nature*, 122, 415, 1955.
5. McGee, E.J., Gallagher, D., Mitchell, P. I., Baillie, M., Brown, D., and Keogh, S.M., Recent chronologies for tree rings and terrestrial archives using ^{14}C bomb fallout history, *Geochim. Cosmochim. Acta*, 68, 2509, 2004.
6. Otlet, R.L., Walker, A.J., Fulker, M.J., and Collins, C., Background carbon-14 levels in UK foodstuffs based on a 1992 survey, *J. Environ. Radioactiv.*, 34, 91, 1997.
7. Froidevaux, P., Geering, J.-J., Pillonel, L., Bosset, J.-O., and Valley, J.-F., ^{90}Sr, [238]U, [234]U, ^{137}Cs, [40]K and [239/240]Pu in Emmental type cheese produced in different regions of western Europe, *J. Environ. Radioactiv.*, 72, 287, 2004.
8. ICRP, *Reference Man: Anatomical, Physiological and Metabolic Characteristics*, Publication no. 23, International Commission on Radiological Protection, Pergamon Press, Oxford, 1976.
9. NCRP, *Exposure of the Population of the United States and Canada from Natural Background Radiation*, NCRP Report 94, National Council on Radiation Protection and Measurements, Bethesda, MD, 1987.
10. Penna-Franca, E., Fiszman, M., Lobao, N., Costa-Ribeiro, C., Trindade, H., Dos Santos, P. L., and Batista, D., Radioactivity of Brazil Nuts, *Health Phys.*, 14, 95, 1968.
11. Ebbs, S., Uranium speciation, plant uptake, and phytoremediation, *Pract. Period. Hazard. Toxic Radioactiv. Waste Manage.*, 5, 130, 2001.
12. Beresford, N.A., Mayes, R.W., Cooke, A.I., Barnett, C.L., Howard, B.J. Stuart Lamb, C., and Naylor, G.P.L., The importance of source-dependent bioavailability in determining the transfer of ingested radionuclides to ruminant-derived food products, *Environ. Sci. Technol.*, 34, 4455, 2000.
13. Rayno, D.R., Estimated dose to man from uranium milling via the beef/milk food chain pathway, *Sci. Total Environ.*, 31, 219, 1983.
14. Lapham, S.C, Millard, J.B., and Samet, J.M., Health implications of radionuclide levels in cattle raised near U mining and milling facilities in Ambrosia Lake, New Mexico, *Health Phys.*, 56, 327, 1989.

15. Betti, M., Aldave de las Heras, L., Janssens, A., Henrich, E., Hunter, G., Gerchikov, M., Dutton, M., van Weers, A.W., Nielsen, S., Simmonds, J., Bexon, A., and Sazykina, T., Results of the European Commission Marina II Study Part II — effects of discharges of naturally occurring radioactive material, *J. Environ. Radioactiv.,* 74, 255, 2004.

16. Kathren, R.L., NORM sources and their origins, *Appl. Radiat. Isot.,* 49, 149, 1998.

17. Smith, K.P., Arnish, J.J., Williams, G.P., and Blunt, D.L., Assessment of the disposal of radioactive petroleum industry waste in nonhazardous landfills using risk-based modeling, *Environ. Sci. Technol.,* 37, 2060, 2003.

18. Pourcelot, L., Louvat, D., Gauthier-Lafaye, F., and Stille, P., Formation of radioactivity enriched soils in mountain areas, *J. Environ. Radioactiv.,* 68, 215, 2003.

19. Schuller, P., Voigt, G., Handl, J., Ellies, A., and Oliva, L., Global weapons' fallout ^{137}Cs in soils and transfer to vegetation in south–central Chile, *J. Environ. Radioactiv.,* 62, 181, 2002.

20. Mitchell, P.I., Sanchez-Cabeza, J.A., Ryan, T.P., McGarry, A.T., and Vidal-Quatras, A., Preliminary estimate of cumulative caesium and plutonium deposition in the Irish terrestrial environment, *J. Radioanal. Nucl. Chem.,* 138, 241, 1990.

21. Hölgye, Z. and Filgas, R., Inventory of [238]Pu and [239/240]Pu in the soil of Czechoslovakia in 1990, *J. Environ. Radioactiv.,* 27, 181, 1995.

22. Wright, S.M., Howard, B.J., Strand, P., Nylén, T., and Sickel, M. A. K., Prediction of 137Cs deposition from atmospheric nuclear weapons tests within the Arctic, *Environ. Pollut.,* 104, 131, 1999.

23. Hardy, E.P., Krey, P.W., and Volchok, H.L., Global inventory and distribution of fallout Pu, *Nature,* 241, 444, 1973.

24. Froidevaux, P., Geering, J.-J., Friedrich-Bénet, K., Schmittler, T., Barraud, F., and Valley, J.-F., Mesure de ^{90}Sr dans les vertèbres et les dents de lait, Environmental Radioactivity and radiation Exposure in Switzerland, Federal Office of Public Health, Division of Radiation Protection, Chemin du Musée 3, 1700 Fribourg, Switzerland, 2002.

25. Geering, J.-J., Friedli, C., and Lerch, P., Method of determination of ^{90}Sr in the environment, *J. Trace Microprobe Techniq.,* 8, 211, 1990.

26. Friedli, C., Geering, J.-J., and Lerch, P., Some aspect of the behaviour of ^{90}Sr in the environment, *Radiochim. Acta,* 52, 237, 1991.

27. UNSCEAR, *Sources, Effects and Risks of Ionizing Radiation,* Report to the General Assembly, United Nations, New York, 1988.

28. Strebl, F., Gerzabek, M.H., Bossew, P., and Kienzl, K., Distribution of radiocaesium in an Austrian forest stand, *Sci. Total Environ.,* 226, 75, 1999.

29. Mück, K., Sustainability of radiologically contaminated territories, *J. Environ. Radioactiv.,* 65, 109, 2003.

30. Jonsson, B., Forseth, T., and Ugedal, O., Chernobyl radioactivity persists in fish, *Nature,* 400, 417, 1999.

31. Smith, J.T., Comans, R.N.J., Beresford, N.A., Wright, S.M., Howard, B.J., and Camplin, W.C., Chernobyl's legacy in food and water, *Nature,* 405, 141, 2000.

32. Nilsson, A. and Huntingdon, H., *Arctic Pollution 2002,* Arctic Monitoring and Assessment Programme, Norway, 2002.

33. McCubbin, D., Leonard, K.S., Bailey, T.A., Williams, J., and Tossell, P., Incorporation of tritium (3H) by aquatic organisms and sediment in the Severn estuary/Bristol Channel (UK), *Mar. Pollut. Bull.,* February 2001, 1, 2001.

34. Ham, G.J., Ewers, L.W., and Wilkins, B.T., *Variations in Concentrations of Naturally-Occurring Radionuclides in Foodstuffs*, NRPB-M892, National Radiological Protection Board, Chilton, UK, 1998.
35. Howard, B.J., Livens, F.R., and Walters, C.B., A review of radionuclides in tidewashed pastures on the Irish Sea coast in England and Wales and their transfer to food products, *Environ. Pollut.*, 93, 63, 1996.
36. Environmental Radiation Ambient Monitoring Systems (ERAMS) Sampling Program, available at www.epa.gov/narel/erams/programms.html.
37. Commission of the European Communities, Commission recommendation on the application of Article 36 of the Euratom Treaty concerning the monitoring of the levels of radioactivity in the environment for the purpose of assessing the exposure of the population as a whole, *Offic. J. Eur. Communities*, July 27, 2000, 2000/473/Euratom, 2000.
38. Environment Agency, Environment and Heritage Service, Food Standards Agency and Scottish Environment Protection Agency, *Radioactivity in Food and the Environment, 2003*, RIFE-9, Environment Agency, EHS, Food Standards Agency and SEPA, Bristol, Belfast, London, and Stirling, 2004.
39. Ministry of Agriculture, Fisheries and Food, *National Food Survey 1997*, Stationery Office, London, 1998.
40. Mondon, K.J. and Walters, C.B., Measurements of radiocaesium, radiostrontium and plutonium in whole diets following deposition of radioactivity in the UK originating from the Chernobyl power plant accident, *Food Addit. Contam.*, 7, 837, 1990.
41. Capar, S.G. and Cunningham, W.C., Element and radionuclide concentrations in food: FDA Total Diet Study 1991–1996, *J. AOAC Int.*, 83, 157, 2000.
42. Sanchez, A.L., Singleton, D.L. Dodd, B.A., Davis, J., Benzing, R., and Sarsby, H., *Analysis of the Food Groups In the Total Diet Study*, CEH Project No. C01141, CEH, Cumbria, 2001.
43. Al-Masri, M.S., Mukallati, H., Al-Hamwi, A., Khalili, H., Hassan, M., Assaf, H., Amin, Y., and Nashawati, A., Natural radionuclides in Syrian diet and their daily intake, *J. Radioanal. and Nucl. Chem.*, 260 (2), 405-412, 2004.
44. Green, N., Hammond, D.J., Davidson, M.F., Wilkins, B.T., and Williams, B., *The Radiological Impact of Naturally-Occurring Radionuclides in Foods from the Wild*, NRPB-W30, National Radiological Protection Board, Chilton, 2002.
45. Food Standards Agency and Scottish Environment Protection Agency, *Radioactivity in Food and the Environment, 2000*, RIFE-6, Food Standards Agency and SEPA, London and Stirling, 2001.
46. Green, N., Hammond, D.J., Davidson, M.F., Wilkins, B.T., Richmond, S., and Brooker, S., *Evaluation of the radiological impact of free foods found in the vicinity of nuclear sites*, NRPB-M1018, Chilton, 1999.
47. Fulker, M.J., Jackson, D., Leonard, D.R.P., McKay, K., and John, C., Dose due to man-made radionuclides in terrestrial wild foods near Sellafield, *J. Radiol. Protect.*, 18, 3, 1998.
48. Food and Agriculture Organization of the United Nations, *Rice Market Monitor*, United Nations, New York, December 2004.
49. Muramatsu, Y., Uchida, S., and Ohmomo, Y., Root-uptake of radioiodine by rice plants, *J. Radiat. Res.*, 34, 214, 1993.

50. Uchida, S., Muramatsu, Y., Sumiya, M., and Ohmomo, Y., Biological half-life of gaseous elemental iodine deposited onto rice grains, *Health Phys.*, 60, 675, 1991.

51. Martin, P. and Ryan, B., Natural-series radionuclides in traditional Aboriginal foods in tropical northern Australia: a review, *Sci. World*, 4, 77, 2004.

52. Iyengar, G.V., Kawamura, H., Dang, H.S., Parr, R.M., Wang, J.W., Perveen Akhter, Cho, S.Y., Natera, E., Miah, F.K., and Nguyen, M.S., Estimation of internal radiation dose to the adult Asian population from the dietary intakes of two long-lived radionuclides, *J. Environ. Radioactiv.*, 77, 221, 2004.

53. Altman, J., The dietary utilisation of flora and fauna by contemporary hunter-gatherers at Momega Outstation, north-central Arnhem Land, *Aust. Aboriginal Stud.*, 1, 35, 1984.

54. Thomas, P.A. and Gates, T.E., Radionuclides in the lichen-caribou-human food chain near uranium mining operations in northern Saskatchewan, Canada, *Environ. Health Perspect.*, 107, 527, 1999.

55. OSPAR, *Quality Status Report 2000*, OSPAR, London, 2000.

56. Camplin, W.C., Rollo, S., and Hunt, G.J., Surveillance related assessments of sea-to-land transfer, In *Proceedings of the Second RADREM – TESC Workshop held in London 21 January 1999*, Ould-Dada, Z., ed., DETR/RADREM/00.001, DETR, London, 2000.

57. Ajdacic, N. and Martic, M., Contamination of some important kinds of plants by fission products, *J. Radioanal. Nucl. Chem.*, 131, 311, 1989.

58. Jackson, D. and Edwards M., *Effect of domestic food preparation processes on radionuclide concentrations,* Proc. 6th SRP International Symposium (edited M Thorne), P8-14, 1999, Published by the Society for radiological Protection, ISBN 0-7058-1784-9.

59. Travnikova, I.G., Gazjukin, A.N., Bruk, G.J., Shutov, V.N., Balonov, M.I., Skuter-land, L., Mehli, H., and Strand, P., Lake fish as the main contributor of internal dose to lakeshore residents in the Chernobyl contaminated area., *J. Env. Radio-activity.*, 77, 63, 2004.

60. Byrom, J., Robinson, C., Simmonds, J.R., Walters, B., and Taylor, R.R., Food consumption rates for use in generalised radiological dose assessments, *J. Radiol. Prot.*, 15, 335, 1995.

61. McColl, N.P. and Prosser, S.L., *Emergency Data Handbook*, NRPB-W19, National Radiological Protection Board, Chilton, UK, 2002.

62. Dell, A.N. and Lally, A.E., The approach towards NAMAS accreditation for a radiochemical laboratory, *Sci. Total Environ.*, 130/131, 331, 1993.

63. Hodson, P.C. and Dell, A.N., 10 years later — practical experience of NAMAS accreditation — was it worth it? in *Environmental Radiochemical Analysis*, Newton, G.W.A., ed., Royal Society of Chemistry, London, 1999.

64. Morris, J.A., After effects of the Chernobyl accident, *Br. Vet. J.*, 144, 179, 1988.

65. De Ruig, W.G. and van der Struijs, T.D., Radioactive contamination of food sampled in the areas of the USSR affected by the Chernobyl disaster, *Analyst*, 117, 545, 1992.

66. Giovani, C., Garavaglia, M., and Scruzzi, E., Radiocaesium in mushrooms from north-east Italy, 1986–2002, *Radiat. Prot. Dosim.*, 111, 377, 2004.

67. Gallelli, C., Panatto, D., Perdelli, F., and Pellegrino, C., Long-term decline of radiocaesium concentration in seafood from the Ligurian sea (Northern Italy) after Chernobyl., *Sci. Total Environ.*, 196, 163, 1997.

68. Assikamakpoulos, P.A., Ionnides, K.G., and Paradopoulou, C.V., Transport of radioisotopes ^{131}I, ^{134}Cs and ^{137}Cs from the fallout following the accident at the Chernobyl nuclear reactor into cheese and other cheese making products, *J. Dairy Sci.*, 70, 1338, 1987.

69. Rantavaara, A., Nygren T., Nygren K., and Hyvonen, T., Radioactivity of game meat in Finland after the Chernobyl accident in 1986: Supplement 7 to Annual report STUK-55., *Report No.STUK-A62, Finnish Centre for Radiation and Nuclear Safety,* Helsinki, 1987.

70. Bunzl, K. and Kracke, W., Transfer of Chernobyl-derived ^{134}Cs, ^{137}Cs, ^{131}I and ^{103}U from flowers to honey and pollen., *J. Environ. Radioactiv.*, 6, 261, 1988.

71. Prohl, G., Muller, H., Voigt, G., and Vogel, H., The transfer of ^{137}Cs from barley to beer, *Health Phys.*, 72 ,111, 1997.

72. Ahman, B. and Ahman, G., Radiocaesium in Swedish reindeer after the Chernobyl fallout: seasonal variations and long-term decline, *Health Phys.*, 66, 503, 1994.

73. Rosen, K., Andersson, I., and Lonsjo, H., Transfer of radiocaesium from soil to vegetation and to grazing lambs in a mountain area in northern Sweden, *J. Environ. Radioactiv.*, 26, 237, 1995.

74. Ahman, B., Wright, S., and Howard, B., Effect of origin of radiocaesium on the transfer from fallout to reindeer meat, *Sci. Total. Environ.*, 278, 171, 2001.

75. Lally, A.E. and Morris, J., Monitoring and surveillance, *Rev. Sci. Tech. Off. Int. Epiz.*, 7, 155, 1988.

76. Fisk, S, and Sanderson, D.C.W., Chernobyl-derived radiocaesium in heather honey and its dependence on deposition patterns, *Health Phys.*, 77, 431, 1999.

77. Food Standards Agency and Scottish Environment Protection Agency, *Radioactivity in Food and the Environment, 1998*, RIFE-4, Food Standards Agency and SEPA, London and Stirling, 1999.

78. Swift, D.J., *Radioactivity in uncommon seafoods,* CEFAS contract C1022, Environmental Report RL 16/02, CEFAS, Lowestoft, 2002.

79. Ministry of Agriculture, Fisheries and Food, *Incident Surveillance Report: Radioactive Contaminated Pigeons in Seascale Village*, available at www.archive.food. gov.uk/maff/archice/food/incid_1/bnfp23.htm, 1998.

80. Strand, P., Brown, J.E., Drozhko, E., Mokrov, Y., Salbu, B., Oughton, D., Christensen, G.C., and Amundsen, I., Biogeochemical behaviour of ^{137}Cs and ^{90}Sr in the artificial reservoirs of Mayak PA, Russia, *Sci. Total Environ.,* 241, 107, 1999.

81. Akleyev, A.V. and Lyubchansky, E.E., Environmental and medical effects of nuclear weapon production in the southern Urals, *Sci. Total Environ.*, 142, 1, 1994.

82. Chesnokov, A.V., Govorun, A.P., Linnik, V.G., and Shcherbak, S.B., ^{137}Cs contamination of the Techa river flood plain near the village of Muslumovo, *J. Environ. Radioactiv.,* 50, 179, 2000.

83. Shutov, V.N., Travnikova, I.G., Bruk, G.Y., Golikov, V.Y., Balonov, M.I., Howard, B.J., Brown, J., Strand, P., Kravtsova, E.M., Gavrilov, A.P., Kravtsova, O.S., and Mubasarov, A.A., Current contamination by ^{137}Cs and ^{90}Sr of the inhabited part of the Techa river basin in the Urals, *J. Environ. Radioactiv.,* 61, 91, 2002.

84. Chesnokov, A.V., Govorun, A.P., Ivanitskaya, M.V., Liksonov, V.I., and Shcherbak, S.B., ^{137}Cs contamination of Techa river flood plain in Brodokalmak settlement, *Appl. Radiat. Isot.,* 50, 1121, 1999.

85. Marshall, E., Health research: U.S., Russia to study radiation effects, *Science*, 275, 1062, 1997.

86. Williams, L., Russ, R.M., McCubbin, D., and Knowles, J.F., An overview of tritium behaviour in the Severn Estuary (UK), *J. Radiol. Prot.*, 21, 337, 2001.

87. International Commission on Radiological Protection, *Age-Dependent Doses to Members of the Public from Intake of Radionuclides, Part 5 — Compilation of Ingestion and Inhalation Dose Coefficients*, Elsevier Science, Oxford, 1996.

88. Food Standards Agency and Scottish Environment Protection Agency, *Radioactivity in Food and the Environment, 1997*, RIFE-3, Food Standards Agency and SEPA, London and Stirling, 1998.

89. Food Standards Agency and Scottish Environment Protection Agency, *Radioactivity in Food and the Environment, 1999*, RIFE-5, Food Standards Agency and SEPA, London and Stirling, 2000.

90. Food Standards Agency and Scottish Environment Protection Agency, *Radioactivity in Food and the Environment, 2001*, RIFE-7, Food Standards Agency and SEPA, London and Stirling, 2002.

91. Environment Agency, Environment and Heritage Service, Food Standards Agency and Scottish Environment Protection Agency, *Radioactivity in Food and the Environment, 2002*, RIFE-8, Environment Agency, EHS, Food Standards Agency and SEPA, Bristol, Belfast, London and Stirling, 2003.

92. Warwick, P. E., Croudace, I.W., Morris, J.E., Dyer, F.M., Howard, A.G., and Cundy, A.B., *Organically-bound tritium (OBT) dispersion and accumulation in Severn Estuary sediments,* Project Report for MAFF Contract R01034, Southampton Oceanography Centre, Southampton, 2002.

93. Food Standards Agency, *Radiological Survey of Foodstuffs from the Cardiff Area*, Food Survey Information Sheet no. 18/01, Food Standards Agency, London, 2001.

94. Seaber, W.M., Barium as a normal constituent of Brazil nuts, *Analyst*, 58, 575, 1933.

95. Turner, R.C., Radley, J.M., and Mayneord, W.V., The naturally occurring alpha-ray activity in foods, *Health Phys.*, 1, 268, 1958.

96. Penna-Franca, E., *Anais 2 Simpósio Interamericano sôbre la Application de la Energia Nuclear para Fines Pacificos*, Buenos Aires, 1959.

97. UNSCEAR, *Sources and Effects of Ionizing Radiation*, Report to the General Assembly, United Nations, New York, 1977.

98. Codex Alimentarius Commission, ALINORM 04/27/12, Appendix 12, Codex Alimentarius Commission, Rome, April 2004.

99. Yoshitome, R., Kunito, T., Ikemoto, T., Tanabe, S., Zenke, H., Yamauchi, M., and Miyazaki, N., Global Distribution of Radionuclides (^{137}Cs and [40]K) in Marine Mammals, *Environ. Sci. Technol.,* 37, 4597, 2003.

100. Wang, J.-J., Wang, C.-J., Lai, S.-Y., and Lin, Y.-M., Radioactivity concentrations of ^{137}Cs and [40]K in basidiomycetes collected in Taiwan, *Appl. Radiat. Isot.,* 49, 29, 1998.

101. Svadlenková, M., Konesný, J., and Smutný, V., Model calculation of radiocaesium transfer into food products in semi-natural forest ecosystems in the Czech Republic after a nuclear reactor accident and an estimate of the population dose burden, *Environ. Pollut.,* 92, 173, 1996.

102. Aarkrog, A., Baxter, M.S., Bettencourt, A.O., Bojanowski, R., Bologa, A., Charmasson, S., Cunha, I., Delfanti, R., Duran, E., Holm, E., Jeffree, R., Livingston, H.D., Mahapanyawong, S., Nies, H., Osvath, I., Pingyu, L., Povinec, P.P., Sanchez, A., Smith, J.N., and Swift, D., A comparison of doses from ^{137}Cs and [210]Po in marine food: A major international study, *J. Environ. Radioactiv.,* 34, 69, 1997.

103. Alonso-Hernandez, C., Diaz-Asencio, M., Munos-Caravaca, A., Suarez-Morell, E., and Avila-Moreno, R., ^{137}Cs and [210]Po dose assessment from marine food in Cienfuegos Bay (Cuba), *J. Environ. Radioactiv.*, 61, 203, 2002.

104. Badran, H.M., Sharshar, T., and Elnimer, T., Levels of ^{137}Cs and [40]K in edible parts of some vegetables consumed in Egypt, *J. Environ. Radioactiv.*, 67, 181, 2003.

105. Rusconi, R., Forte, M., Abbate, G., Gallini, R., and Sgorbati, G., Natural radioactivity in bottled mineral waters: a survey of northern Italy, *J. Radioanal. Nucl. Chem.*, 260, 421, 2004.

106. Kuo, Y.-C., Lai, S.-Y., Huang, C.-C., and Lin, Y.-M., Activity concentrations and population dose from radium-226 in food and drinking water in Taiwan, *Appl. Radiat. Isot.*, 48, 1245, 1997.

107. Al-Masri, M.S., Nashawati, A., Amin, Y., and Al-Akel, B., Determination of [210]Po in tea, mate and their infusions and its annual intake by Syrians, *J. Radioanal. Nucl. Chem.*, 260, 27, 2004.

9 Radiation Detection Methods

Ashraf Khater

CONTENTS

9.1 INTRODUCTION

Sources of ionizing radiation are inside and surrounding us all the time and everywhere. This radiation comes from radionuclides which occur naturally as trace elements in rocks and soils of the earth as a consequence of radioactive decay. Radionuclides also exist in the atmosphere, lithosphere, hydrosphere, and biosphere. Since the middle of the last century, and the discovery of nuclear radiation, much attention has been focused on the different sources of ionizing radiation and their useful applications and harmful effects on the human body and its environment. In addition to naturally occurring radioactive materials (NORMs), technologically enhanced naturally occurring radioactive materials (TENORMs) and man-made (artificially produced) radionuclides have been introduced into the environment from the proliferation of different nuclear applications. All of these sources have contributed to the increase in the levels of environmental radioactivity and radiation doses.

Radioecology is concerned with the behavior of radionuclides in the environment. It deals with the understanding of where radioactive materials originate and how they migrate, react chemically, and affect the ecosphere after their release into the environment. All these aspects are very dynamic processes where the environment greatly affects and is affected by the fate of radioactive substances. So the main goals of studying radioactivity in the environment and food are to provide a scientific basis for the effective utilization of radioactivity, such as geochronology, and to predict the impacts to man and his environment due to different radionuclides.

Radiation detection and radioactivity analysis are the main topic of this chapter. The different types of radiation sources (NORMs, TENORMs, and man-made) are summarized in detail in Chapter 1 and Chapter 2 of this book. This chapter deals with three main themes: interactions of radiation with matter, radiation detectors, and radioactivity analysis of environmental and food samples.

Heat and light are radiations that you can feel or see directly, but there are other kinds of radiation, such as γ, X-ray, and neutrons, that humans cannot recognize or feel directly. Radiation can be classified into two categories: nonionizing, such as visible light, and ionizing, such as γ rays and X-rays. Ionizing radiation has the ability to ionize the atoms and molecules of the media it passes through. Ionizing radiation can be classified into two categories: directly ionizing and indirectly ionizing. Based on their electrical properties, ionizing radiation can be classified into charged radiations, such as α and β particles, and uncharged radiations, such as γ rays and neutrons. Also, according to their penetration power, radiation can be classified as soft or hard radiation.

Radiations are mainly classified into four groups:

- Heavy charged particles, including all particles with a mass greater than or equal to one atomic mass unit (amu), such as α particles, protons, and fission products.
- Charged particles, including β particles (negative electrons), positrons (positive electrons), internal conversion electrons, and auger electrons.
- Electromagnetic radiations, including γ-rays (following β particles decay or nuclear reactions), characteristic x-rays, annihilation radiation and bremsstrahlung.
- Neutrons, including fast neutrons, intermediate neutrons, epithermal neutrons, thermal neutrons, and cold neutrons. Neutrons can be generated from spontaneous fission, radioisotope (alpha-neutron) sources, photo-neutron sources, or reactions from accelerated charged particles.

The backbone of studying environmental radioactivity and radioecology is radiation detection and radioactivity analysis. The radiation detectors are one of the main components of radiation detection and measurement systems, which include the detector, the signal processing unit, and the output display device, such as a counter or spectrometer. Radiation detectors basically depend on the interaction of incident radiation with the detector material, which produces a detectable output signal. For each type of radiation, there is one or more suitable type of detector or detection system; each has advantages and disadvantages.

9.2 RADIATION INTERACTION WITH MATTER

Knowledge of the mechanisms by which ionizing radiation interacts with matter is fundamental to an understanding of specific radiation topics such as instrumentation, dosimetry, and shielding. Recall that the basic building block of matter is the atom, which consists of a nucleus, a positively charged central core containing protons and (with one exception) neutrons, surrounded by orbiting electrons. In a neutral atom, each electron supplies a negative charge to counter the positive charges found within the nucleus. Ionizing radiations, those radiations that possess sufficient energy to eject electrons from neutral atoms, include α particles, β particles, γ-rays, and x-rays. These radiations transfer energy to matter via interactions with the atom's constituent parts.

Radiation detection is based on the different mechanisms of radiation's interaction with matter. These mechanisms depend on both the physical properties of the radiation and the physical and structural properties of the detector materials. The interaction of radiation with matter will be explained here on two levels: the microscopic level, to understand the mechanisms of losing radiation energy inside the matter, and the macroscopic level, to understand the effect of different absorber materials on the intensity of radiation during and after passing through an absorber.

The following expressions are related to the interaction of radiation with matter and should be defined first:

- Radiation stopping power (specific energy loss): the average energy loss per unit path length, usually expressed in megaelectron volts per centimeter (MeV/cm).
- Radiation range: the linear distance behind which no particle passes through the absorber material. It depends on the type and energy of the particle and on the material through which the particle passes.
- Radiation range straggling: the variation in the path length for individual particles that have the same initial energy.
- Radiation path length: the total distance traveled by the particle in the absorber material, where it is linear for heavy charged particles and nonlinear for charged particles.
- Mean free path: the average length of the path the radiation travels without interaction with the absorber material.
- Specific ionization: the average number of ion pairs (electron and positive ion pairs) formed per centimeter in the radiation track.
- Mean ionization energy: the average energy required to form one ion pair in the matter. It is nearly independent of the energy of the radiation, its charge, and its mass.

9.2.1 Heavy Charged Particles

On the microscopic level, when charged particles travel through the absorber material, they undergo elastic and inelastic collisions with the orbital electrons of the absorbing material. Heavy charged particles interact with the matter under the effect of the Coulomb force (electrostatic force) between the positively charged particles, such as α particles and protons, and the negative orbital electrons of the constituent atoms of the absorber material. Rutherford scattering (i.e., interactions with nuclei of the matter atoms) are possible, but they are rare and are not normally significant in the response of radiation detectors. Under the effect of the Coulomb force, the heavy charged particle interacts simultaneously with many orbital electrons of the absorbing medium atoms. Because of the large mass differences between the charged particles and the electrons, the energy transfer from the charged particles per collision is very small. The maximum energy transfer in one collision is about 1/500 of the particle energy per nucleon. The charged particles lose their energies after many collisions within the matter. The particle's energy is decreased with increasing path length and finally stops within the matter after losing its energy. During the energy transfer process, after decreasing the particle's energy and velocity, the charged particles pick up electrons from the surrounding medium, reduce their charge, and finally become neutral atoms at the end of their track.

The heavy charged particles have a linear path and a definite range in a given absorbing material. Depending on the energy transferred to the orbital electrons, either it brings the electrons to a higher orbit with less binding energy (atom excitation) or it remove the electrons, called primary electrons, from the atoms (primary atom ionization). Atomic ionization produces ion pairs where each ion pair is composed of an electron and a positive ion of an absorber atom from which one electron has been removed. The energetic primary electrons, known as δ electrons or δ rays, interact with the absorber atoms and lose their energy via secondary ionization. Secondary ionization is very important for radiation detection and radiation protection, because it indirectly increases the energy transfer to the absorbing medium.

The Bethe formula (Equation 10.1) describes the specific energy loss for charged particles:

$$-\frac{dE}{dx} = \frac{4.\pi.e^4.z^2}{m_0.\upsilon^2} N.B \tag{9.1}$$

$$B \equiv Z.\left[\ln.\frac{2m_0.\upsilon^2}{I} - \ln.\left(1 - \frac{\upsilon^2}{c^2}\right) - \frac{\upsilon^2}{c^2} \right] \tag{9.2}$$

where
ez = charge of the primary charged particle,
Z = atomic number of the absorber material,
m_0 = electron rest mass,
υ = velocity of the primary charged particle,
c = speed of light in a vacuum,
I = average excitation and ionization energy of the absorber,
N = density of the absorber atoms (number of electrons per unit volume).

Equation 9.1 is generally valid for the charged particles where the velocity remains larger than that of the orbital electrons in the absorbing atoms. It begins to fail at low particle energies, where the charge exchange between the particles and the absorber atoms becomes significant. The specific energy loss, linear stopping power (dE/dx), varies as $1/\upsilon^2$ or inversely with particle energy ($1/E$). The rate of energy transfer is increased with decreasing charged particle velocity because it spends a greater amount of time in the vicinity of any given electron. For different charged particles that have the same velocity, the particle with the greatest charge (ze) will have the largest energy loss per track length. For different absorber materials, dE/dx depends on the product NZ, linear stopping power increases with the increasing atomic number of the absorber material (i.e., a higher density material).

9.2.2 BETA PARTICLES

The interaction of β particles with matter is similar to that of heavy charged particles, where the Coulomb force is the dominant force between the constitutes. β particles interact with the matter and lose their energy through collisions of incident particles with orbital electrons and consequently either excite or ionize the absorber atoms. Because both β particles and electrons have the same mass, the energy loss per collision is larger compared to that for heavy charged particles. Because of the large deviation in the direction of β particles after collision, they follow a much more tortuous path. For fast electrons, the specific energy loss due to collisions has also been derived by Bethe and is written as

$$-\frac{dE}{dx} = \frac{2\pi \cdot e^4}{m_0 \cdot \upsilon^2} Z \cdot B \tag{9.3}$$

$$B = \tag{9.4}$$

$$\left[\ln \frac{m_0 \cdot \upsilon^2 \cdot E}{2.I^2(1-\frac{\upsilon^2}{c^2})} - (\ln 2)\left(2\sqrt{1-\frac{\upsilon^2}{c^2}} - 1 + \frac{\upsilon^2}{c^2} \right) + (1-\frac{\upsilon^2}{c^2}) + \frac{1}{8}\left(1-\sqrt{1-\frac{\upsilon^2}{c^2}} \right)^2 \right]$$

where the symbols have the same meaning as in Equation 9.1.

In addition to the energy loss due to atom excitation or ionization, particle energy may be lost by another radiative process, bremsstrahlung "braking" radiation. When high-speed charged particles pass close to the intense electric field of the absorber nuclei, the particle suffers strong deceleration and bremsstrahlung radiation are emitted. The energy loss due to bremsstrahlung radiation is minor compared to that from atom excitation and ionization collision processes. It is more significant in absorber materials of high atomic number. The ratio of the contribution of radiative processes and collision processes is given by

$$\left(\frac{dE}{dx} \right)_{radiative} \Bigg/ \left(\frac{dE}{dx} \right)_{collision} \cong \frac{EZ}{700} \tag{9.5}$$

where

    Z = atomic number of absorber material,
    E = energy of the incident particle.

Finally, β particles lose their energy inside the absorber and stop at the end of their tracks. Negative β particles act as free electrons in the absorber, while positive β particles interact with free electrons (i.e., matter-antimatter interaction). Annihilation radiation begins with two photons, having an energy of 511 keV for each are generated, which are very penetrable compare to the range of positron. These photons interact with matter and may lead to energy deposition in other locations.

The β particle energy spectrum is different from that of α- or γ-rays, where β particles can have values from zero to the maximum (endpoint) energy value. For the majority of β particles, the absorption curves (number of β particles as a function of absorber thickness) have a near exponential shape and are represented by

$$\frac{I}{I_0} = e^{-nt} \tag{9.6}$$

where

I_0 = counting rate without absorber,
I = counting rate with absorber,
t = absorber thickness (in g/cm^2),
n = absorption coefficient.

Backscattering is a very important process that can significantly affect the specific energy lost in the matter, and consequently the radiation detection. Some particles undergo large angle deflections along their track that lead to backscattering. Backscattered particles on the absorber surface or inside the absorber itself can reemerge from the absorber surface without depositing all their energy in the absorbing medium, which will significantly affect the detection process. Also, backscattering of β particles that reemerge from the surface of some β particle sources due to the thick backing could increase the number of emitted particles from the source surface.

9.2.3 Gamma and X-Rays

The electromagnetic radiations, such as γ and x-rays, interact with matter in a completely different way. The concepts of range and specific energy loss are not applicable as for charged particles. Electromagnetic radiations have no electric charge and no mass, and their rest mass is zero. They can pass through an absorber without energy loss (i.e., they have a high penetration power). The relationship between energy (E), frequency (ν), and wavelength (λ) is

$$E = h\nu = h\frac{c}{\lambda} \tag{9.7}$$

where h is Planck's constant.

When electromagnetic radiations, γ-rays, x-rays, and bremsstrahlung radiation, travel with the velocity of light, they are called photons. γ rays and x-rays have well-defined energies (i.e., monoenergetic) and have different origins. γ-rays originate from the nucleus, while x-rays originate from atoms. Bremsstrahlung radiation is produced by accelerating and decelerating charged particles and has a continuous energy spectrum.

There are three main mechanisms of interaction of γ-rays and x-rays with matter that play an important role in radiation detection processes: photoelectric absorption, Compton scattering, and pair production. These interaction mechanisms lead to the partial or complete transfer of γ-ray photon energy to electron energy which leads to indirect ionization of the absorber atoms.

9.2.3.1 Photoelectric Absorption

This mechanism of interaction is very important for γ- and x-ray measurements. The photon interacts with the absorber atoms and disappears (i.e., photon absorption occurs). Depending on the photon energy, the most bonded orbital electron in the K or L shell will absorb the photon energy to be removed from the atom with a kinetic energy given by

$$E_e = h\nu - E_b,\qquad(9.8)$$

where

E_e = photoelectron kinetic energy,
$h\nu$ = photon energy,
E_b = electron binding energy.

The photoelectrons are energetic electrons and interact with matter exactly like β particles. These electrons leave the atom and create an electron vacancy in their inner orbit, where either a free electron or an electron from a higher orbit fills this vacancy and generates x-rays. The generated x-rays interact with the absorber and can produce another photoelectron (i.e., photoelectric absorption) with less binding energy (known as an auger electron) than the original photoelectron.

The photoelectric coefficient (τ), the probability of photoelectric absorption per unit length, depends on the photon energy (E) and the absorber atomic number (Z). Photoelectric absorption is the predominant mechanism of interaction for low-energy photons (E_γ). It is enhanced with increasing absorber atomic number (Z). A rough approximation is given by

$$\tau\left(m^{-1}\right) \cong \text{Constant } \frac{Z^n}{E_\gamma{}^m},\qquad(9.9)$$

where n and m are constant values that range between 3 and 5.

9.2.3.2 Compton Scattering

Compton scattering is an inelastic collision between the incident photon and the weak-bonded electron in the outer shell of the absorber atoms. The incident photon dissipates a part of its energy and deflects with a scattering angle of θ. The recoil electron is removed from the atom with a kinetic energy that depends on the amount of energy transferred from the photon. The energy transfer varies from zero, when $\theta = 0$, to a maximum value, when $\theta = \pi$. The Compton coefficient decreases with increasing energy and increases linearly with the atomic number Z of the absorber material. The energy of the recoil electron and the scattered photon are given by

$$E_\gamma = E_0 \left(\frac{1}{1 + \left(E_0/m.c^2 \right).\left(1 - \cos\theta \right)} \right), \tag{9.10}$$

$$E_e = E_0 - E_\gamma = E_0 \left[\frac{\left(E_0/m_0.c^2 \right).\left(1 - \cos\theta \right)}{1 + \left(E_0/m_0.c^2 \right).\left(1 - \cos\theta \right)} \right], \tag{9.11}$$

where
  E_0 = incident photon energy,
  E_γ = scattered photon energy,
  E_e = recoil electron energy,
  m_0 = electron rest mass.

The Compton scattering coefficient (σ), the probability of occurrence per unit length, is approximated and given by

$$\sigma\left(m^{-1} \right) = NZf\left(E_\gamma \right), \tag{9.12}$$

where $f(E_\gamma)$ is a function of E_γ.

9.2.3.3 Pair Production

Pair production is the main interaction mechanism for the energetic photon. Practically, it becomes significant for the few megaelectron volt energy photons. Theoretically it is possible for photons with energy (E_γ) of 1.022 MeV, which is equivalent to the energy of two electron rest masses ($2\ m_0C^2$). The photon disappears in the nucleus field of the absorber atoms and one electron-positron pair is generated. The kinetic energy of the electron (E_{e-}) and the positron (E_{e+}) is given by

$$E_{e^-} = E_{e^+} = 0.5\left(E_\gamma - \left(m_0C^2 \right)_{e^-} - \left(m_0C^2 \right)_{e^+} \right) = 0.5\left(E_\gamma - 1.022 MeV \right). \tag{9.13}$$

The pair production coefficient (κ), the probability of occurrence per unit length, is a complicated function of Z and E which changes slightly with Z and increases with E:

$$\kappa\left(m^{-1}\right) = NZ^2 f\left(E_\gamma, Z\right),\qquad(9.14)$$

where $f(E_\gamma, Z)$ is a function of E and Z.

Both electrons and positrons interact with the absorber as β particles and finally come to rest after losing their kinetic energy. Then the electron acts as a free electron and the positron interacts with the electron (i.e., matter-antimatter inter-action) and generates two inhalation photons, each with an energy of 0.511 MeV.

At the macroscopic level, the incident photons interact with the absorber material and their numbers decrease with increasing thickness of the absorber (known as radiation attenuation). Photon attenuation is due to the main interaction mechanisms of photons (photoelectric effect, Compton effect, and pair produc-tions effect), that is, photons are completely absorbing or scattering. There are other mechanisms of photon interaction with matter, but they are insignificant in γ- and x-ray measurement. The linear attenuation coefficient (μ) is the probability per unit length that the photon is interacted with and removed from the beam. The linear attenuation coefficient is the sum of the probabilities of the three main interaction mechanisms (photoelectric, Compton scattering, and pair production) and is given by

$$\mu = \tau(photoelectric) + \sigma(compton) + \kappa(pair) .\qquad(9.15)$$

The mean free path (λ) of a γ-ray photon is related to the linear attenuation coefficient and the half-value thickness ($X_{1/2}$), and is given by

$$\lambda = \frac{1}{\mu} = 1.4 \ X_{1/2}.\qquad(9.16)$$

The mass attenuation coefficient (μ_m) is much more widely used because of the variation in the absorber density (ρ) and is the same regardless of the physical state of the absorber. It is given by

$$\mu_m = \frac{\mu}{\rho}.\qquad(9.17)$$

The number of transmitted γ-ray photons (I) through an absorber of thickness t from the incident γ-ray photons (I_0) is given by

$$I = I_0 \, e^{-\mu t},\qquad(9.18)$$

$$I = I_0 e^{-\mu_m \rho t}, \tag{9.19}$$

where ρt (in m²/kg) is the mass thickness.

The kinetic energy of the electrons and positrons produced as a result of photoelectric and pair production effects is absorbed completely inside the absorber, while the x-ray and Compton scattered photons may escape. For radiation measurements, it is more practical to use the absorption coefficient to calculate the absorption fraction, which relates directly to the incident γ-ray photons and to the output response of the detector. The γ-ray energy absorption coefficient (μ_a) is the probability of photon energy absorption inside the absorber material and is given by

$$\mu_a = \tau(photoelectric) + \frac{E_e}{E_\gamma}\sigma(compton) + \kappa(pair), \tag{9.20}$$

where μ_a may be linear (in m−1) or the mass (in m²/kg) energy absorption coefficient, E_e is the kinetic energy of the recoil electron, and E is the energy of the incident photon.

9.3 RADIATION DETECTORS

A radiation detection system is composed of a detector, signal processor electronics, and a data output display device such as a counter or multichannel analyzer. The backbone of any radiation detection system is the radiation detector. The physical properties and characteristics of the detector control the features of the detection system. A radiation detector is composed of three main components:

- A sensitive volume where the radiation interactions occur
- Structural components that enclose the sensitive volume to maintain the proper conditions for its optimum operation
- A signal output display device that extracts the information from the sensitive volume and transfers it to the signal processing device

This section deals with the main radiation detector properties and aspects of radiation detection. There are three main radiation detectors categories: gas-filled detectors, scintillation detectors, semiconductor detectors. Radiation detectors and detection systems are also classified according to their physical form (gas, liquid, and solid), according to the nature of the detector output signal (current [ions] and light), and according to their function (counting, pulse height spectrometry, dosimetry, imaging, and timing).

There are two approaches to studying this subject. The first approach is to study the different detector types in terms of their characteristic properties, such as structure, theory of operation, response to different incident radiations, and output signals. All these determine the possible functions of the detection system. The second approach is to know the required detection system functions, then determine the detector types and modes of operation. Both approaches are complementary and depend on the researcher's interests and knowledge of the scientific principles of radiation detection and the practical aspects of radioactivity analysis.

Some of the operating characteristics for radiation detection include detection efficiency, energy resolution, background, proportionality of the signal to the energy deposited, pulse shape, and time resolution or dead time. The functions and applications of the different radiation detection systems are dependent on these parameters.

Detection efficiency is defined as the ratio of the number of particles or photons recorded by the detector to the number of particles or photons emitted by the source, known as the absolute efficiency (ε). It is also defined as the ratio of the number of particles or photons recorded by the detector to the number of particles or photons striking the detector, known as the intrinsic efficiency (η), which depends on the solid angle (δ) of the source-detector geometric arrangement and is given by

$$\eta = \delta\varepsilon. \tag{9.21}$$

Energy resolution is defined as the capability of the detector to distinguish between two particles or photons with different but close energies.

Resolving time is defined as the minimum time required by the detection system to recover from one event or interaction so it is able to record another event. It is defined also as the minimum time in which the detection system cannot record any radiation interaction or signal because it is busy processing the previous signal, also known as the dead time.

9.3.1 GAS-FILLED DETECTORS

A gas-filled detector is composed of an enclosed gas volume between two electrodes (anode and cathode) (see Figure 9.1). Gas-filled detectors have different shapes — two parallel electrodes, cylindrical with a central rod as an anode, and spherical — but they work based on the same principles. When the incident radiation travels through the gas (the sensitive volume of the detector) and interacts with the gas atoms and molecules, atom excitation and ionization occur. The gas ionization produces electron-ion pairs; their number depends on the energy deposited during the radiation-gas interaction. The average energy required to form one ion pair is about 35 eV, including excitation energy. Ion pairs are recombined locally after their formation inside the gas volume, if the applied voltage is low or zero. The electric field (E) between the detector electrodes exerts electric forces to move the negative electrons toward the anode and the positive ions toward the cathode. The strength of the electric field $E(r)$ at point P between the cylindrical detector electrodes is given by

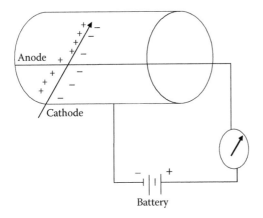

FIGURE 9.1 Basic structure of the gas-filled detector.

$$E(r) = \frac{V}{r \ln(b/a)} , \qquad (9.22)$$

where

r = distance of point P from the center of the cylinder,
a = radius of the anode,
b = inner radius of cylinder.

Both electrons and positive ions of the gas atom have the same charge and different masses, where the positive ions are much heavier than the electrons. The acceleration, a (electric force/mass, in m/s²), of an electron is thousands of times higher than that of the positive ion. The drift velocity of the electrons is thousands of times faster than that of the positive ion. The output signal is based on the collected charges (electron and positive ions) and, depending on the operating mode, the output signal is either a current signal due to the collected charges (a resistance circuit) or a pulse due the drop in external circuit voltage at the current saturation condition (a resistance-capacitance circuit). There is a time difference between the output current signal due to electron collection on the anode and positive ions collection on the cathode. Practically, the output signal depends on the electrons charge collection to have a short responding time.

The structural material and design of gas field counters affect the counting efficiency of different radiation types. For charged particles, the counter windows should be thin to avoid particle absorption within the counter window. For β particles, the counter is designed to stand a higher gas pressure, which is necessary to stop incident β particles with the gas volume of the counter. For γ-rays, the counter walls are constructed from high atomic number materials, where the counter response to γ-rays comes through its interaction with the counter walls. As the applied voltage increases, the electric field strength increases and the recombination rate decreases to zero (i.e., all created ions are collected). Up

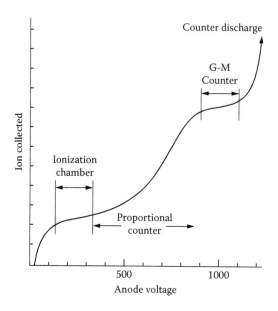

FIGURE 9.2 Gas-filled detector response curve as a function of the applied voltage.

to this voltage, the region is known as the partial recombination region. The response curve of gas-filled detectors is shown in Figure 9.2. It is divided into five regions: recombination, ionization, proportional, Geiger-Muller, and continuous discharge. A gas-filled detector may operate in any of these regions, depending on the gas type, gas pressure, applied voltage, and counter size.

9.3.1.1 Ionization Chambers

The applied voltage, less than 1000 V, is high enough to collect electrons before recombination with positive ions. The recombination rate is zero, and even with an increase in the applied voltage, the collected charge rate stays constant, known as the ionization chamber plateau. The detector output signal, cither current or pulse, is exactly equivalent to the energy deposited divided by the energy required to ionize one gas atom (i.e., no amplification). To maintain the ionization chamber conditions, both the electric field strength (E) and the gas mixture must be controlled. α particles have a higher specific ionization than that of electrons or γ rays because of its higher linear energy transfer (energy loss per unit length of the path). Therefore the ionization chamber has the ability to distinguish between the different types of radiation and the same radiation with different energies. The energy resolution (the ability to distinguish between two photons or particles having different but close energies) of an ionization chamber is quite good. Ionization chambers are very useful for the measurement of high-radiation fields and intensities of extended photon emitters. The ionization chamber structure changes according to the radiation type. It is basically a metal cylinder with a central anode and its inner walls are usually lined by an air equivalent material.

For β particle detection, the entrance window of the detector should be thin to decrease particle absorption. For β particles, the gas pressure increases to stop all particles inside the active volume of the chamber to ensure complete particle energy deposit. For γ-rays, the detector should be lined with a high atomic number material to increase the probability of γ-ray interaction. Ionization chamber detectors operate in different modes, depending on the output signal: current mode, charge integration mode, or pulse mode. There are many applications of radiation detection systems based on ionization chambers, including calibration of radioactive sources and measurement of gases such as radon.

9.3.1.2 Proportional Counters

As the applied voltage increases (range 800 to 2000 V), the electric field strength will be strong enough to not only remove the electrons and positive ions of the primary ionization, but also to accelerate the primary ionization electrons and positive ions. The accelerated electrons gain a relatively higher kinetic energy and produce a secondary ionization in the region closed to the anode due to their collisions with the gas atoms. Also, the accelerated positive ions strike the cathode and create a secondary ionization. This multiplication process (i.e., primary ionization multiplication) is known as a Townsend avalanche or Townsend cascade. The height of the output signals is linearly proportional to the energy dissipated and the primary ionization inside the counter. Thus radiation detection and energy measurement are possible. As the applied voltage increases, the proportionality of the output signal to the dissipated energy and the primary ionization decreases. This range of voltage is known as the limited proportional region. It is very practical to operate the counter in this range for high-level radiation measurements. The proportional counter can distinguish between α-particles and β electron particles, where the signal from the α particle is larger than that due to the β signal. In studying the characteristic curve for a proportional gas counter with an α/β emitter mixed source, as the high voltage increases, only α particle signals are large enough to pass the discriminator of the counting channel. The α signal count rate will increase to reach a plateau, known as the α plateau. The length of the plateau depends on the source properties, being thin or thick, and the source-detector geometric arrangement, being an internal (located inside the counter) or external source. As the high voltage increases, the count rate increases due to β particle signals, until they reach another plateau where both α and β particles are counted (Figure 9.3). Proportional counters usually operate in pulse mode.

One of the most important environmental applications of proportional counters is the low-background total α/β gas flow proportional counter. Generally, gross counting is very useful for environment sample screening to compare the radioactivity content of many environmental samples. Proportional counters with α/β particle discrimination are useful to measure gross α and gross β particles separately. α/β discrimination is based on the applied voltage and the different pulse shape, where α particles can be counted in a lower voltage gradient.

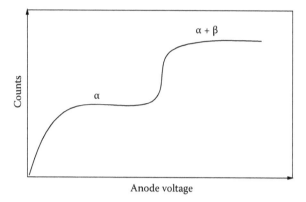

FIGURE 9.3 Proportional counter response curve for α and α/β particles as a function of the applied voltage.

α particles have a different pulse shape due to their high specific ionization. The pulses due to α particles can be discriminated in the presence of β particles, but β particles cannot be discriminated in the presence of α particles due α-β-cross talk. It is possible to use gross α/β to determine specific radionuclides such as ^{137}Cs, ^{210}Pb, and ^{90}Sr after radiochemical separation. The detection systems based on proportional counters have different geometries and applications such as 2π α-β counters and 4π α-β gas flow counters.

9.3.1.3 Geiger-Muller Counters

As the applied voltage increases (range 1000 to 3000 V), gas multiplication increases greatly due to the strong applied electric field between the electrodes. Geiger-Muller counters work in the same manner as proportional counters, the main difference being that ion pairs form along the radiation track and produce avalanche. In Geiger-Muller counters, one avalanche can produce another avalanche within the counter sensitive volume and spreads as a chain reaction. So the output pulses of Geiger-Muller counters are correlated with the original radiation properties (i.e., all pulses are the same regardless of the initial number of ion pairs produced by radiation). Geiger-Muller counters can operate as simple counters and not as spectrometers because it is impossible to differentiate between the different radiation energies.

Geiger-Muller counters are used as simple, economical radiation counters with a single electronic process where it does not need amplification of the large amplitude output signal. One of the main disadvantages of the Geiger-Muller counter is its long dead time compared to other counters. This limits its use to low count rate (a few thousand pulses per second) situations. Also the dead time correction should be considered.

Geiger-Muller counter quenching is another problem that appears as a continuous output of multiple pulses. The negative ions are collected and produce the primary discharge of the counter, and then the positive ions slowly drift toward the cathode where they hit the cathode and produce free electrons. At the cathode surface, the positive ions are neutralized by combining with an electron released from the cathode, and the rest of the electrons move toward the anode, leading to a second discharge. Counter quenching is handled in two ways: externally through an electronic circuit to decrease the high voltage after the primary discharge, or internally by mixing quench gas with lower ionization energy to decrease the production of electrons at the cathode surface and to prevent counter quenching.

9.3.2 SCINTILLATION DETECTORS

Luminescence processes play a very important role in radiation detection. The interaction of different radiations with a scintillator will ionize and excite its atoms and molecules. A large percentage of the absorbed energy is transferred to heat. After a short time, a small percentage of the deposited energy is released due to scintillator atom deexcitation that produces fluorescence light, visible light pulses, known as scintillation. The light pulses (scintillations) are converted to photoelectrons that are magnified through the photomultiplier tube to electric signals.

The prompt emission of visible light from a scintillator following its excitation due to energy absorption is known as the fluorescence process. Delayed fluorescence has the same emission spectrum as prompt fluorescence, but with a much longer emission time. The phosphorescence process corresponds to the emission of longer wavelength visible light than that of fluorescence and generally with much slower emission times. The quality and suitability of a scintillator as a radiation detector depends on its ability to convert as large a fraction as possible of the incident radiation energy to prompt fluorescence and to minimize the delayed fluorescence and phosphorescence processes.

The quality of the scintillator as a radiation detector depends on the following properties:

- Linear response between the deposited energy and the output light pulse.
- Decay time between the energy absorption and the light emission.
- Radiation energy absorption efficiency, specially for γ rays and neutrons.
- Scintillation efficiency, efficiency of conversion of absorbed energy to light.
- Transparency to its fluorescence light.
- Its index of refraction.

A high-quality scintillator has a liner response, short decay time, high absorption and scintillation (emission) efficiencies, a high transparency to its fluorescence photons, good optical quality, and an index of refraction near that of glass (1.5) to permit efficient coupling to the photomultiplier tube.

Radiation detection systems based on scintillation detectors consist of three main components: a scintillator (including the sensitive volume of the detector),

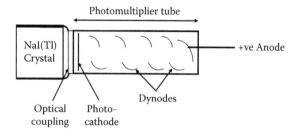

FIGURE 9.4 Cross section of NaI(Tl) inorganic scintillator crystal with photomultiplier tube (PMT).

an optical coupling system, and a photomultiplier tube and signal possessing electronic. The NaI(Tl) scintillation detector structure is shown in Figure 9.4. The outer surface of the scintillator (the sensitive volume of the detector) is optically isolated inside a holding vessel where the outer surfaces are constructed from reflecting materials. The side of the scintillator facing the photomultiplier tube is transparent to allow the passage of the produced light pulses — scintillation — due to the interaction of radiation within the scintillator. The light is emitted isotropically and somehow has to be channeled toward the photomultiplier tube. Any loss at this stage reduces the signal pulse height, decreases the low-energy sensitivity, and degrades the energy resolution. The optical coupling system may vary from virtually nothing to a highly sophisticated arrangement to ensure the efficient transfer of the light pulse from the scintillator to the photomultiplier tube. The photomultiplier tube consists of a photosensitive layer (photocathode) and 9 to 12 dynodes where the applied positive voltage increases gradually by about 100 to 200 V for each dynode and anode. The photons produced in the scintillator hit the photocathode and release a number of electrons that gain kinetic energy, due to the potential difference between the photocathode and the first dynode, and hit the first dynode and release five to eight electrons. The maximum values of quantum efficiency, the fractional number of electron released per photon, are 0.2 to 0.3 and depend on the wavelength of the light. The produced photoelectrons are internally multiplied due to an increase in the applied voltage on the dynodes that generate a relatively large electric pulse output at the anode, which is nearly proportional to the energy absorbed in the scintillator. Therefore the radiation detection process with a scintillation detector includes energy absorption in the scintillator, conversion of the absorbed energy to light photons, loss of photons in the scintillator, collection of photons and emission of electrons by the photocathode, electron multiplication in the photomultiplier tube (PMT), and finally output electric pulse analysis.

The number of electrons, n_e, released at the photocathode per absorbed energy (in keV), E_a, is given by

$$n_e = E_a S T_p G C, \tag{9.23}$$

where

S = scintillation efficiency (the number of photons converted to light per keV),

T_p = fraction of photons not absorbed in the scintillator,

G = light collection efficiency (the fraction of photons that fall on the photocathode),

C = quantum efficiency (the fractional number of electrons released per photon hitting the photocathode).

Scintillation detectors allow the measurement of radiation intensity, with a higher efficiency than that of Geiger-Muller counters, especially for γ-rays, and the determination of deposited energy. They can be used to measure radiation intensity and as a spectrometer to measure the energy spectrum of radiation.

9.3.2.1 Inorganic Scintillators

The inorganic crystal scintillators are mainly alkali halides such as sodium iodide or cesium iodide. They have a high atomic number, high densities, and high light output, so they are the most widely used especially for γ-ray detection. There are two types of inorganic crystal scintillators: pure or intrinsic crystals such as NaI and CsI and doped or extrinsic crystals such as NaI(Tl), CsI(Tl), and CaI_2(Tl). Thallium is a high atomic number element, which is added to the pure crystal as impurities and is known as activator.

The scintillation mechanism in inorganic materials depends on the energy states or bands determined by the crystal lattice of the material. Normally electrons are bound at lattice sites. The lower energy band is known as the valence band. The next energy band is the conduction band, which is usually empty. Energy dissipated in the material removes electrons from the lattice sites to the conduction band, which becomes free to move anywhere in the lattice and leaves a positive hole in the valence band, which can also move. Sometimes the absorbed energy is not enough to elevate the electron to the conduction band. Instead, the electron remains electrostatically bound to the positive hole in the valence band (i.e., excitation). Energy gaps, in which electrons can never be found in the pure crystal, exist between the valence and conduction bands. As a result of the interaction of radiation with the scintillator crystal, the electron can gain enough energy to rise from the valence band to the higher energy level of the conduction band and leave a positive hole in the valence band. In the pure crystal, after a certain decay time, an electron returns to the valence band with the emission of a photon. This process is inefficient and the librated photon energy is too high to lie in the visible range where most photomultiplier tubes respond best. A small amount of an impurity (i.e., activator) is added to enhance the probability of visible light photon emission during the deexcitation process. Activators such as thallium will change the energy band arrangement in some lattice sites where additional energy bands exist in the forbidden energy band of the pure crystal,

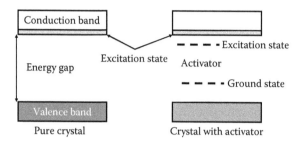

FIGURE 9.5 Energy bands for pure crystal and crystal with activator material.

as shown in Figure 9.5. The deexcitation of electrons through the activator energy bands, which have a lower energy gap, will produce photons, which lie in the visible range and are the basis for an efficient scintillation process. So the output light pulse is produced as a result of activator atom transitions (i.e., deexcitation), with typical half-lives on the order of 10^{-7} sec.

There are other processes that compete with the scintillation process, such as phosphorescence and quenching. Phosphorescence can often be a significant source of background light. Quenching represents a loss mechanism in the conversion of radiation energy to scintillation light due to certain radiationless transitions. The magnitude of the light output (i.e., the scintillation efficiency) and the wavelength of the emitted light are the most important characteristics of any scintillator. Scintillation efficiency and the wavelength of the emitted light affect the number of photoelectrons released from the photocathode and the pulse height at the output of the detection system.

The most widely used inorganic scintillator for γ-ray measurement uses a NaI(Tl) crustal. It has an excellent light yield, a linear response to electrons and γ-rays over most of the significant energy range, and a high atomic number. It can be manufactured in large sizes and different shapes. NaI(Tl) is hygroscopic, somewhat fragile, and can be easily damaged by mechanical or thermal shock. Various experimental data have shown that the absolute efficiency of NaI(Tl) is about 12%.

Other inorganic scintillators, including CsI(Tl), CsI(Na), CaF_2(Eu), LiI(Eu), bismuth germanate, BaF_2, ZnS(Ag), and CaF_2(Eu) have different densities, light conversion efficiencies, and wavelength ranges of the emission spectra. Details can be found in various references [1–3].

9.3.2.2 Organic Scintillators

Organic scintillators belong to the class of aromatic compounds and consist of an organic solvent such as toluene or xylene with low concentrations of one or more additives known as solutes. Organic scintillators are either used as pure organic crystals or as liquid organic solutions or polymers known as plastic scintillators.

The scintillation process in organic scintillators is the result of molecular transitions and is not affected by the physical state of the scintillator (i.e., crystalline solid, vapor, or liquid). A more detailed description of the scintillation process can be found in various references [1–3]. The main advantage of organic scintillators over inorganic scintillators is their fast response time, which is less than 10 nsec for organic scintillators and about 1 μsec for inorganic scintillators. This makes organic scintillators suitable for fast timing measurements. The scintillation efficiency for inorganic scintillators is generally higher than that of organic scintillators. For example, the scintillation efficiency of anthracene, which has the highest scintillation efficiency of all organic scintillators, is only about one third that of NaI(Tl) crystals. Beside the scintillation of the organic molecule following deexcitation, there are other radiationless deexcitation processes, called quenching. Quenching increases with increasing impurities, such as dissolved oxygen, in liquid scintillators. Although prompt fluorescence represents most of the observed scintillation, delayed fluorescence is also observed in many cases. Delayed fluorescence often depends on the nature of the exciting radiation and the rate of energy loss (dE/dx) of the exciting particle. The α and β particle pulse shapes are shown in Figure 9.6. Pulse shape analysis or discrimination is used to differentiate between different kinds of radiation particles, where the decay time of the pulse due to α particles is longer than that due to β particles.

There are different types of organic scintillators, including pure organic crystal, liquid organic solution, and plastic scintillators. Each has certain advantages and disadvantages for particular applications. The dissipated energy in pure organic scintillators transfers between molecules before deexcitation occurs. The energy dissipated in liquid and plastic scintillators is primarily absorbed by the solvent then transferred to the solute molecules, which are the efficient scintillation molecules where light emission occurs. Anthracene and stilbene are most common and are used as pure organic crystal scintillators. Anthracene has the highest scintillation efficiency of any organic scintillator. Stilbene has lower

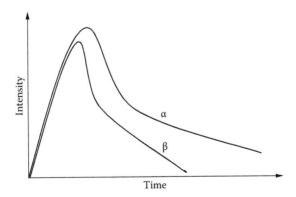

FIGURE 9.6 α and β particle pulse shapes.

scintillation efficiency, but is more suitable to differentiate between different kinds of radiation particles by pulse shape discrimination. Both materials are relatively fragile and difficult to obtain in large sizes.

Liquid organic scintillators and plastic scintillators have the same composition, but different physical forms. They are composed of solvent, which is a liquid for liquid organic scintillator and a polymer for plastic scintillators, and one or more solutes. One of the solutes is sometimes added to serve as a wave shifter. It absorbs the light produced by the primary solute and reradiates it at a longer wavelength to match the spectral sensitivity of the photomultiplier tube or to minimize bulk self-absorption in large liquid or plastic scintillators. Liquid organic scintillators have many applications in nuclear and environmental field measurements, especially for α and β particles. Liquid scintillators are used in sealed containers, which can reach few meters in size, and are handled in the same manner as solid scintillators. Liquid scintillators can be mixed with liquid samples for 4π configuration measurement, with nearly 100% counting efficiency.

9.3.3 SEMICONDUCTOR DETECTORS

Semiconductors are materials that do not have enough free charge carriers to behave as electrical conductors or a high resistivity to act as electrical insulators. As we mentioned before, the solid crystal has three energy bands: the valence band, the conduction band, and the forbidden band. For electrical conductors, the width of the forbidden energy band is very small. This allows the movement of valence electrons to the conduction band under the effect of any electric field strength higher than zero, where the electrons can move freely in the crystal lattice and carry electric current. For electrical insulators, the width of the forbidden energy band is large (about 10 eV) enough to prevent the movement of valence electrons to the conduction band, which is completely empty. For semiconductor materials, the forbidden energy band is relatively narrow, to prevent the movement of electrons to the conduction band at low temperatures (i.e., the conductivity of the semiconductors is zero). As temperature increases, some electrons gain enough energy to cross the forbidden band to the conduction band, where electrons can carry electric current under the influence of an electric field in the same way as conductors.

Semiconductor crystals as a detector material should have the capability of supporting large electric field gradients, high resistivity, and exhibit long life and mobility for both electrons and holes. If the mobility is too small and lifetime is too short, most electrons and holes will be trapped in crystal lattice imperfections or recombine before they can be collected. The group IV elements silicon and germanium are the most widely used semiconductor crystal as radiation detectors. Some of the key characteristics of various semiconductors for radiation detectors are shown in Table 9.1. The conductivity of semiconductors increases with an increase in the concentration of impurities, which create new energy levels that facilitate the movement of the carrier within the crystal. The ideal semiconductor material is "intrinsic" or "low effective impurity" material that is produced by a

TABLE 9.1
Some Key Characteristics of Various
Semiconductors as Detector Materials

Material	Z	Band gap (eV)	Energy/E_h pair (eV)
Si	14	1.12	3.61
Ge	32	0.74	2.98
CdTe	48–52	1.47	4.43
HgI_2	80–53	2.13	6.5
GaAs	31–33	1.43	5.2

process called "doping," which involves the addition of an impurity to reduce the charge carrier concentration (i.e., adding an electron-accepting impurity to compensate for electron donor impurities). Although doping increases the resistivity of the material, it also increases the probability of electron hole trapping or recombination. Prior to the mid-1970s, the required purity level of silicon and germanium could be achieved only by lithium ion drifting, counterdoping P-type (electron acceptor) crystals with N-type (electron donor) impurity to produce Ge(Li) and Si(Li) crystals. Since 1976, sufficient pure germanium has been available, but the doping process is still widely used in the production of Si(Li) x-ray detectors.

Semiconductors have four valence electrons in the upper energy level of the valence band. If they are doped with atoms, as crystal impurity, with three valence electrons, such as gallium, positive holes will be created in the crystal, known as P-type crystal, and the holes are the major current carrier. If they are doped with atoms with five valence electrons, such as arsenic, excess electrons will be created in the crystal, known as N-type crystal, and the electrons are the major current carrier. Semiconductors have a P-N diode structure and radiation detection is based on the favorable properties of the intrinsic region, the region near the junction between N- and P-type semiconductor materials, which is created by the depletion of charge carriers. The depletion region is the sensitive volume of the semiconductor detector where the ionizing radiation interacts and the dissipated energy produces electron hole pairs in the same way as gas-filled detectors. Electron-hole pairs are swept to the P and N regions. The produced charge is linearly correlated to the energy deposited in the detector. Semiconductors might be considered as solid state ionization chambers, with several advantages over gas devices. An unbiased P-N junction can act like a detector, but only with very poor performance, because the depletion region thickness is quit small, the junction capacitance is high, and the spontaneous electric field strength across the junction is low and not enough to collect the induced charge carriers that could be lost due to trapping and recombination. The performance of the P-N junction as a radiation detector is improved by applying an external voltage that causes

TABLE 9.2
Energy Resolution (FWHM)
for Different Detector Types

Energy (keV)	59	122	1332
Proportional counter	1.2	—	—
X-ray NaI(Tl)	3.0	12.0	—
3 × 3 NaI(Tl)	—	12.0	60
Si(Li)	0.16	—	—
Planar Ge	0.18	0.5	—
Coaxial Ge	—	0.8	1.8

the junction to be reversed biased. As the applied voltage increases, the width of the depletion region and the sensitive volume increase and the performance of the detection is improved. The applied voltage should be kept below the breakdown voltage of the detector to avoid catastrophic deterioration of the detector properties.

Because of the narrow energy band gap, 0.74 eV for germanium and 1.12 eV for silicon, semiconductor detectors are thermally sensitive. Both germanium and silicon photon detectors are cooled with liquid nitrogen during operation to reduce the thermal charge carrier generation (noise) to an acceptable limit, where the reverse leakage currents are in the range of 10^{-9} to 10^{-12} amp at liquid nitrogen temperature (77°K). The narrow energy band gap of semiconductor materials is 1/10 that required to produce an electron hole pair in a gas. This gives them the advantage of better energy resolution over gas-filled and scintillation detectors, where the increase in the number of charge carriers in the semiconductor detector leads to improved statistics and better energy resolution. The excellent energy resolution of semiconductor detectors is due to the much larger number of charge carriers per pulse (i.e., they produce a much larger number of charge carriers for a given incident radiation than is possible with any other detector type). The energy resolutions of different radiation detectors are given in Table 9.2. A comparison of different detector energy resolution is shown in Figure 9.12. Germanium is widely used for γ- and x-rays, while silicon is used for x-rays as Si(Li) and charged particles as silicon surface barrier detectors. NaI(Tl) scintillator has a relatively greater detection efficiency than that of semiconductor detectors because of its high atomic number. Semiconductor detectors for γ- and x-ray spectroscopy have several advantages over NaI(Tl) scintillators; among these are high energy resolution, compact size, relatively fast timing characteristics, and an effective thickness. Their disadvantages include the limitation to small sizes, some of them need to be cooled, and their relative sensitivity to performance degradation from radiation-induced damage.

9.3.3.1 Germanium Detectors

Germanium detectors are made of hyperpure germanium (HPGe) crystal that is mounted in a vacuum chamber. They are cooled by a liquid nitrogen cryostat to reduce the leakage current to an acceptable level. The preamplifier is located near the detector as part of the cryostat package to reduce electronic noise. A cross section of a typical HPGe detector with the liquid nitrogen cryostat is shown in Figure 9.7. There are different types of germanium detectors: coaxial, planar, and well. Their geometry and construction features are shown in Figure 9.8. The geometry and construction features of the detector affect its detection features, such as detection efficiency for γ- and x-rays, energy range, and energy resolution. Variations in detector efficiency and energy resolution as a function of incident radiation energy for the different detector types are shown in Figure 9.9 and Figure 9.10. Coaxial P-type germanium detectors are used for γ-rays, with an energy range of 100 keV to about 10 MeV, and cannot be used for low-energy γ- and x-rays because they cannot penetrate the aluminum detector window and high-energy γ-rays might pass through the sensitive volume without interaction. For x-ray spectroscopy, N-type and planar germanium detectors can be used because of the thin beryllium entrance windows. At low energies, detector effi-

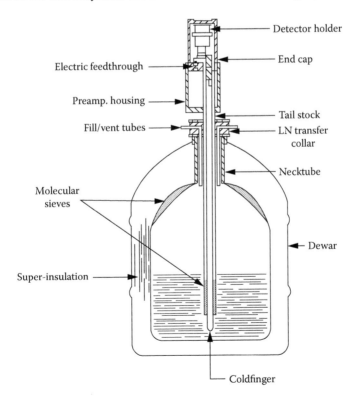

FIGURE 9.7 Cross section of a HPGe detector with liquid nitrogen cryostat.

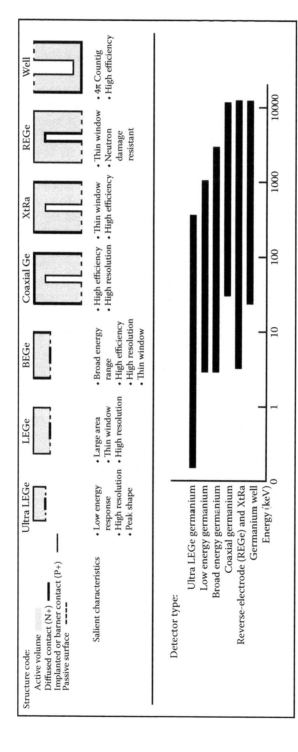

FIGURE 9.8 The different geometries of HPGe detectors and their operational energy ranges.

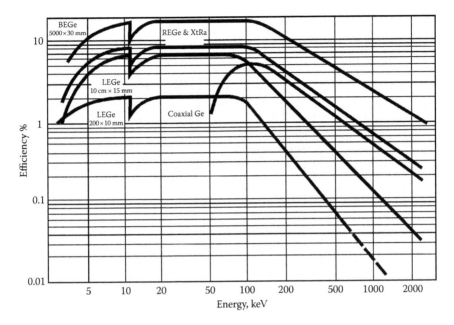

FIGURE 9.9 Typical absolute efficiency curves for various germanium detector types as a function of the incident radiation energy.

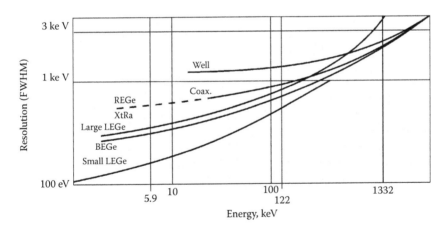

FIGURE 9.10 The energy resolution curves of the different HPGe detector types as a function of the incident radiation energy.

ciency is a function of the cross-sectional area and window thickness, while at higher energies, total active detector volume determines counting efficiency. Coaxial germanium detectors are specified in terms of their relative full-energy peak efficiency compared to that of the 3 in. × 3 in. NaI(Tl) scintillation detector

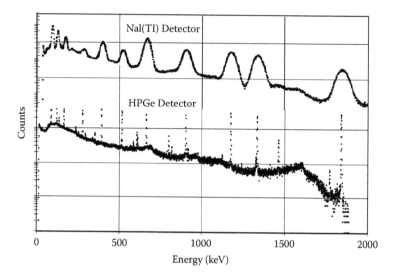

FIGURE 9.11 γ-ray spectra for the same source measured using NaI(Tl) scintillation and HPGe detectors.

at a detector-to-source distance of 25 cm. Germanium detectors of greater than 100% relative efficiency have been produced. NaI(Tl) scintillation and germanium detector spectra for the same source are shown in Figure 9.11.

9.3.3.2 Silicon Detectors

9.3.3.2.1 Si(Li) X-Ray Detectors

P-type silicon crystal is doped with lithium atoms (the lithium drifting process) to produce a very stable Si(Li) crystal that can be stored at room temperature. It is only useful for x-ray detection in the energy range of 4 to 50 keV. The signal:noise ratio is a very significant parameter that affects the resolution and the performance of any radiation detector, especially in low-level radioactivity measurement (Figure 9.12). It is a critical problem with silicon detectors because the energy deposited in silicon by x-rays and the produced electric signals are small. That is why the proper electronics must be used to reduce the noise and to amplify the signal. Both Si(Li) and planar germanium detectors can be used for x-ray spectroscopy, but the Si(Li) detector is better because its escape peaks are very low. The planar germanium detector can be very useful in high x-ray and very low energy γ-ray measurements. x-rays interact with the silicon mainly by photoelectric effect, and the spectrum looks simpler than that produced by using germanium detectors.

The Si(Li) detector window is usually made of low-Z (atomic number) materials such as beryllium. In addition to the detector window thickness, x-ray energy will affect the detection efficiency, where the efficiency increases with an increase in the x-ray energy to a maximum level and then decreases with increasing energy because at the high energy the x-rays might pass through the active volume

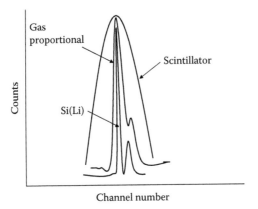

FIGURE 9.12 Comparison of the energy resolution (FWHM) of gas-filled, scintillation, and semiconductor detectors.

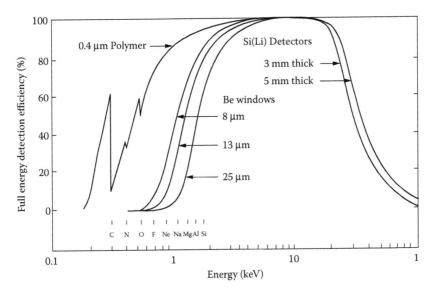

FIGURE 9.13 The efficiency curve of the Si(Li) detector as a function of the incident radiation energy.

without interaction. The detection efficiency as a function of incident x-ray energy is shown in Figure 9.13.

9.3.3.2.2 Silicon Charged Particle Detectors

These are also know as silicon diode detectors or surface barrier (SSB) detectors and the modern versions are known as passivated implanted planar silicon (PIPS) detectors. They have become the detectors of choice for heavy charged particle measurements, including α particles and fission fragments spectroscopy. They have a P-N structure in which a depletion region is formed by applying reverse bias. In the SSB detector, a surface barrier junction is formed by oxidizing the surface of the N-type silicon. Electric contact is made to the P-type oxidized surface by a thin layer of gold and to the N-type surface by a layer of aluminum. The depletion region is the sensitive volume of the detector and is formed by to the migration of electrons toward the P-type region and the hole toward the N-type region. The width of the depletion region increases with an increase in the bias voltage and can extend to the limit of the breakdown voltage. The resistivity of the silicon must be high enough to allow a large enough depletion region at a moderate bias voltage. PIPS detectors employ implanted rather than surface barrier contacts and are therefore more rugged and reliable than SSB detectors. Detectors are generally available with depletion layer depths of 100 to 700 μm and active areas of 25 to 5000 mm².

9.3.4 OTHER TYPES OF RADIATION DETECTORS

There are other types of detectors that are used for radiation detection and dosimetry, such as thermoluminescence detectors (TLDs), Cerenkov counters, nuclear track detectors, neutron detectors, and others. Details about these detectors are described in various references [1,4].

9.4 BASIC RADIATION DETECTION SYSTEM

The previous sections discussed the main aspects of radiation detector operation principles for the different radiation types. The choice of detector type for a specific radiation measurement should be based on the detector properties, such as counting efficiency, energy resolution, signal rise time, dead time, and signal:noise ratio. Generally a simple radiation detection system consists of a detector, a pulse processing electronic unit, and an output device such as a counter, single-channel analyzer, or multichannel analyzer. A diagram of a basic radiation detection system is shown in Figure 9.14.

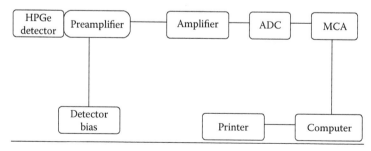

FIGURE 9.14 Diagram of the basic radiation detection system.

9.4.1 PREAMPLIFIER

The preamplifier has three essential functions: conversion of the charge (the electric output pulse of the detector) to a voltage pulse, signal amplification, and pulse shaping. In addition, the preamplifier also matches the high impedance of the detector and the low impedance of the coaxial cables to the amplifier. Most detectors can be represented as a capacitor into which a charge is deposited as a result of radiation interaction within the active volume of the detector. During the charging process, a small current flows and the voltage drops across the bias resistor, which is the pulse voltage. The rise time of the preamplifier output pulse is related to the collection time of the charge and ranges from a few nanoseconds to a few microseconds, while its decay time is the resistance-capacitance time constant characteristic of the preamplifier itself, usually set at about 50 µsec. Most preamplifiers are charge sensitive (i.e., the output voltage pulse is proportional to the input charge).

9.4.2 AMPLIFIER

The amplifier reshapes the pulse as well as amplifies it. Details can be found in various references [1,2,5]. Typical preamplifier and amplifier pulse forms are shown in Figure 9.15.

9.4.3 PULSE HEIGHT ANALYSIS AND COUNTING TECHNIQUES

Pulse height analysis consists of a simple discriminator that can be set above the noise level of the detection level and produces a standard logic pulse for use in a pulse counter or as a gating signal. The detection system signal output device can be either a single-channel analyzer or counter or a multichannel analyzer. The single-channel analyzer has a lower-level discriminator (LLD) and an upper-level discriminator (ULD) and produces an output logic pulse whenever a voltage input pulse falls between the discriminated levels. Counters and rate meters are used to record the number of logic pulses, either on an individual basis (as in a counter) or as an average count rate (as in a rate meter). The multichannel analyzer, which can be considered a series of single-channel analyzers with incrementing narrow windows, basically consists of an analog-to-digital converter (ADC), control logic, memory, and a display device. The display device reads the memory content versus memory location, which is equivalent to the number of pulses and appears as an energy spectrum.

9.4.4 SHIELDING

The principle role of detector shielding is to reduce the number of background counts. The accuracy of the radioactivity measurement process is affected significantly by the background contribution to the measured count. The lower limit of detection in counts is proportional to the square of the number of background

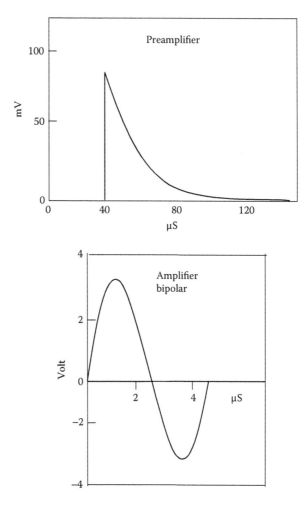

FIGURE 9.15 Typical preamplifier and amplifier (bipolar and unipolar) output signal and logic pulse.

counts. The minimum detectable activity (MDA) is defined as the smallest concentration of a radionuclide that can be determined reliably with a giving detection system. For low-level radioactivity measurements, it is essential to reduce the background count and increase detection efficiency. Counting efficiency can be improved by using a larger amount of source sample and a larger detector volume, and by improving the source-detector geometry. The detection limit (L_d) and MDA are given by the following equations:

$$L_d = 2.71 + 4.65 \sqrt{B} \,, \tag{9.24}$$

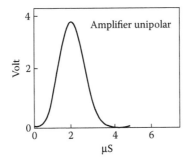

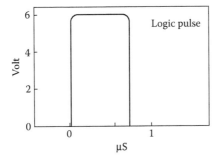

FIGURE 9.15 (continued).

$$MDA = 2.71 + 4.65 \, \frac{\sqrt{B}}{t \cdot \varepsilon}, \tag{9.25}$$

where

B = background counts in the region of interest or of the counting system,
t = counting time (in sec),
ε = counting efficiency.

Sources of background radiation exist everywhere, but at different levels, and the following sources are considered as the most common sources:

- Environmental radioactivity due to natural radionuclides that exist in different concentration levels around the detection system, such as ^{238}U series, ^{232}Th series, and ^{40}K radionuclides.
- Radioactive impurities in the detector components and shielding material.
- Cosmic radiation, which is composed mainly of neutrons, electromagnetic radiation, protons, and electrons.
- Instrument electronic noise, which affects the output pulse height and quality.

In addition to these sources, the environmental sample itself can be another source of background radiation.

There are two types of shielding, passive shielding and active shielding. Passive shielding is where heavy materials such as lead and iron are used as shielding materials and entirely surround the γ-ray detector. For γ-ray spectrometry, background radiation can be reduced to 1/100 by a 10 cm thickness of lead. Old lead is preferred because of its low content of ^{210}Pb (22.2 yr half-life) that decays to an energetic β emitter ^{210}Bi (E_{max} = 1.17 MeV). The interaction of β particles within the lead shield result in bremsstrahlung, which may contribute to an increase in background rate. Lead shielding is also used as a passive shield in the low background liquid scintillation counters. For γ-ray spectrometers, usually the lead shield is lined with a few millimeters of cadmium and copper, where the characteristic K x-rays (approximately 73 keV) excited by scattered radiation emerging from the lead can be stopped by the cadmium layer and the cadmium K x-rays (22 keV) in turn are stopped in the innermost liner of copper. Active shielding is another detection system surrounding the main detection system, where the output pulses of both are going through an electronic circuit (such as anticoincident circuit) to eliminate the background pulses which are counted simultaneously in both detectors. Plastic and inorganic scintillators are used as passive shielding for γ-ray spectrometry, liquid scintillation counters and gas flow counters in what is known as the electric guard technique. More details can be found in various references [1,6].

9.5 RADIOACTIVITY ANALYSIS

Radioactivity analysis of food and environmental samples is a very significant task in any radioecological study and the accuracy of the measured natural and artificial radionuclide concentrations affects the study conclusions and the consequent recommendations for environmental and human protection. Radioecology studies include the following main tasks:

- Sampling planning and sample collection.
- Sample preparation.
- Radioactivity analysis.
- Quality control measures.
- Data evaluation.
- Study conclusions and recommendations.

In principle, the sample preparation is a process in which samples are taken through several steps to reach the most appropriate form for radioactivity measurement. It serves to preserve the sample and keep it in a more homogenized form, including drying, crushing, homogenization, and sieving of the soil and sediment samples. Sample preparation serves also to increase the counting efficiency, and sometimes it is essential for performing the radioactivity analysis itself, such as for α emitter analysis (e.g., uranium isotopes, plutonium isotopes, and ^{210}Po), where the source sample should be a thin layer to reduce the self-absorption of α particles and the counting process is impossible without source sample chemical preparation.

The radioactivity analysis process includes source sample preparation: choosing the counting techniques that fulfill the analysis objectives; counting system adjustments, such as reducing electronic noise and background counts; energy and efficiency calibration; MDA calculation; radioactivity measurements; and calculation of the radioactivity concentration and its associated error. Radioactivity measurements are classified into relative measurements, where the standard sources are used for measurement system calibration, and absolute measurements, which do not need any standard sources for radioactivity analysis. Absolute measurement methods include the defined solid angle method, the 4π counting method, the internal gas counting method, and other methods based on the coincidence technique. The most often used radioactivity analysis methods for food and environmental samples include 2π α/β gas flow counters, liquid scintillation spectrometers, γ-ray spectrometers, β particle spectrometers, and α particle spectrometers.

9.5.1 2π α/β COUNTING WITH A GAS FLOW COUNTER

A low background gas flow proportional counter is a very useful radioactivity counting system for environmental samples. Many laboratories use total α/β measurements as a rapid method to estimate the activities of α and β radionuclides in water, air, soil, sludge, and wastewater. The main purpose of gross α/β measurement is to provide adequate information concerning the activity within samples, and thus to determine if further detailed analysis is required. This counting technique is based on the ability of proportional counters to differentiate between the ionization events due to α and β particles, which depends on the voltage bias applied on the counter. There are a variety of available counters that offer simultaneous separate α and β measurement, where for each sample there are two separate measuring channels for α and β activities. The ultraflat flow proportional counter tubes are located above the source sample planchets, as shown in Figure 9.16. To reduce the background, the measuring counters are covered at the top by a large-area flow counter tube acting as a common guard counter (i.e., active shielding), in addition to 10 cm of lead (i.e., passive shielding).

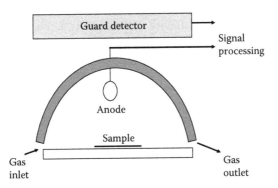

FIGURE 9.16 Layout of a low background gas flow proportional gas counter.

Gross α/β measurement techniques are applicable for α particle emitters having energies greater than 3 MeV and for β particle emitters having energies greater than 0.1 MeV. The solids concentration in the source sample is a limiting factor in determining the sensitivity of gas flow proportional counting because of self-absorption of α and β particles by the sample itself. Because α and β particles are attenuated or scattered by the sample solids, calibration curves for self-absorption and scattering must be established if there is mass in a sample. Sample density on the planchet area should not exceed 10 mg/cm² for gross α and 20 mg/cm² for gross β for a 2-in. diameter counting planchet. Moisture absorbed by the dried sample residue is an interferant because it enhances self-absorption [7].

The 2-in. diameter gas proportional detectors have a manufacturer-measured α background of 0.05 counts/min and a β background of 1.0 counts/min. An instrument with 1.0 counts/min β background will have an LLD of 37 mBq for a 60 min. count at the 95% confidence level, with 30% detection efficiency, whereas an instrument with an α background of 0.05 counts/min will have an LLD of 67 mBq for the same count time and detection efficiency [3].

When measuring α and β particle activity using a gas flow proportional system, counting at the α voltage plateau discriminates against β particle activity, whereas counting at the β voltage plateau is somewhat sensitive to the α particle activity present in the sample. This phenomenon is termed "cross talk" and is compensated for during instrument calibration. The cross talk factors are determined using α (^{238,239}Pu or ^{241}Am) and β (^{90}Sr or ^{137}Cs) solutions of known activity concentrations counted over a range of absorber thicknesses (in mg/cm²) encountered during routine sampling and counting [7].

For gross α and gross β measurements, the detector must be calibrated to obtain the counting efficiency (i.e., the ratio of the counting rate to the disintegration rate). α-emitting radionuclides such as ^{241}Am, ^{230}Th, and ^{238}Pu and β-emitting radionuclide such as ^{90}Sr/^{90}Y reference standard are prepared in the same sample geometries and weight ranges used for efficiency calibration where both self-absorption and backscattering of the α and β particles are considered. Sample weight stability, which can be obtained by heating the sample to high temperature to convert the hygroscopic salts to oxides, is essential to ensure the accuracy of the self-absorption counting efficiency factor for the samples [7] and to overcome the possible uncertainty in the gross α/β counting of soil samples due to the lack of well-characterized soil standards for calibrations and the unpredictable absorption effects that soil has on counting results. Burnett et al. [8] proposed an alternative approach based on direct counting of pressed soil wafers to estimate total α/β activities.

In addition to gross α/β screening measurements, a gas flow proportional counter is used also for analysis of some α-emitting radionuclides such as ^{226}Ra and β-emitting radionuclides such as ^{210}Pb and ^{90}Sr/^{90}Y in different environmental samples after proper radiochemical analysis to separate the radionuclides of interest. More details can be found in various references [3,4,7,9].

9.5.2 LIQUID SCINTILLATION SPECTROMETER

Since the early applications of liquid scintillation counting, the liquid scintillation counting systems have been designed mainly to detect low-energy β particle emitters (e.g., ^{3}H, ^{14}C). Their applications have been extended to detect high-energy β particle emitters (e.g., ^{90}Y, ^{210}Bi), and some of the new versions of liquid scintillation counters are able to detect α particle emitters (e.g., uranium isotopes, $^{239+240}$Pu). Conversion electrons or Auger electrons can be detected and quantified using variations of the liquid scintillation counting techniques. Liquid scintillation counters play the role of an energy transducer, converting energy from nuclear decay into light. The light is sensed by photomultiplier tubes and generates electric pulses, which are coincidence gate discriminated and are analyzed by means of integrated electronic circuits and logic according to their timing and amplitude. Then they are recorded and displayed as counts (i.e., count rate or energy spectrum). A liquid scintillation counting system diagram is shown in Figure 9.17. The liquid scintillation measurement method is a quantitative technique to determine radioactivity, but not a qualitative one to find radiation energy or the sort of nuclide.

Liquid scintillation consists of a solvent and organic scintillators (the liquid scintillation cocktail) that may be composed of one, two, or three solutes. Usually the samples are incorporated in the LS cocktail to be assayed, which results in either a homogeneous or heterogeneous sample, depending on the solubility of

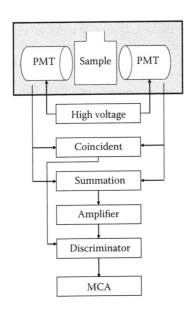

FIGURE 9.17 Layout of a liquid scintillation spectrometer.

the sample in the cocktail. Homogeneous sample counting is the preferred modality, where the counting efficiency is 4π counting geometry and relatively high. Consequently additives or solubilizers are often used to promote sample homogeneity. Since the sample comes into intimate contact with the scintillation components, it interferes with the energy transfer process (quenching) and reduces the scintillation counting efficiency. Quenching processes are either chemical or color quenching, which reduce the maximum light output of the scintillation system. In heterogeneous sample counting, the sample to be assayed is finely dispersed or suspended, or is counted on a solid support by immersion in a liquid scintillation where the counting geometry may not be 4π geometry (i.e., relatively low counting efficiency and the quenching process has only a slight effect or none at all on scintillation efficiency).

The three classes of liquid scintillations used for internal sample counting are

- Toluene- or xylene-based scintillators. These are the most efficient light transducers, provided that their energy transfer process is not disturbed by the presence of impurities. Toluene-based scintillators are relatively stable and easy to prepare using scintillation grade chemicals.
- P-dioxane-based scintillators. These were introduced to meet the need for measuring aqueous samples. P-dioxane is miscible with water, but is an inefficient scintillator solvent. When supplemented with a high concentration (50 to 100 g/l) of naphthalene, a dioxane-based scintillator may attain an efficiency that is about 70% of a toluene-based scintillator. They have obvious disadvantages, such as their high cost and the solvent p-dioxane is readily oxidized during storage, forming peroxides, which cause sever quenching and give rise to intense chemiluminescence (chemical quenching) in the presence of alkaline tissue solubilizers.
- Emulsion or colloid scintillators. These have a high capacity for holding aqueous samples, high counting efficiency and the advantage of low cost and great flexibility. The emulsion scintillators are not stable counting systems (i.c., not thermodynamically stable), and with slight changes in composition, the appearance and counting efficiency can undergo abrupt changes.

Depending on the liquid scintillation cocktail, the α-particle detection efficiency is generally greater than 95%, whereas the β-particle detection efficiency is dependent on energy, spectral shape, and cocktail. Typically β particles with maximum energies (E_{max}) greater than 0.250 MeV are detected with greater than 90% counting efficiency. The counting efficiency is reduced due to different interferences (i.e., quenching) that result in photon quenching, chemical quenching and color quenching; these are processes in which the maximum photon yield is not achieved for a given radioactive source due to sample inhomogeneity, adverse energy transfer, and nontransparency of the liquid scintillation solution to the photon emitted, respectively, therefore quenching correction and efficiency determination are identical. Since samples vary in quench characteristics, their efficiency must be determined individually. The most frequently used methods for quenching correction are

- Internal standard method. When properly carried out, it is the most accurate method for quenching correction, in which a calibrated standard of the measured radionuclide is added to a sample that has been previously counted for efficiency determination:

$$Counting\ efficiency\ =\ \varepsilon\ =\ \frac{C_2 - C_1}{A}, \tag{9.26}$$

  where
  C_1 = count rate of the sample (in cps),
  C_2 = count rate of the sample plus the added internal standard (in cps),
  A = calibrated activity of the added internal standard (in Bq).

- Quenched and unquenched standard methods. A series of liquid scintillation samples have the same calibrated standards activity as ^3H and ^{14}C, and each sample has successively increasing amounts of a quencher or nonradioactive equivalent of the material to be assayed. A relationship between the loss in count or counting efficiency and the quenching level can be computed and used for counting efficiency correction.
- Channels ratio method. This is based on a downward shift of the pulse height spectrum of the radionuclides in the presence of a quencher. The extent of the shift is related to the counting efficiency of the liquid scintillation system.
- External standard method. This method uses Compton recoil electrons from high-energy γ-rays, photoelectrons from low-energy γ-rays (less than 60 keV), or x-rays, or a combination of these, for quenching correction. It is an integral part of all modern liquid scintillation spectrometer. A correlation curve between the count rate of the γ-ray standard and the sample counting efficiency is obtained using a set of quenched standards.

The α particle-emitting radionuclides can be measured by a liquid scintillation counter where pulse-shape discrimination is used, as the characteristics of pulses from β particles differ from those derived from α particles. α particle emitters may be counted by direct incorporation of aqueous samples containing the nuclide in an emulsion-type scintillator or by extracting the nuclide of interest from the aqueous sample with an extractive scintillator. The liquid scintillation counter spectrum of electroplated $^{236+239+240}PU$ (α-emitting radionuclides) and ^{241}Pu (β-emitting radionuclides) is shown in Figure 9.18. More details of liquid scintillation counter operation and α particle emitter analysis can be found in various references [10].

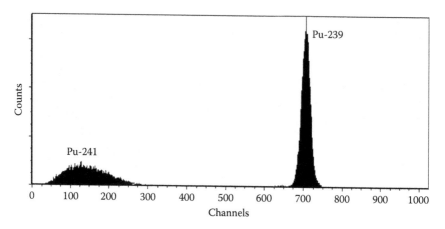

FIGURE 9.18 α/β spectra of a liquid scintillation counter with pulse shape analyzer.

9.5.3 γ-Ray Spectrometry

γ-ray measurement techniques are the backbone of radionuclide concentration estimation in environmental samples because most radionuclides emit γ-rays, the high penetration of γ-rays permits comparatively simple source preparation, and γ-ray spectrometry gives good selectivity in discriminating among radionuclides. The most important detection media for γ-ray spectrometry are inorganic scintillators such as NaI(Tl), CsI(Na), and CaI$_2$(Eu), and semiconductors such as HPGe. The most often used γ-ray detectors are NaI(Tl) and HPGe.

The probability of the various types of interactions depends upon the dimensions and the nature of the detecting medium and upon the energy of the incident photon. The total intrinsic detection efficiency is dependent upon the geometric arrangement. The photopeak/total ratio (or photofraction) is relatively independent of geometry for a given detector. The selection of γ ray spectrometer is based on its photopeak counting efficiency, energy resolution, and cost. γ-ray spectrometry based on an HPGe detector is preferred for the determination of radionuclides in food and environmental samples because of the higher resolving power (energy resolution = full width at half maximum [FWHM]) of the HPGe detector than that of the NaI(Tl) detector; high-energy resolution is essential for analysis of the complex γ-spectra. NaI(Tl) scintillation is preferred when high-energy resolution is not essential. The energy resolution of NaI(Tl) crystal (3 in. $\times$ 3 in.) is about 6% for the photopeak of ^{137}Cs at 661.6 keV (i.e., it is about 40 keV) and about 60 keV for the photopeak of ^{60}Co at 1332 keV, while the energy resolution of HPGe detectors is about 1.9 keV for the photopeak of ^{60}Co at 1332 keV (see Figure 9.19). The main advantages of NaI(Tl) are that they can be obtained in larger sizes, they have a high efficiency, and they cost less than semiconductor detectors. The disadvantages of HPGe detectors are their lower efficiency than that of NaI(Tl) and the necessity to cool them to liquid nitrogen temperature.

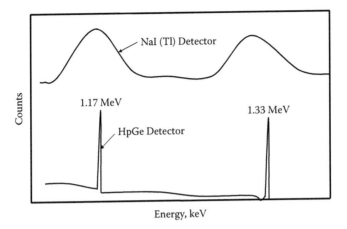

FIGURE 9.19 ^{60}Co γ-ray spectra for HPGe and NaI(Tl) detectors.

Low-level γ-ray spectrometry is a very useful technique, but it needs great care and a highly skilled person to avoid the different sources of interference. Only a brief description of γ-ray spectrometry will be given here; more details can be found in various references [1,2,5,11]. The detector size, the source sample geometry (source-detector geometric arrangement), the contents of γ-ray emitters in the source sample, and the number and energy of the γ-rays emitted produce a complex γ-ray spectrum in which γ-ray photopeak should be carefully identified and analyzed. The γ-ray spectrum includes (see Figure 9.20)

- The photopeak (full absorption energy peak) at energy E. This is the characteristic energy for the measured radionuclides
- The Compton edge. The scattered (Compton) electrons have an energy from zero up to a maximum energy E_{max}, which corresponds to the energy of the Compton edge and is given by

$$E_{max} = E - \frac{E}{1 + \left(\dfrac{2E}{m_0 c^2} \right)}. \tag{9.27}$$

- Backscatter peak. Sometimes Compton interactions occur very close to the surface of the detector, where there is a possibility that electrons can escape outside the detector sensitive volume and only the scattered photon will be detected. The minimum energy of the scatted photon corresponds to the energy of the backscattered peak and is given by

$$E_{min} = \frac{E}{1 + \left(\dfrac{2E}{m_0 c^2} \right)}. \tag{9.28}$$

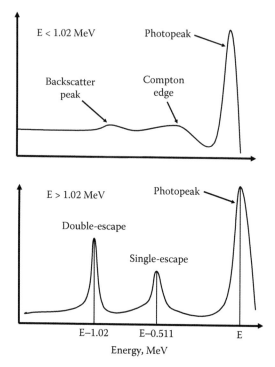

FIGURE 9.20 γ-ray spectrum showing the full absorption peak, Compton edge, and backscatter peak for γ-ray energy less than 1.02 MeV, and full absorption peak with the single and double escape peaks for γ-ray energy greater than 1.02 MeV.

- The single-escape peak with energy = $E - 0.511$ MeV. This corresponds to the escape of one annihilation photon.
- The double-escape peak with energy = $E - 1.02$ MeV. This corresponds to the escape of both annihilation photons.
- Peak at 511 keV. This appears when the pair production reaction occurs near the detector surface and corresponds to the possibility that only one of the annihilation photons is detected in the counter.

For high-quality γ-ray spectrometry using HPGe detectors, there are different aspects that should be very carefully considered, such as

- Detector type and specifications. Choosing the suitable detector type depends on the detector counting efficiency, energy resolution, and cost, and the right choose of detector size, shape, and peak to Compton ratio (the ratio of the peak height at 1.33 MeV γ-ray line of ^{60}Co to the height of the Compton continuum between 1040 and 1096 keV).
- Detector shields and background reduction
- Cosmic ray contribution to the background

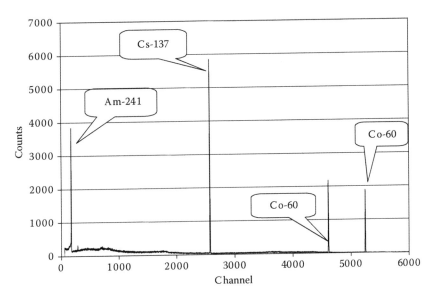

FIGURE 9.21 γ-ray spectrum of different radionuclides used for HPGe energy calibration.

- Radon gas concentrations in the surrounding counting room environment
- Electronic settings, such as amplifier time constant and shaping, pole-zero (P/Z) cancellation, and pulse pileup
- Energy calibration and efficiency calibration of the γ-ray spectrometer for certain source sample geometries
- Spectrum analysis, and activity and error calculation

Energy calibration of the γ-ray spectrometer is a relationship between the channel number of the multichannel analyzer and the γ-ray energy, which is essential for γ-ray spectrum analysis. Mixed standard γ-ray sources, of known radionuclides (such as ^{241}Am [59.5 keV], ^{137}Cs [661.6 keV], and ^{60}Co [1173.2 and 1332.5 keV]) and defined γ-ray energy lines with at least three different γ-ray energies to cover the energy range of interest are used for energy calibration (see Figure 9.21 and Figure 9.22).

Photopeak efficiency is a function of γ-ray energy, the source sample geometry, and the source sample detector arrangement. Any slight change in these factors affects the counting efficiency and thus the accuracy of the calculated activity concentration of the different radionuclides in the measured sample. Experimentally peak efficiency is a function of γ-ray energy. Efficiency calibration of the spectrometer can be carried out using different methods. The simplest method is using a standard source of the same radionuclides of interest, such as ^{134}Cs/^{137}Cs, and the same sample geometry and sample-detector arrangement. The counting efficiency and the activity concentration (A_i) of a radionuclide (J) are given by

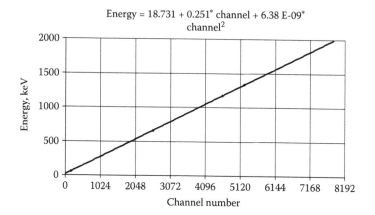

FIGURE 9.22 Energy calibration curve for a HPGe γ-ray spectrometer.

$$\varepsilon_{ij} = \frac{C/t}{A} \, 100 \, , \qquad (9.29)$$

$$A_i = \frac{C_{ij}}{t \, \varepsilon_{ij} \, w} \, , \qquad (9.30)$$

where

ε_{ij} = peak efficiency,

C/t = count rate (in cps),

A_i = activity concentration (in Bq/kg or Bq/l),

C_{ij} = total count of the photopeak of radionuclide i at energy j (in keV),

t = counting time (in sec),

w = weighing factor (equivalent to 1/sample weight in kilograms or 1/sample volume in liters),

A = activity concentration of the standard sample (in Bq).

Another efficiency calibration method is performed using a standard mixed radionuclide source (a list of radionuclides is given in Table 9.3) of a known radionuclide concentration and their main energy lines that cover the energy range of interest. The γ-ray spectrum and the full peak efficiency curve are given in Figure 9.23 and Figure 9.24.

Another efficiency calibration method (in the energy range of 186 to 2450 keV) is performed in two stages. In the first stage, the relative efficiency curve of the HPGe detector is determined using a ^{226}Ra point source where the most intensive γ-rays of ^{226}Ra in equilibrium with its daughters have been used. The relative intensities (the intensity of line x divided by the intensity of 609 keV γ-energy line) of the photopeaks corresponding to these γ-ray lines have been measured

TABLE 9.3
List of Radionuclides and Their
Half-Lives and Photon Energies
for a Mixed Standard γ Source

Nuclide	Half-Life, Days	Photon Energy, keV
^{241}Am	157,850	59.54
^{109}Cd	462.1	88.03
^{57}Co	271.83	122.06
		136.47
^{139}Ce	137.66	165.86
^{203}Hg	46.604	279.20
^{113}Sn	115.09	391.69
^{85}Sr	64.849	514.01
^{137}Cs	11,000	661.66
^{60}Co	1925.3	1173.23
		1332.49
^{88}Y	106.63	898.04
		1836.06

by the detector and calculated. The photopeak relative efficiency is found by dividing the relative intensity of the photopeak with energy (E) by the reference relative intensity of the same photopeak:

$$\varepsilon(E) = I_M(E)/I_R(E), \tag{9.31}$$

where
   $\varepsilon(E)$ = relative efficiency at energy (E),
   $I_M(E)$ = relative intensity measured by the detector for the photopeak
         with energy (E),
   $I_R(E)$ = reference relative intensity of the same photopeak [12].

The relative efficiency curve of the detector was made of 17 different energy values covering the energy range from 186 KeV to 2450 KeV. The efficiency curve is plotted in Figure 9.25. The relative efficiency of the detector corresponding to any photopeak energy can be obtained using this averaged curve.

In the second stage, the average relative efficiency curve of the detector is normalized to an absolute efficiency figure. The normalization was done using standard solutions of potassium chloride. Potassium containing 0.0118% of ^{40}K has specific activity of about 850 pCi/g (31.45 Bq/g). Pure potassium chloride is an excellent low-level reference source in many respects: low-level specific activity, wide availability at high purity, and relatively simple branching decay. The normalizing factor for any radionuclide was calculated relative to the potassium chloride solution normalizing factor using the following equation:

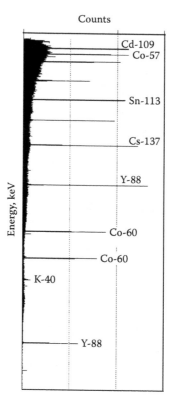

FIGURE 9.23 γ-ray spectrum of mixed standard source for efficiency calibration of a HPGe γ-ray spectrometer.

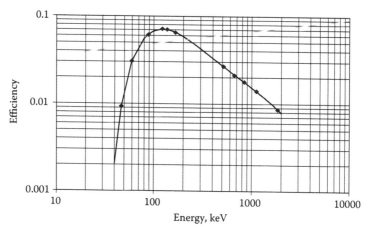

FIGURE 9.24 Full peak efficiency curve of a HPGe γ-ray spectrometer.

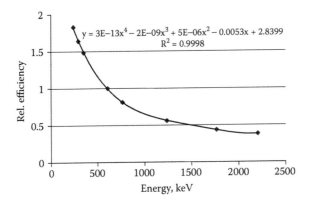

FIGURE 9.25 Relative full peak efficiency curve of a HPGe γ-ray spectrometer.

$$N.F_{(Y)} = \frac{R.E_{(1460\,keV)} \times P.D_{(K)}}{R.E_{(Y)} \times P.D_{(Y)}} \times N.F_{(K)}, \qquad (9.32)$$

where

$NF_{(y)}$ = normalizing factor for y radionuclide (in Bq/kg/cps),

$RE_{(1460\,keV)}$ = relative efficiency of ^{40}K,

$RE_{(y)}$ = relative efficiency of radionuclide y,

$PD_{(K)}$ = percentage of photon per disintegration of ^{40}K,

$PD_{(y)}$ = percentage of photon per disintegration of y radionuclide,

$NF_{(K)}$ = normalizing factor of ^{40}K (in cps of potassium chloride solution divided by ^{40}K concentration in Bq/l or Bq/kg).

The counting efficiency varies with variations in sample density, chemical composition, geometry, and sample-detector arrangement. The effects of sample density and chemical composition on the counting efficiency are energy dependent. To avoid the possible effects of sample density and composition on the counting efficiency, it is preferred that the counted samples be similar or close to that of the efficiency calibration samples.

9.5.4 β Particle Spectrometry

When the radionuclides emit no or very low intensity γ- or x-rays, α or β particle measurement is a necessity. β particle-emitter radionuclides (maximum β particle energy in MeV) that are frequently assayed include ^{3}H (0.0186), ^{14}C (0.156), ^{32}P (1.71), ^{35}S (0.167), ^{45}C (0.257), ^{85}Kr (0.84), ^{89}Sr (1.49), ^{90}Sr (0.546), and ^{90}Y (2.28). Because of the continuous nature of a β particle energy spectrum, spectrometric identification and quantification of a sample containing several β particle emitters are generally difficult. Thus radiochemical separation of the different β particle emitters in environmental samples is essential. Except for the conversion electron emitters, they have a sharp energy spectrum. The most often used counting systems for β particle emitter assays are the gas-filled counters, operating in either the proportional or Geiger-Muller voltage range, and the liquid scintillation counters. Both techniques were discussed previously. Often the counting systems that are based on gas-filled detectors can be more sensitive because of lower background than that of liquid scintillation counters. The counting efficiency of the β particle counting system is given by

$$\eta = \frac{n}{f_a A} \, , \tag{9.33}$$

where

n = count rate (in cps),
f_a = absorption correction factor, including the correction factors due to counting geometry factor, source self-absorption, and source-mount backscattering,
A = activity of the radionuclide of interest.

It is essential in the sample source preparation to have the source sample as a thin layer and to prepare it in a reproducible manner to minimize the uncertainty due to changes in the absorption correction factor.

Semiconductor detectors can be used for β particle spectrometry, especially spectrometry measurement of conversion electron (EC) emitters, such as the assay of ^{137}Cs by measuring the 624 keV EC of its [137m]Ba daughter. Details of β particle counting and spectrometry can be found in various references [1,3].

9.5.5 α Particle Spectrometry

Many naturally occurring radionuclides, particularly members of the uranium, thorium, and actinium decay series, and the transuranic elements are mainly α emitters. α particle spectrometry is a very sensitive technique with a very low counting background. There is a clear difference between α particles and other kinds of radiation with a high linear energy transfer and high energy range typically between 4 and 9 MeV. The counting background of the spectrometer may be either due to the α particle active materials in their construction material or due to contamination. The background count rates, counting efficiencies, and MDA values for different α particle counting techniques are given in Table 9.4. To increase the sensitivity of the α particle counting system one can use a detector with a large active area or concentrate the α particle active material in a source sample. The thickness of the α source affects the quality of α particle counting and spectrometry methods. α gross counting can be performed using a gas-filled detector or liquid scintillation counter. For high α particle spectrometry, a very thin source sample preparation is essential to reduce the self-absorption of the α particles in the source itself. Source sample counts in a vacuum chamber can

TABLE 9.4
**Background Count Rate, Counting Efficiency, and Minimum Detectable
Activity (MDA) for Different α Particle Measurement Techniques**

	Background (cpm)	Counting Efficiency (%)	MDA (Bq/l) in 100 min.
Gas flow proportional counting	0.05–0.5	35	2.1
Liquid scintillation counting with PSA	0.1–1.0	95	0.5
α spectrometry	0.003–0.01	25	0.4

reduce the absorption of α particles in the air between the sample and the detector. A semiconductor detector (PIPS detector) is used for α spectrometry because of its high-energy resolution and its compact size (see Figure 9.26). Counting efficiency and energy resolution can be checked using a mixed standard α emitter electroplated source that contains ^{239}Pu, ^{241}Am, and ^{244}Cm, or ^{234}U, ^{238}U, ^{239}Pu, and ^{241}Am. The α spectrum of the mixed standard α source is shown in Figure 9.27. The counting efficiency does not change with α particle energies (i.e., it is constant over the α particle energy range of 4 to 9 MeV). The energy resolution is given as the FWHM of the ^{241}Am α peak at 5.49 MeV. Counting efficiency and energy resolution are affected by the detector active area and the source-to-detector distance. Some α particle spectrometers are based on the Frisch grid ionization chamber, which usually has a larger active area and a lower energy resolution (FWHM = 40–50 keV) than that of a PIPS detector.

The main advantage of α spectrometry is its high sensitivity due to the high-yield α decay process, low background, and elimination of other possible interferences by chemical separation. Also it is applicable to a wide range of radionuclides and environmental samples. The main disadvantage is the lengthy chemical separation and source preparation procedure.

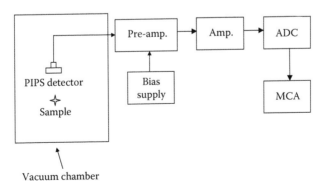

FIGURE 9.26 Diagram of an α particle spectrometer with PIPS detector.

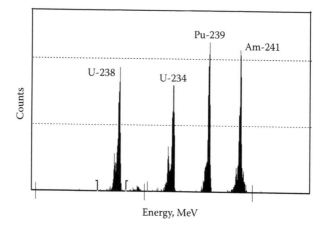

FIGURE 9.27 α spectrum of mixed standard source.

9.5.6 RADIOCHEMICAL ANALYSIS

Radiochemical analysis becomes essential when the activity concentration of the radionuclides is close to the detection limit of the direct measuring technique or when the levels of interference in the radionuclide assay process cannot be tolerated. The interference may be due to matrix interference, in which the sample matrix absorbs the emitted particles, or spectral interferences, where the spectra of other radionuclides prevent the accurate measurement of the radionuclides of interest. Radiochemical analysis is essential for quantitative α and β particles spectrometry of the different natural (such as uranium isotopes, thorium isotopes, ^{210}Pb, ^{210}Po, ^{226}Ra, and ^{228}Ra) and artificial radionuclides (such as $^{239+240}$Pu, ^{238}Pu, ^{241}Am, and ^{244}Cm) in the different environmental matrixes. Also, improving sensitivity in radiochemical separations usually entails a more through elimination of interfering components. A diagram of the different radiochemical analysis steps is shown in Figure 9.28.

In general, it is necessary to add isotopic or nonisotopic carriers before any radiochemical analysis is commenced. Isotopic carriers serve two functions: to provide additional mass of the element, which aids in the separation process, and to provide a means of measuring the chemical yield. Nonisotopic carriers serve only to aid in the separation of the desired nuclides. The sample preparation step includes drying, ashing, and scavenging, while the sample solubilization and equilibrium step includes dissolution and leaching. Radiochemical concentration and separation includes coprecipitation, ion exchange, and solvent extraction. After the separation step, the radionuclides of interest exists in a pure portion and are used for counting the source preparation by autoplating (as for polonium isotopes), electroplating, or coprecipitation (as for uranium, plutonium, and thorium isotopes). As an example, radiochemical analysis of uranium and plutonium isotopes are discussed.

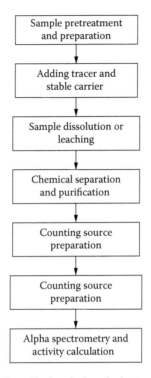

FIGURE 9.28 Flowchart of the radiochemical analysis steps.

9.5.6.1 Determination of Uranium Isotopes

9.5.6.1.1 Principles of the Analytical Procedure

The ashed sample is spiked with uranium tracer (^{232}U) for chemical yield and activity calculation. The ashed sample is dissolved using HNO_3, HCl and HF acids. Uranium in the dissolved sample solution is extracted from most of the matrix elements with trioctylphosphine oxide (TOPO) and back-extracted with 1 M $NH_4F/0.1$ M HCl solution. The uranium fraction is purified by coprecipitation with LaF_3 and anion exchange. Finally, the pure uranium fraction is electrodeposited on a stainless steel disk from HCl/oxalate solution and measured by means of α spectrometry. The flowchart of uranium isotope analysis is shown in Figure 9.29.

9.5.6.1.2 Sample Preparation

9.5.6.1.2.1 Soil and Sediment Samples

1. Dry the sample at 110°C until the weight remains constant, then grind, homogenize, and sieve the dried sample through a 2-mm sieve.
2. Weigh about 10 g of dried sample and moisten it with HNO_3 until no further reaction occurs. Dry the sample on a sand bath.
3. Ash the dried sample at 550°C for at least 6 to 8 h. Grind and homogenize the sample ash. If the residue is not free of organic carbon, which

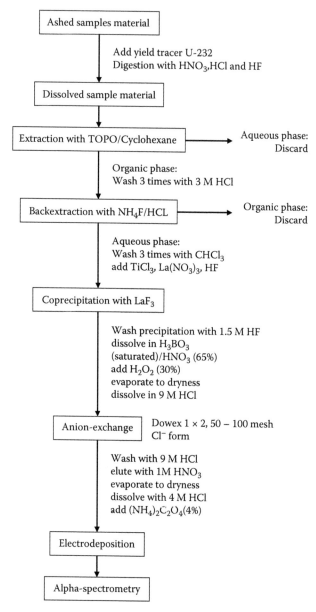

FIGURE 9.29 Flowchart of uranium isotope radiochemical analysis.

can be recognized by a dark brown- or black-colored ash, repeat the ashing process.

4. Weigh up to 5 g ashed sample into a platinum or Teflon dish and add ^{232}U tracer (50 to 100 mBq) for chemical yield determination.

5. Add 40 ml HNO_3 and 10 ml HF and digest on a medium temperature (70°C to 80°C) hot plate.
6. Repeat step 5 until no further dissolution takes place (white residue).
7. Add 3 ml HNO_3 (65%) three times and evaporate to near dryness.
8. Dissolve the sample residue in 100 ml of 8 M HNO_3 in a 250-ml glass beaker and cover it with a watch glass.
9. Boil the sample solution for 30 min., cool it to room temperature, and adjust the solution volume to 100 ml.
10. Continue with separation and source preparation.

9.5.6.1.2.2   Biological Samples (Plants, Milk, Meat, and Fish)

1. Dry the sample at 110°C until the weight remains constant, then grind and homogenize the dried sample.
2. Ash the dried sample material at 550°C for at least 6 to 8 h. Grind and homogenize the sample ash. If the residue is not free of organic carbon, which can be recognized by a dark brown- or black-colored ash, repeat the ashing process.
3. Weigh 20 to 50 g of ashed sample material into an Erlenmeyer flask (1 L) and add ^{232}U tracer (50 to 100 mBq) for chemical yield determination.
4. Add 100 ml of HNO_3 and digest on a medium temperature (70 to 80°C) hot plate and stir using a Teflon-coated magnetic bar.
5. Repeat the addition of HNO_3 and digestion until you have a clear solution.
6. Evaporate the solution to near dryness and dissolve the sample residue in 100 ml of 8 M HNO_3 in a 250-ml glass beaker and cover it with a watch glass.
7. Boil the sample solution for 30 min., cool it to room temperature, and adjust the solution volume to 100 ml.
8. Continue with separation and source preparation.

9.5.6.1.3   Separation and Source Preparation

1. Transfer the dissolved sample into a 250-ml separation funnel.
2. Extract uranium isotopes with 25 ml 0.2 M TOPO/cyclohexane by shaking for 15 min. each.
3. After phase separation, transfer the organic phase into another 250-ml separation funnel.
4. Extract uranium isotopes with 25 ml 0.2 M TOPO/cyclohexane by shaking for 15 min. each. Combine the organic phases in the 250-ml separation funnel. Discard the aqueous phase.
5. Wash the organic phase three times with 50 ml of 3 M HCl by shaking for 5 min. each. Discard the washing solution.
6. Back-extract uranium isotopes two times with 25 ml of 1 M NH_4F/0.1 M HCl by shaking for 15 min. each. Combine the aqueous phases and discard the organic phase.

7. Wash the aqueous phase two times with 50 ml $CHCl_3$ by shaking for 2 min. each. Discard the organic phase.
8. Transfer the solution into a 100-ml polyethylene centrifuge tube. Add drop-wise 2 to 3 ml of $TiCl_3$ (15%) until you have a violet color. The color should stay visible for 10 min.
9. Add 20 ml HF (40%) and 2 ml $La(NO_3)_3$ (25 mg La^{3+}/ml). After a short interval of agitation, centrifuge the sample solution for 5 min. at 3000 rpm to separate the fine crystalline precipitate.
10. Repeat the addition of 2 ml $La(NO_3)_3$ (25 mg La^{3+}/ml) two times, then centrifuge the sample solution for 5 min. at 3000 rpm and discard the aqueous phase after decanting.
11. Wash the precipitate carefully with 15 ml of 1.5 M HF and centrifuge the sample solution for 5 min. at 3000 rpm. Discard the aqueous phase after decanting.
12. Dissolve the precipitate in 10 ml hot saturated HBO_3 and 10 ml concentrated HNO_3.
13. Add 1 ml H_2O_2 (30%) and leave the sample solution for 15 min.
14. Evaporate the sample solution to dryness.
15. Dissolve the sample residue in 10 ml of 9 M HCl by heating. Cool the sample solution to room temperature.

9.5.6.1.4 Column Preparation

1. Transfer about 1 g Dowex (1×2, 50 to 100 mesh, Cl form) with distilled water into a glass column 15 cm in length with an inner diameter of 8 mm. Condition the column by passing 50 ml of 9 M HCl at a rate of 1 ml/min.
2. Pass the sample through the conditioned anion exchanger column at a rate of 1 ml/min.
3. Wash the column with 50 ml of 9 M HCl at a rate of 1 ml/min. Discard the washing solution.
4. Elute uranium isotopes with 50 ml of 1 M HNO_3 in a crystallizing dish.
5. Evaporate to dryness. Add 1 ml HCl (32%) twice and fume to dryness each time.
6. Carefully rinse the crystallizing dish with 0.4 ml of 4 M HCl and transfer the solution into a cleaned electrolytic cell for electrodeposition on a stainless steel plate.
7. Rinse the crystallizing dish again three times with 1 ml $(NH_4)_2C_2O_4$ (4%) each and transfer the solutions into the cell.
8. Rinse the crystallizing dish again with 0.6 ml of distilled water and transfers the solution into the cell.
9. Perform electrodeposition for 3 h at 300 mA.
10. Before switching off the current, add 1 ml NH_3 (25%) and continue the electrolysis for 1 min.

11. Discard the solution, then rinse the cell with distilled water. Discard the water and then disconnect the current.
12. Remove the stainless steel disk from the cell and rinse it with distilled water and then ethanol.
13. Measure the α activity on the stainless steel disk by means of α spectrometry.

9.5.6.1.5 Calculation of the Results

9.5.6.1.5.1 Calculation of the Chemical Yield

$$\eta = \frac{C_{n,U-232}}{C_{Ex,U-232}} \cdot 100 , \tag{9.34}$$

where

η = chemical yield (in percent),
$C_{n,U-232}$ = measured net count rate in the ^{232}U peak (per sec),
$C_{Ex,U-232}$ = expected count rate in the ^{232}U peak (per sec).

$$C_{Ex,U-232} = A_{U-232} \cdot t_M \cdot \varepsilon , \tag{9.35}$$

where

A_{U-232} = added ^{232}U activity (in Bq),
t_M = time of measurement of the sample (in sec),
δ = counting efficiency of the measuring device.

9.5.6.1.5.2 Calculation of Uranium Isotope Specific Activities in the Sample

The activities are calculated as is commonly done for isotope dilution analysis:

$$A_{U-238} = \frac{A_{U-232}}{M \cdot (C_{U-232} - C_{0,U-232})} \cdot \left[C_{U-238} - C_{0,U-238} - C_{T,U-238} \right] , \tag{9.36}$$

$$A_{U-235} = \frac{A_{U-232}}{\rho_{U-235} \cdot M \cdot (C_{U-232} - C_{0,U-232})} \cdot \left[C_{U-235} - C_{0,U-235} - C_{T,U-235} \right], \tag{9.37}$$

$$A_{U-234} = \frac{A_{U-232}}{M \cdot (C_{U-232} - C_{0,U-232})} \cdot \left[C_{U-234} - C_{0,U-234} - C_{T,U-234} \right], \tag{9.38}$$

where

A_{U-238} = specific activity or concentration of ^{238}U (in Bq/g or Bq/l),
A_{U-235} = specific activity or concentration of ^{235}U (in Bq/g or Bq/l),
A_{U-234} = specific activity or concentration of ^{234}U (in Bq/g or Bq/l),
M = amount of sample taken for analysis (in g or l),
C_{U-238} = count rate in the ^{238}U peak (per sec),
$C_{0,U-238}$ = background count rate in the ^{238}U peak (per sec),
C_{U-235} = count rate in the ^{235}U peak (per sec),
$C_{0,U-235}$ = background count rate in the ^{235}U peak (per sec),
C_{U-234} = count rate in the ^{234}U peak (per sec),
$C_{0,U-234}$ = background count rate in the ^{234}U peak (per sec),
C_{U-232} = count rate in the ^{232}U peak (per sec),
$C_{0,U-232}$ = background count rate in the ^{232}U peak (per sec),
$C_{T,U-238}$ = background in the ^{238}U peak (per sec) (count rate that is not produced by the decay of ^{238}U, but is a consequence of peak tailing),
$C_{T,U-235}$ = background from peak tailing in the ^{235}U peak (per sec),
$C_{T,U-234}$ = background from peak tailing in the ^{234}U peak (per sec),
A_{U-232} = activity of ^{232}U, added for yield determination (in Bq),
ρ_{U-235} = emission probability for α decay of ^{235}U ($\rho_{U-235} = 0.816$).

9.5.6.1.5.3 Calculation of Standard Deviation

The standard deviations of the uranium activities are obtained with the following equations:

$$s_{D,U-238} = \frac{A_{U-232}}{M \cdot C_{n,U-232}} \cdot$$

$$\sqrt{\frac{C_{U-238}}{t_M} + \frac{C_{0,U-238}}{t_0} + \frac{C_{T,U-238}}{t_M} + \left(\frac{C_{n,U-238}}{C_{n,U-232}}\right)^2 \cdot \left(\frac{C_{U-232}}{t_M} + \frac{C_{0,U-232}}{t_0}\right)} \quad , \quad (9.39)$$

$$s_{D,U-235} = \frac{A_{U-232}}{\rho_{U-235} \cdot M \cdot C_{n,U-232}} \cdot$$

$$\sqrt{\frac{C_{U-235}}{t_M} + \frac{C_{0,U-235}}{t_0} + \frac{C_{T,U-235}}{t_M} + \left(\frac{C_{n,U-235}}{C_{n,U-232}}\right)^2 \cdot \left(\frac{C_{U-232}}{t_M} + \frac{C_{0,U-232}}{t_0}\right)} \quad , \quad (9.40)$$

$$s_{D,U-234} = \frac{A_{U-232}}{M \cdot C_{n,U-232}} \cdot \quad (9.41)$$

$$\sqrt{\frac{C_{U-234}}{t_M} + \frac{C_{0,U-234}}{t_0} + \frac{C_{T,U-234}}{t_M} + \left(\frac{C_{n,U-234}}{C_{n,U-232}}\right)^2 \cdot \left(\frac{C_{U-232}}{t_M} + \frac{C_{0,U-232}}{t_0}\right)} \quad ,$$

where

$s_{D,U-238}$ = standard deviation of the ^{238}U specific activity or concentration
         (in Bq/g or Bq/l),

$s_{D,U-235}$ = standard deviation of the ^{235}U specific activity or concentration
         (in Bq/g or Bq/l),

$s_{D,U-234}$ = standard deviation of the ^{234}U specific activity or concentration
         (in Bq/g or Bq/l),

$C_{n,U-238}$ = net count rate in the ^{238}U peak,

$C_{n,U-235}$ = net count rate in the ^{235}U peak,

$C_{n,U-234}$ = net count rate in the ^{234}U peak,

C_{U-232} = net count rate in the ^{232}U peak,

t_M = time of measurement of the sample (in sec),

t_0 = time of measurement of the background (in sec).

9.5.6.2 Determination of Plutonium Isotopes

9.5.6.2.1 *Principle of the Analytical Procedure*

The ashed sample is spiked with plutonium tracer (^{236}Pu or ^{242}Pu) for chemical yield determination and activity calculation. The ashed sample is leached twice using HNO$_3$/HF and HNO$_3$/Al(NO$_3$)$_3$ solution mixtures, with the addition of NaNO$_2$, which transfers Pu^{3+} to Pu^{4+}. Plutonium is extracted from the leached sample solution with TOPO and back-extracted with ascorbic acid in HCl solution. The plutonium fraction is purified by coprecipitation with LaF$_3$ and anion exchange. Finally, the pure plutonium fraction is electrodeposited on a stainless steel disk from HCl/oxalate solution and measured using α spectrometry. The flowchart of plutonium isotopes analysis is shown in Figure 9.30.

9.5.6.2.2 *Sample Preparation*

9.5.6.2.2.1 *Soil and Sediment Samples*

1. Dry the sample at 110°C until the weight remains constant, then grind, homogenize, and sieve the dried sample through a 2-mm sieve.
2. Weigh about 120 g of dried sample and moisten it with HNO$_3$ until no further reaction occurs. Dry the sample on a sand bath.
3. Ash the dried sample at 550°C for at least 6 to 8 h. Grind and homogenize the sample ash. If the residue is not free of organic carbon, which can be recognized by a dark brown- or black-colored ash, repeat the ashing process.
4. Weigh up to 100 g ashed sample into an Erlenmeyer flask (1 l) and add plutonium tracer (50 to 100 mBq) for chemical yield determination.
5. Add 290 ml of 8 M HNO$_3$/0.9 M HF and boil while stirring on a hot plate for 30 min.
6. Carefully add 2.5 g NaNO$_2$ to the hot solution. Cool the solution to room temperature.

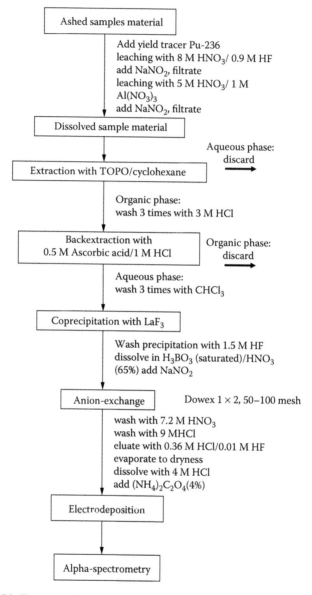

FIGURE 9.30 Flowchart of plutonium isotope radiochemical analysis.

7. Filter the leached solution under pressure reduced using a Buchner funnel with a Whatman no. 42 filter paper. Transfer the solution into a 600-ml glass beaker. Transfer the filter with the ashed sample residue back into the Erlenmeyer flask (1 l).

8. Add 250 ml of 5 M HNO_3/1 M $Al(NO_3)_3$ and boil the sample solution while stirring on a hot plate for 30 min.
9. Carefully add 2.5 g $NaNO_2$ to the hot solution. Cool the solution to room temperature.
10. Filter the leached solution under reduced pressure using a Buchner funnel with a Whatman no. 42 filter paper. Combine the leaching solutions. Discard the filter paper and the sample residue.
11. Continue with separation and source preparation.

9.5.6.2.2 Biological Samples (Plants, Milk, Meat, and Fish)

1. Dry the sample at 110°C until the weight remains constant, then grind and homogenize.
2. Ash the dried sample material at 550°C for at least 6 to 8 h. Grind and homogenize the sample ash.
3. Weigh 20 to 50 g of ashed sample material into an Erlenmeyer flask (1 l) and add plutonium tracer (50 to 100 mBq) for chemical yield determination.
4. Add 100 ml of HNO_3 and digest on a medium temperature (70 to 80°C) hot plate and stir using a Teflon-coated magnetic bar.
5. Repeat the addition of HNO_3 and digestion until you have a clear solution.
6. Evaporate the solution to near dryness and dissolve the sample residue in 100 ml of 8 M HNO_3.
7. Boil the sample solution and carefully add 2.5 g $NaNO_2$ to the hot solution. Cool the solution to room temperature.
8. Continue with separation and source preparation.

9.5.6.2.3 Separation and Source Preparation

1. Transfer the dissolved sample into a separation funnel (250 or 1000 ml).
2. Extract plutonium isotopes with 25 ml of 0.2 M TOPO/cyclohexane by shaking for 15 min.
3. After phase separation, transfer the organic phase into another 250-ml separation funnel.
4. Extract plutonium isotopes again with 25 ml of 0.2 M TOPO/cyclo-hexane by shaking for 15 min., then combine the organic phases in the 250-ml separation funnel. Discard the aqueous phase.
5. Wash the organic phase three times with 50 ml of 3 M HCl by shaking for 5 min. each. Discard the washing solution.
6. Back-extract plutonium isotopes two times with 25 ml of 0.5 M ascorbic acid/1 M HCl by shaking for 15 min. each. Combine the aqueous phases in a 250-ml separation funnel and discard the organic phase.
7. Wash the aqueous phase two times with 50 ml $CHCl_3$ by shaking for 2 min. each. Discard the organic phase.
8. Transfer the solution into a 100-ml polyethylene centrifuge tube.

9. Add 20 ml HF (40%) and 2 ml La(NO$_3$)$_3$ (25 mg La^{3+}/ml). After a short interval of agitation, centrifuge the sample solution for 5 min. at 3000 rpm to separate the fine crystalline precipitate.
10. Repeat the addition of 2 ml La(NO$_3$)$_3$ (25 mg La^{3+}/ml) two times, centrifuge the sample solution for 5 min. at 3000 rpm, then discard the aqueous phase after decanting.
11. Wash the precipitate carefully with 15 ml of 1.5 M HF and centrifuge the sample solution for 5 min. at 3000 rpm. Discard the aqueous phase after decanting.
12. Dissolve the precipitate in 10 ml hot saturated HBO$_3$ and 10 ml concentrated HNO$_3$.
13. Add 0.25 ml of 1.5 M NaNO$_2$ (freshly prepared).

9.5.6.2.4 Column Preparation

1. Transfer about 1 g Dowex (1 × 2, 50 to 100 mesh, NO$_3$ form) with distilled water into a glass column 15 cm in length with inner an diameter of 8 mm. Condition the column by passing 50 ml of 7.2 M HNO$_3$ at a rate of 1 ml/min.
2. Pass the sample solution through the conditioned anion exchanger column at a rate of 1 ml/min.
3. Wash the column with 50 ml of 7.2 M HNO$_3$ at a rate of 1 ml/min. Discard the washing solution.
4. Wash the column with 10 ml of 9 M HCl at a rate of 1 ml/min. Discard the washing solution.
5. Elute plutonium isotopes with 10 ml of 0.36 M HCl/0.01 M HF in a crystallizing dish.
6. Evaporate the eluted solution to dryness. Add 1 ml HCl (32%) twice and fume to dryness each time.
7. Carefully rinse the crystallizing dish with 0.4 ml of 4 M HCl and transfer the solution into a cleaned electrolytic cell for electrodeposition on a stainless steel plate.
8. Rinse the crystallizing dish three times with 1 ml (NH$_4$)$_2$C$_2$O$_4$ (4%) each and transfer the solution into the cell.
9. Rinse the crystallizing dish again with 0.6 ml distilled water and transfer the solution into the cell.
10. Perform electrodeposition for 2 h at 300 mA.
11. Before switching off the current, add 1 ml NH$_3$ (25%) and continue the electrolysis for 1 min.
12. Discard the solution, then rinse the cell with distilled water. Discard the water and then disconnect the current.
13. Remove the stainless steel disk from the cell and rinse it with distilled water and then ethanol.
14. Measure the α activity on the stainless steel disk by means of α spectrometry.

9.5.6.2.5 Calculation of the Results

9.5.6.2.5.1 Calculation of the Chemical Yield

$$\eta = \frac{C_{n,Pu-236}}{C_{Ex,Pu-236}} \cdot 100 \ , \tag{9.42}$$

where

η = chemical yield (in percent),

$C_{n,Pu-236}$ = measured net count rate in the ^{236}Pu peak (per sec),

$C_{Ex,Pu-236}$ = expected count rate in the ^{236}Pu peak (per sec).

$$C_{Ex,Pu-236} = A_{Pu-236} \cdot t_M \cdot \varepsilon \ , \tag{9.43}$$

where

A_{Pu-236} = added ^{236}Pu activity (in Bq),

t_M = time of measurement of the sample (in sec),

ε = counting efficiency of the measuring device.

9.5.6.2.5.2 Calculation of Plutonium Isotope Specific Activities

The activities are calculated as is commonly done for isotope dilution analysis:

$$A_{Pu-239+240} = \frac{A_{Pu-236}}{M \cdot (C_{Pu-236} - C_{0,Pu-236})} \cdot$$
$$\left[C_{Pu-239+240} - C_{0,Pu-239+240} - C_{T,Pu-239+240} \right] \ , \tag{9.44}$$

$$A_{Pu-238} = \frac{A_{Pu-236}}{M \cdot (C_{Pu-236} - C_{0,Pu-236})} \cdot \left[C_{Pu-238} - C_{0,Pu-238} - C_{T,Pu-238} \right], \tag{9.45}$$

where

$A_{Pu-239+240}$ = specific activity or concentration of $^{239+240}$Pu (in Bq/g or Bq/l),

A_{Pu-238} = specific activity or concentration of ^{238}Pu (in Bq/g or Bq/l),

M = amount of sample taken for analysis (in g or l),

$C_{Pu-239+240}$ = count rate in the $^{239+240}$Pu peak (per sec),

$C_{0,Pu-239+240}$ = background count rate in the $^{239+240}$Pu peak (per sec),

C_{Pu-238} = count rate in the ^{238}Pu peak (per sec),

$C_{0,Pu-238}$ = background count rate in the ^{238}Pu peak (per sec),

C_{Pu-236} = count rate in the ^{236}Pu peak (per sec),

$C_{0,Pu-236}$ = background count rate in the ^{236}Pu peak (per sec),

$C_{T,Pu-239+240}$ = background in the $^{239+240}$Pu peak (per sec) (count rate that is not produced by the decay of $^{239+240}$Pu, but is a consequence of peak tailing),

$C_{T,Pu-238}$ = background from peak tailing in the ^{238}Pu peak (per sec),

$C_{T,Pu-236}$ = background from peak tailing in the ^{236}Pu peak (per sec),

A_{Pu-236} = activity of ^{236}Pu, added for yield determination (in Bq).

9.5.6.2.5.3 Calculation of Standard Deviation

The standard deviations of the plutonium activities are obtained with the following equations:

$$s_{D,Pu-239+240} = \frac{A_{Pu-236}}{M \cdot C_{n,Pu-236}} \cdot \tag{9.46}$$

$$\sqrt{\frac{C_{Pu-239+240}}{t_M} + \frac{C_{0,Pu-239+240}}{t_0} + \frac{C_{T,Pu-239+240}}{t_M} + \left(\frac{C_{n,Pu-239+240}}{C_{n,Pu-236}}\right)^2 \cdot \left(\frac{C_{Pu-236}}{t_M} + \frac{C_{0,Pu-236}}{t_0}\right)}$$

$$s_{D,Pu-238} = \frac{A_{Pu-236}}{M \cdot C_{n,Pu-236}} \cdot$$

$$\sqrt{\frac{C_{Pu-238}}{t_M} + \frac{C_{0,Pu-238}}{t_0} + \frac{C_{T,Pu-238}}{t_M} + \left(\frac{C_{n,Pu-238}}{C_{n,Pu-236}}\right)^2 \cdot \left(\frac{C_{Pu-236}}{t_M} + \frac{C_{0,Pu-236}}{t_0}\right)} \tag{9.47}$$

where

$s_{D,Pu-239+240}$ = standard deviation of the $^{239+240}$Pu specific activity or concentration (in Bq/g or Bq/l),

$s_{D,Pu-238}$ = standard deviation of the ^{238}Pu specific activity or concentration (in Bq/g or Bq/l),

$C_{n,Pu-239+240}$ = net count rate in the $^{239+240}$Pu peak,

$C_{n,Pu-238}$ = net count rate in the ^{238}Pu peak,

t_M = time of measurement of the sample (in sec),

t_0 = time of measurement of the background (in sec).

9.5.6.2.5.4 Quality Control

Quality control measurements are necessary to provide documentation to show the reliability of the achieved results. The results' reliability is a function of precision (reproducibility) and accuracy (the closeness to the true value). Precision can easily be determined by additional internal determinations. The accuracy of the results can be determined through performing control analysis with reference materials that are as similar as possible to the analyzed material samples, and through participating in intercomparisons or proficiency measurements at least once a year. After performing 10 to 12 assays, a blank has to be performed with the same equipment and the same chemicals to ensure that there is no cross contamination. A blank is always recommended when samples with high activity content have been analyzed or when there are symptoms of a contamination of the laboratory, the equipment, or the chemicals.

The status of the equipment should be checked routinely by measuring background, blanks, and standards. These results often give the first indication of analytical difficulties. Analytical control samples generally constitute about 10% to 15% of the total samples [9,13].

ACKNOWLEDGMENT

I would like to express my deep gratitude to Dr. M.H. Abou-Taleb, Dr. Yasser Ebaid, and Dr. Tareq Youssif for reviewing the manuscript and fruitful discussion. Also, I wish to acknowledge the assistance of Dr. Max Pimpl and Dr. Randa Higgy in the radiochemical analysis section, and of Mr. W. Christoph in γ-ray analysis. Finally, I acknowledge the support I received from Canberra Co. to make most of the figures and tables available to be used in this chapter.

REFERENCES

1. Knoll, G.F., *Radiation Detection and Measurement*, 2nd ed., John Wiley & Sons, New York, 1989.
2. Tsoulfanidis, N. *Measurement and Detection of Radiation*, 1st ed., Hemisphere Publishing, New York, 1983.
3. NCRP, *A Handbook of Radioactivity Measurement Procedures*, NCRP report no. 58, National Council on Radiation Protection and Measurement, Bethesda, MD, 1985.
4. L'Annunziata, M.F., *Handbook of Radioactivity Analysis*, 2nd ed., Academic Press, Amsterdam, 2004.
5. Gilmore, G. and Hemingway, J., *Practical Gamma-Ray Spectrometry*, 1st ed., John Wiley & Sons, New York, 1995.
6. Theodorsson, P., *Measurement of Weak Radioactivity*, 1st ed., World Scientific, Singapore, 1996.
7. Scarpitta, S.C., *Preparation and Validation of Gross Alpha/Beta Samples Used in EML's Quality Assessment Program*, Report EML-592, U.S. Department of Energy, New York, 1997.
8. Burnett, W.C., Wong, R., Clark, S.B., and Crandall, B., Direct counting of soil wafers: An improved total alpha/beta screening analysis. *Radioanal. Nucl. Chem.*, 235, 173, 1998.
9. Valkoic, V., *Radioactivity in the Environment*, 1st ed., Elsevier Science, Amsterdam, 2000.
10. McDowell, W.J. and McDowell, B.L., *Liquid Scintillation Alpha Spectrometry*, 1st ed., CRC Press, Boca Raton, FL, 1994.

11. IAEA, *X-ray and Gamma-Ray Standards for Detector Calibration*; IAEA-TEC-DOC-619, International Atomic Energy Agency, Vienna, 1991.

12. Farouk, M.A. and Souraya, A.M., Ra-226 as a standard source for efficiency calibration of Ge(Li) detector. *Nucl. Instrum. Meth.*, 200, 593, 1982.

13. IAEA, *Measurement of Radionuclides in Food and the Environment: A Guidebook*, Technical Reports Series no. 295, International Atomic Energy Agency, Vienna, 1989.

Stuart Thomson, Mark Reinhard, Mike Colella, and Claudio Tuniz

CONTENTS

10.1 INTRODUCTION

10.1.1 THE NUCLEAR AND RADIOLOGICAL TERRORIST THREAT

In the last 15 years we have seen vast changes in the worldwide political landscape. The end of the Cold War and the subsequent dissolution of the Soviet
Union saw a reshuffling of international alliances and the disintegration of former
political ties. With the end of the Cold War, many envisaged a new world order
and hoped security would be rooted within the United Nations. Clearly, this has
not occurred.

The reawakening of ethnic and religious tensions and the exacerbation of
global socioeconomic issues are causing conflicts in a number of critical regions
of the world. One phenomenon of particular concern is the upsurge in global
terrorist activity. The appalling events of the Tokyo subway attack (1995), Okla-
homa City bombing (1995), September 11 attacks (2001), Bali bombings (2002),
and recent attacks in Madrid, Russia, and Jakarta (2004) exemplify the considerable threat small, well-organized groups can pose to the safety of a civilian
population. Moreover, these events show that terrorism is fast becoming a considerable threat to global security.

While terrorist groups continue to use primarily conventional weapons to
conduct their operations, there is concern that several may be considering the use
of radiological weapons [1,2]. Relevant to this discussion are both nuclear (fissionable) and other radioactive materials, which although disparate in terms of
their potential to cause destruction, are both of increasing concern to the worldwide community.

10.1.2 RADIOACTIVE AND NUCLEAR MATERIALS

Radioactive materials may be either naturally occurring or anthropogenic (man-
made). Naturally occurring radioactive materials (NORMs) include isotopes produced via the uranium series, the actinium series, and the thorium series, and the
low-abundance isotope of potassium, ^{40}K. Besides the NORMs of primordial
origin, there is a very weak (but measurable) concentration of natural radionuclides, such as ^3H, ^{14}C, and ^{10}Be, produced by nuclear reactions of highly
energetic cosmic rays.

Anthropogenic radioactive materials are produced via appropriate nuclear
reactions. Examples include the production of ^{60}Co via neutron capture in a

nuclear reactor and the production of ^{18}F in a medical cyclotron via the (p,n) reaction. Many anthropogenic short-lived isotopes are commonly used in industrial and medical applications.

Nuclear materials form a special subset of radioactive materials. In addition to being radioactive, nuclear materials can undergo nuclear fission. The two most important nuclear materials from the point of view of weapons manufacture, and therefore nuclear safeguard controls, are enriched uranium and plutonium.

10.1.3 CATEGORIZATION OF NUCLEAR AND RADIOLOGICAL MATERIALS

The International Atomic Energy Agency (IAEA) classifies radioactive materials into five separate categories: unirradiated direct use nuclear materials, irradiated direct use nuclear materials, alternative nuclear materials, indirect use nuclear materials, and radioactive sources [3].

Unirradiated direct use nuclear material does not contain substantial quantities of fission products and can be readily used to construct a nuclear weapon or improvised nuclear device (IND) [3]. This is primarily because these materials require little or no further processing. Examples of such materials are highly enriched uranium (HEU), containing the isotope ^{235}U at a concentration greater than 20%, or plutonium containing less than 7% ^{240}Pu [3]. Irradiated direct use nuclear materials contain substantial quantities of fission products and require further processing to produce materials capable of being used to fabricate a nuclear device. Irradiated direct use nuclear materials can be found in spent reactor fuels [3].

Alternative nuclear materials include radionuclides such as ^{241}Am and ^{237}Np, which are fissionable and may have the potential to be used in a nuclear device [3]. Indirect use materials are those that require significant processing to enable them to be used in a nuclear weapon. Examples of indirect use materials include uranium containing ^{235}U in quantities less than 20% and plutonium containing ^{238}Pu in quantities greater than 80% [3]. The processing of such material is technically challenging and requires specific facilities and expertise. Hence indirect use nuclear materials pose less of a threat than direct use materials.

Radioactive sources is the classification given to nonfissionable radioactive materials. These sources are used in industry, medicine, agriculture, research and education. The IAEA classifies radioactive sources based on the risk they pose to health [4]. Table 10.1 details the nomenclature typically used to categorize nuclear and radioactive materials. There is no separate international classification system to categorize materials according to the potential for malevolent use, however, parameters to consider include those based on the radiological hazards, in addition to issues related to portability, dispersability, and the potential for theft. Table 10.2 details the results of a Monterey Institute of International Studies report commissioned to determine the radioactive materials that pose the greatest risk to public health and safety, focusing on the potential consequences of their malevolent use [5]. More detailed guidance on the categorization of nuclear material is available from the IAEA [3,4].

TABLE 10.1

The Categorization of Nuclear and Other Radioactive Materials: Examples of Materials and Their Application (Adapted from IAEA [28])

Category	Type of Material	Examples of Radioactive Isotopes
Unirradiated direct use nuclear material	Highly enriched uranium (HEU)	>20% ^{235}U
	Plutonium and mixed uranium/plutonium oxides (MOX) ^{233}U	<80% ^{238}Pu
Irradiated direct use nuclear material	Irradiated nuclear fuel material	In irradiated nuclear fuel
Indirect use nuclear material	Depleted uranium (DU)	<0.7% ^{235}U
	Natural uranium (NU)	0.7% ^{235}U
	Low enriched uranium (LEU)	>0.7% ^{235}U and <20% ^{235}U
	Plutonium (^{238}Pu)	>80% ^{238}Pu
Radioactive sources	Thermoelectric generators	^{238}Pu and ^{90}Sr
Category 1 (most dangerous)	Irradiators/sterilizers	^{60}Co and ^{137}Cs
	Teletherapy sources	^{60}Co and ^{137}Cs
Radioactive sources	Industrial γ radiography	^{192}Ir
Category 2	High/medium dose rate brachytherapy	^{103}Pd, ^{60}Co, ^{137}Cs, and ^{125}I
Radioactive sources	Fixed industrial gauges	^{60}Co, ^{137}Cs, ^{241}Am
Category 3	Well logging gauges	^{241}Am, ^{137}Cs, and ^{252}Cf
Radioactive sources	Thickness/fill level gauges	^{241}Am
Category 4	Portable gauges (e.g., moisture, density)	^{137}Cs and ^{60}Co
Radioactive sources	Medical diagnostic sources	^{131}I
Category 5 (least dangerous)	Fire detectors	^{241}Am, ^{238}Pu

10.1.4 RADIOLOGICAL SCENARIOS

In recent publications, four mechanisms by which terrorists can exploit current nuclear and radioactive stockpiles and obtain suitable weapons have been discussed [1,6]. The mechanisms are

- The theft and detonation of an existing nuclear weapon.
- The theft or purchase of fissile material for the purpose of manufacturing and detonating an IND.
- Attacks on nuclear facilities leading to widespread release of radioactive material.
- The illegal acquisition of radioactive materials for the manufacture of either a radiological dispersal device (RDD) or a radiation emission device (RED).

TABLE 10.2
Radioactive Sources of Greatest Concern (Adapted from Ferguson et al. [5])

Isotope	Common Use	Form	Half-Life	Emissions
^{137}Cs	Teletherapy, blood irradiations, and sterilization facilities	Solid, chloride powder	30.1 yr	β and γ radiation
^{60}Co	Teletherapy, industrial radiography, and sterilization facilities	Solid, metal	5.3 yr	β and γ radiation
^{192}Ir	Industrial radiography and low dose brachytherapy	Solid, metal	74 days	β and γ radiation
^{226}Ra	Low dose brachytherapy	Solid, metal	1600 yr	α and γ radiation
^{90}Sr	Thermoelectric generators	Solid, oxide powder	28.8 yr	β radiation
^{241}Am	Well logging, thickness, moisture and conveyor gauges	Solid, oxide powder	433 yr	α radiation
^{238}Pu	Heat sources for pacemakers and research sources	Solid, oxide powder	88 yr	α radiation

The first two scenarios relate to the detonation of a nuclear device, while the latter scenarios relate to the use of radioactive materials to impart a radiation dose to a civilian population and contaminate an area and its inhabitants with radioactive material.

The detonation of a nuclear warhead or an IND within a city would result in a significant loss of life, loss of buildings and infrastructure, and would have an enormous environmental and economic impact. Civilians who survive the blast would endure both short- and long-term health effects due to radiation exposure [1]. Although this scenario is the most devastating, it is considered the most unlikely due to the high security most states use to guard their nuclear stockpiles [1].

The technical requirements in manufacturing a nuclear device are significant and require considerable infrastructure, expertise, and financial resources. While some commentators do not see these hurdles as insurmountable to terrorists, it is generally accepted that the most likely method by which terrorists could obtain nuclear material and technical information would be via existing state-owned facilities [1]. For this reason, the proliferation of nuclear materials, particularly in the last 15 years, has been a great concern to the international community, as it may increase the probability of such technology falling into the wrong hands [7,8].

An attack on a nuclear facility is a means by which terrorists could expose the public to radiation and cause contamination of the surrounding area. However, all states require strict security for such facilities, particularly larger establishments such as nuclear power plants. The large structural mass surrounding a reactor core would facilitate the need for a large catastrophic event to cause a reactor core breach. With this in mind, it would be extremely difficult for terrorists to achieve such a feat. Nonetheless, some of the latest reactor construction techniques are incorporating extra security measures to further limit the possibility of a successful terrorist attack.

The final terrorist scenario listed involves the use of an RDD or RED. This scenario is deemed the most probable form of terrorist attack. This is because many radionuclides are widely used in medicine, industry, and science and are accessible to criminals and terrorists [9]. An RDD requires radioactive material that is capable of dispersal into the surrounding environment. The resulting contamination would present a potential health hazard and would require significant decontamination to be undertaken. An RED works primarily by stealth and utilizes a radioactive source to expose potential victims to radiation. A source placed in a location where it can impart a dose to a target may go undetected for long periods. While the use of either an RDD or RED is considered the most plausible terrorist act, the consensus is that such acts would generally result in a small number of immediate deaths [9]. The benefit to terrorists using such a device is the disruption it is likely to cause. A device used in a city is likely to result in hysteria from the public, based on the fear that they may have been exposed to radiation [1]. In the case of an RDD, the consequent contamination from such a device would take considerable time to clean up, resulting in long-term evacuation of the area, which is likely to have significant economic and social impacts [1,9].

Protecting and accounting for both nuclear and other radioactive materials is a major concern of the international community and there have been significant efforts to modernize physical protection and accounting systems throughout the world [9]. Individual states and international organizations have also been providing both technical and financial support to less wealthy nations. One example is the recent commitment of the G8 group of nations to provide US$20 billion over 10 years to help former Soviet Union states manage and secure their radioactive materials [6]. However, the problem of securing radioactive materials is a worldwide dilemma. In the past, many security measures applied to nonfissionable radioactive sources aimed to prevent accidental access or petty theft of the sources [10]. Any thought of terrorists using radionuclides as weapons were not persuasive enough to enforce a move to more regulated systems. While many states are now acting to address this issue, there still exist many thousands of unaccounted for sources worldwide. These sources are termed "orphaned sources," an expression used by the IAEA to denote radioactive sources that are outside official regulatory control, which may have been lost, discarded, or stolen [4]. Therefore orphaned sources represent potential weapons for terrorists.

10.1.5 THE ILLICIT TRAFFICKING OF RADIOACTIVE MATERIALS

Since 1993 there have been 540 confirmed cases (Table 10.3) of illicit trafficking of nuclear and radioactive materials registered on the IAEA's illicit trafficking database [11]. The majority of the confirmed incidents involved some form of criminal intent. This figure most probably represents a conservative estimate of the true problem, and there are growing concerns that more organized and sophisticated

TABLE 10.3
Confirmed Incidents Involving Illicit Trafficking
of Nuclear Materials and Radioactive Sources
By Participating Member States

Illicitly Trafficked Material	Confirmed Incidents (1993 to 2003)
Nuclear material	182
Other radioactive material	300
Nuclear and other radioactive material	23
Radioactively contaminated material	30
Other	5

trafficking of radioactive materials may be occurring undetected [12]. These figures illustrate the need for comprehensive programs worldwide to both secure existing sources and to recover orphaned sources.

10.1.6 THE ROLE OF SCIENTIFIC PRACTITIONERS

The need to develop strategic programs aimed at preventing, recovering, and responding to terrorist acts involving nuclear and other radiological materials requires a high level of involvement from the scientific community. The utilization of existing technology and the development of improved methods of detection and characterization are required to ensure the security of all radioactive materials.

For the purposes of this discussion, the primary focus will be on some of the scientific methods and procedures currently used to track illicit radioactive materials. Of particular relevance are the fields of radiation detection and analytical techniques used for nuclear and radiological forensic science.

10.2 RADIATION DETECTION STRATEGIES

10.2.1 INTRODUCTION

The use of radiation detectors to identify the presence of radioactive materials is essential to any program aimed at minimizing the potential threat that such materials may pose. In recent years there has been significant interest in the development of new radiation detector strategies for uncovering radioactive materials. These strategies range from the development of "simple to use" radiation detection devices for emergency responders to the development of new detector systems that give detailed information on relevant radionuclides and their quantities.

In developing these new capabilities, the scientific community has become more closely involved with agencies such as law enforcement, fire, medical, and customs [13–15]. Clearly the operational needs of each agency involve the use of different instrumentation and strategies, requiring both instrument companies and scientists to become more conscious of the challenges that each of these agencies face. Another requirement is the need for distributing information about new detector technologies to user groups in a form that is easily interpreted and not overwhelmingly technical.

The global need for solutions in this area also necessitates the sharing of any new capabilities or techniques between states. To this end, the IAEA has supported international technical initiatives to explore suitable technologies and novel solutions for user groups. (The relevant programs include the coordinated research project (CRP) "Improvement of Technical Measures to Detect and Respond to Illicit Trafficking of Nuclear and Other Radioactive Materials" and the "Illicit Trafficking Radiation Detection Assessment Program" (ITRAP), and the International Technical Working Group's (ITWG) Nuclear Forensic Laboratories (INFL) program. These programs have enabled cooperative research to be undertaken, allowing the pooling of available knowledge and resources.

Much of the focus of recent detector research has been on the development and implementation of instrumentation for international border monitoring. Examples include [13] fixed, automated portal monitors; personal radiation detectors (PRDs); handheld /neutron detectors; and multipurpose handheld radioisotope identifiers. Much of today's detection equipment is based on well-established technology developed to meet the needs of the scientific and industrial communities. Evidently the ability to use existing "off-the-shelf" technology is attractive, as it has enabled the relatively quick distribution of hardware in response to the heightened security threats following the terrorist attacks of recent years. Two drawbacks to this approach are evident. The first is that many of the off-the-shelf instruments are not optimized to address the needs of border monitoring agencies. Second, a rush to deploy existing radiation detection instruments has failed to address more strategic questions concerning the detection of radioactive materials at border control points. Part of the solution to providing the best instrumentation and detector strategies is to design equipment to suit the required applications of user agencies.

10.2.2 RADIONUCLIDES OF INTEREST TO BORDER MONITORING

Of the thousands of radionuclides associated with NORMs or anthropogenic production, only a few are liable to be encountered by border monitoring staff. These materials include isotopes produced in significant quantities for designated applications in medicine or industry, and NORMs that are prevalent in many substances commonly traded (e.g., ceramics, stoneware, and fertilizers).

The radionuclides of greatest interest, as determined by various agencies associated with the IAEA [13], are listed below:

- Medical radionuclides: ^{18}F, ^{32}P, ^{51}Cr, ^{67}Ga, ^{90}Y, ^{99}Mo, ^{99m}Tc, ^{111}In, ^{123}I, ^{125}I, ^{131}I, ^{133}Xe, ^{153}Sm, ^{198}Au, and ^{201}Tl.
- Industrial or scientific radionuclides: ^{22}Na, ^{57}Co, ^{60}Co, ^{75}Se, ^{90}Sr, ^{133}Ba, ^{137}Cs, ^{152}Eu, ^{192}Ir, ^{198}Au, ^{207}Bi, ^{226}Ra, ^{238}Pu, and ^{241}Am.

- NORMs: ^{40}K, ^{226}Ra, ^{232}Th, and ^{238}U.
- Nuclear materials: ^{233}U, ^{235}U, ^{237}Np, and ^{239}Pu.

Neutron sources based on mixed radionuclides may also be encountered due to the widespread use of neutron emitters in mining and other underground gauging applications. These include mixed radionuclide neutron sources like ^{241}AmBe and ^{238}PuBe, in which the ^{241}Am and ^{238}Pu produce α particles that interact with beryllium via a (α,n) reaction to form neutrons.

Visual identification is not a reliable means of identifying the presence of radioactive material. The most suitable method for measurement of emitted radiation is the use of dedicated radiation detection instrumentation employed in an appropriate manner. The majority of the radionuclides listed above have γ-ray emissions with energies between 50 keV and 3 MeV, which are measurable by most γ-ray spectroscopy instruments (notable exceptions are the pure β emitters such as ^{32}P, ^{90}Sr, and ^{90}Y). The measurement of γ-ray emissions relies on the transmission of photons through any packaging or shielding material (i.e., lead) placed around the radioactive material. Therefore the ability to detect the material depends on the type and quantity of shielding material surrounding the radioactive material, the type of radionuclides present, and the activity of the source.

10.2.3 RADIATION DETECTION AT BORDER CONTROL POINTS

Border control points are strategic positions along regulatory control boundaries where customs agents can potentially monitor the movements of all people, transport vehicles, and goods through a defined transport corridor. Such points are therefore ideal for monitoring and controlling the movement of radioactive materials.

The techniques and strategies aimed at detecting the presence of radioactive materials in this context differ considerably from those found in the laboratory. Apart from the obvious requirement that the inspection procedures must reliably detect the presence of illicit radioactive materials, there are additional requirements, including

- The inspection system should not unnecessarily impede or disrupt the flow of general traffic.
- The analysis is performed in real time in order to enable customs and law enforcement officers to act rapidly.
- There should be the ability to deal with the wide variety of traffic that may pass through the corridor.

In establishing a system that satisfies this somewhat competing set of criteria, a "staged" or "layered" approach is used. The first stage will typically employ a system for the gross detection of radioactive material. This would consist of an autonomously operated radiation detector system fixed in position along the transport corridor. All traffic passes by the fixed monitor, thereby allowing non-invasive testing for radioactive material. The detector would monitor changes in the ambient radiation level from that attributed to the local background. The system would alarm when levels exceeded a set threshold. An alarm would then initiate a personnel response that would confirm the alarm state. If confirmed, stage two would commence.

The second stage of the detection strategy is to assess the radiological hazards and potential health risks to which an operator may be exposed and then locate the radioactive material. The assessment of radiological hazards is discussed extensively in a number of publications such as those prepared by the International Commission on Radiological Protection (ICRP) [16], the International Commission on Radiological Units and Measurements (ICRU) [17], and the U.S.-based National Commission on Radiation Protection (NCRP) [18]. Locating the radioactive materials is the domain of handheld instrumentation. By scanning the instrument over the vehicle, cargo, or person, the location of the radiation can be determined. Once this has been performed, stage three would commence.

The purpose of stage three is to identity the isotopes that are present in the sample. By measuring the γ-ray spectrum of the suspect sample and comparing it to a library of radionuclide spectra, the identity of the sample can be determined. Border monitoring staff can then determine if the source of the radiation is an innocent event, such as the sanctioned movement of an industrial radiography source, an inadvertent event, such as the presence of residual radioactivity within an individual having recently undergone a medical treatment with a radiopharmaceutical agent, or an illicit event, such as the intentional smuggling of radioactive material.

At present, no single instrument is able to perform all the measurements required for stages one to three. Therefore, instrument selection is crucial to implementing an effective detection strategy within each stage.

10.2.3.1 Gamma Ray Detectors

Advice for the selection and use of detector instrumentation, specifically for border monitoring applications, is detailed in a recent IAEA publication jointly sponsored by the World Customs Organization (WCO), European Police Office (Europol), and International Criminal Police Organization (Interpol) [13]. Similar information regarding detector instrumentation for measuring nuclear materials is also available from the IAEA [19].

The two most important properties of γ radiation detection instrumentation are the "detection efficiency" and the "energy resolution." The detection efficiency relates to the sensitivity of the instrument at detecting radiation emitted by a source, while the energy resolution relates to the ability of the detector to accurately measure the energy of the detected radiation. The border control setting also introduces operational considerations that are not relevant in the industrial or scientific context. These additional considerations include factors such as the ease of use, as perceived by the nonexpert user, and instrument reliability criteria such as ruggedness and the ability to operate in adverse environmental conditions.

Detection efficiency relates to the relative sensitivity of the instrument to respond to a particular intensity of radiation. This is an inherent property of the detector that depends on the γ-ray absorbing properties of the material from which the detector is manufactured, as well as the size or volume of the active region of the detector.

The ability of the detector to absorb γ rays per unit volume increases with the atomic number of the detector material's constituent atoms and the density of the resultant detector material. Solid-state materials such as sodium iodide (NaI) are associated with high detection efficiencies due to the relatively high average atomic numbers of sodium and iodine, that is, 32 ($Z_{Na} = 11$, $Z_I = 53$), and the fact that the material is a dense solid. A lower detection efficiency can be expected in other solid-state detectors, such as those based on silicon, due to the lower atomic number of silicon by comparison ($Z_{Si} = 14$). All gaseous-type detectors suffer from low detection efficiency due to the low density of atoms in the gaseous state.

By increasing the volume of the detector, the overall ability to absorb radiation and thereby contribute to a measurable signal will increase. This can be achieved through the use of large-volume detectors or through the use of a bank of multiple detectors operated in parallel. In addition to the inherent properties of a particular type of detector, the overall sensitivity of the system will also be subject to the operational conditions imposed by the monitoring facility. This will include the distance of separation between the radioactive material and the detector, the length of time of the measurement, and, in the case of a moving item, the speed of the item relative to the detector.

In general, the intensity of radiation at the surface of a detector is inversely proportional to the square of the distance of separation between the material and the detector (assuming the radioactive source is a point source). A doubling of the distance of separation will result in a fourfold decrease in the intensity of radiation at the detector. For this reason, it is important to minimize this distance of separation to achieve the greatest possible signal. Signal intensity will also increase with increasing measurement time. Hence there is a trade-off between the time required for a measurement and the time deemed acceptable in terms of processing objects through a border crossing.

Energy resolution is a measure of a detector's ability to resolve γ rays of different energy. Energy resolution is only relevant to spectroscopic measurements and is therefore only important for identifying a radioisotope. Detectors with the highest energy resolution are those based on elemental semiconductor materials such as high-purity germanium (HPGe) or silicon. However, silicon has a relatively low atomic number and is not suited to spectroscopic measurements of γ rays with energies above 100 keV. Therefore, it is not a suitable material for border monitoring applications.

The high energy resolution of HPGe makes it the detector of choice for γ spectroscopy. An unfortunate limitation of HPGe is the requirement that the detector must operate at low temperatures. This is necessitated by the requirement to reduce thermally generated noise, which at room temperature results in an unacceptably low signal:noise ratio. Cooling of the detector is achieved in the laboratory using liquid nitrogen or electronic cooling devices. In the field, the use of liquid nitrogen is restricted and in many cases not feasible. Recently, however, HPGe-based detectors, cooled via electrically operated Stirling cooling cycles, have become commercially available, albeit at significant financial cost.

Other detectors with moderate to good energy resolution include those based on the compound semiconductors cadmium telluride (CdTe) and cadmium zinc telluride (CdZnTe). Despite the relatively high average atomic number of the constituent atoms and the existence of the material in a solid state, such detectors suffer from relatively low detection efficiency due to technological limitations in the production of detector crystals with volumes greater than 1 cm^3.

The mainstay of handheld room temperature operable γ-ray spectroscopy instruments is the thallium doped sodium iodide scintillation detector, NaI(Tl). Its low energy resolution makes this detector unsuitable for many of the demands of border monitoring. However, subject to the limitations of the other detector types discussed above, it is often the detector of choice for γ-ray spectroscopy in a border monitoring context.

Research efforts directed toward the realization of new detector materials with energy resolutions superior to that of NaI(Tl), but with similar operating characteristics, are currently under way. Some successes have been achieved in lanthanum halide-based scintillator materials such as $LaCl_3$ and $LaBr_3$ [20,21].

10.2.3.2 Stage One: Fixed Portal Monitors

Fixed portal monitors are designed to screen vehicles, cargo, or people for the presence of radioactive material as part of the first stage of any detection strategy. This type of system will typically consist of an array of detectors located in close proximity to the passing traffic, usually within vertical pillars or just below the transport surface. To maximize the ability of the system to detect the presence of radioactive materials, the detectors employed must have high detection efficiency. Energy resolution is not important because this stage of detection is concerned simply with detecting the presence of radioactive material.

Portal monitors are typically produced using inorganic or organic scintillators. Other systems use large-volume halogen-quenched Geiger-Mueller tubes. The associated software of portal monitor systems usually includes functions such as real-time data collection and analysis, data logging for historical analysis, alarm setting, signal communication, and the ability to integrate with other networked security systems.

A major problem encountered with portal monitors is the prevalence of false alarms caused by spikes in the local background radiation or due to the passing of innocuous transports, such as those containing NORMs. Innocuous alarms can be overcome by setting the alarm threshold to a suitable value. However, due to the lack of any spectroscopic data, differentiating between innocuous radioactive materials and those due to inadvertent or malevolent activities is more difficult.

In general, all alarms triggered by the presence of radiation materials need to be investigated further using stage two and stage three strategies.

10.2.3.3 Stage Two: Locating and Isolating the Source of Radioactivity

Following the detection of radioactive material, identification of its exact location becomes important. This is best performed using a handheld instrument operating in either a count rate mode or in a dose rate mode. The advantage of the dose rate mode is the ability to monitor the radiological hazard posed by the radioactive material during the search. The disadvantage of this approach is a reduced instrument response time associated with the long signal integration time required to perform a dose measurement. This may reduce the speed at which the radioactive material is localized.

Handheld search instruments generally possess a wide response range, from background to high radiation levels. A response to low levels of radiation is needed in order to detect small or shielded sources. A response to high levels of radiation is required in order to identify the presence of a large radiological hazard. The response readout of handheld survey instruments is usually in the form of either an analog or digital display. Modern dose rate meters are also equipped with alarms, which can be set at a predetermined dose rate. This alarm is typically set to advise the user of unsafe radiation levels.

10.2.3.4 Stage Three: Isotopic Analysis

The existence of a unique signature for each radionuclide that emits γ-rays allows the measurement of this signature to be used as a means of assaying the isotopic composition of any detected radioactive material. The working basis of all γ-ray spectrometers is collection of the energy deposited by a single γ-ray photon in the active volume of the detector and the conversion of this energy into a voltage pulse, the amplitude of which is proportional to the initial energy of the γ ray. By sorting the voltage pulses according to the amplitude, a spectrum of different γ-ray energy intensities can be displayed. Comparison of the spectrum against reference libraries enables identification of the radionuclides.

A variety of different types of γ-ray detectors are available. This includes those based on scintillator materials, such as thallium-activated sodium iodide, as discussed previously, or those based on semiconductor materials such as HPGe and CdZnTe. Packaging of these detectors into handheld analyzers, complete with the ability to display the isotopic composition of an interrogated item in real time, is highly desired by border control officers. Most handheld analyzers are based on either NaI or CdZnTe.

Instruments with high resolution, typical of HPGe, are most ideally suited to this application. The Stirling engine-cooled HPGe detectors, which have recently become available, offer the desired high energy resolution at the expense of being heavy and somewhat bulky in comparison to the other isotopic analyzers.

10.2.4 MASKING OF ILLICIT MATERIALS

Knowledge of the underlying deficiencies of radiation detection instruments and the inherent difficulties of γ-ray spectrometry can be exploited to circumvent the detection of nuclear and other radioactive materials. The intentional use of lead or dense materials to shield the emissions of radiation from illicit radioactive materials is the simplest approach to masking. The use of single- or dual-energy x-ray machines to detect the presence of shielding materials in combination with radiation monitoring systems is an effective way of circumventing this type of strategy. Of greater concern is the potential use of legal radioisotope shipments, such as radiopharmaceuticals, to mask the presence of illicit nuclear or other radioactive materials. The principle behind masking is to prevent or confuse the handheld isotope analyzers from obtaining the signatures required to unambiguously identify the radionuclides of concern.

A number of research programs are currently studying methods to improve the performance of detector systems or to formulate better methodologies to combat potential masking strategies (e.g., the IAEA's CRP "Improvement of Technical Measures to Detect and Respond to Illicit Trafficking of Nuclear and Other Radioactive Materials"). Such programs administered by the IAEA evaluate the performance of commercially available detector systems under border control conditions. Some of the areas under examination include new algorithms and software techniques to improve the identification of radionuclide γ-ray signatures, the investigations of different scenarios whereby nuclear materials or other radioactive materials can be masked with legitimate γ emitters, and investigations to verify legal shipments based on measurement attributes in standardized testing arrangements. The latter program also has applications in the verification of radioisotope quantities, thus enabling customs agents to authenticate the quantities of radionuclides being transported.

10.2.5 OTHER TYPES OF DETECTORS

10.2.5.1 Neutron Detectors

The lack of any significant neutron-emitting NORMs and limited use of neutron-emitting radionuclides for medical or industrial purposes makes neutron detection a reliable indicator of the presence of nuclear materials. Neutrons are detected through the measurement of ionizing nuclear reaction products, such as protons and α particles, produced when the neutron interacts with agents such as boron trifluoride (BF_3) gas or ^{3}He gas. Neutron coincidence counting is the technique generally used in the nondestructive assay of bulk quantities of nuclear materials, and in particular of plutonium.

10.2.5.2 Radiation Pagers

Pager and pocket γ and γ/neutron monitors are small, lightweight radiation detectors that can be worn on the person of customs officers or border monitoring staff. The units constantly measure the local background radiation level surrounding the instrument and can provide an alarm state when the radiation level exceeds a set threshold. Some units may also include nonvolatile memory, which allows storage of a history of the unit's operation. Access to these data are usually obtained by downloading to a computer.

The detection efficiency of these instruments is generally much less than that of large-volume portal monitors. For this reason, such instruments are not considered as a replacement for the fixed portal monitors described above in "Stage One" of the detection strategy. However, the ability to equip roaming officers with such instruments may provide some additional benefit to border control situations where narrow corridors with fixed portal monitors cannot be established.

In summary, the place of pagers or pocket monitors within the overall framework of detection of illicitly trafficked nuclear or other radioactive materials is dependent on individual user agency operational strategies. In addition to the perceivable benefits the units provide by enabling real-time radiation monitoring, the units may also provide additional coverage in the field to detect illicitly trafficked radioactive material.

10.3 NUCLEAR AND RADIOLOGICAL FORENSICS

10.3.1 INTRODUCTION

The discovery of radioactive material, whether due to malevolent or inadvertent actions, will ultimately result in the initiation of a preplanned emergency response. Strategies to respond to such events should involve representation by experts from emergency services, scene investigators, and technical and scientific experts [14]. Following this initial action, scene investigators and scientific experts begin the identification, documentation, and collection of forensic samples.

The role of the nuclear forensic scientist is to analyze nuclear or other radioactive material for clues that may provide information about a material and its origin. Characteristics that may be of use include physical characteristics such as sample morphology, elemental composition, isotopic composition, trace elements, and the presence of organic solvents.

The use of elemental analysis techniques enables the elemental composition of a sample to be determined. This can be used as a fingerprint, enabling direct comparisons with other samples to be made. The isotopic abundance of the material may yield information on possible enrichment processes or irradiation processes within a nuclear reactor. Isotopic techniques can also yield parent/daughter ratios that provide information on the age of a material, that is, the time that has elapsed since the sample was first purified [22]. By using the oxygen isotope ratio technique, $^{18}O/^{16}O$ (^{18}O), the geographical origin of a sample can sometimes be established. This method has been demonstrated in principle for uranium oxides [23].

While the information obtained by the use of these techniques is indeed valuable, it alone does not yield information on the origin of the material. The process of attribution requires not only experimental data, but also information specific to individual manufacturing facilities. Therefore, the processing methods used will contribute to the creation of products with unique chemical and physical signatures that may assist the nuclear forensic scientist [24]. The rigorous characterization that is required to certify radioactive materials during processing means that extensive datasets exist within each facility. Recording this information within specific forensic databases is a strategy being pursued by organizations such as the IAEA and the Institute of Transuranium Elements (ITU). Other means of identifying radioactive material is via the use of intelligence or regulatory databases. Examples of these include the IAEA's Illicit Trafficking Database (ITDB) [11] and various registers maintained by individual national regulatory authorities. Information from these sources, particularly that relating to missing or stolen radioactive materials, may provide useful information for the purposes of attribution.

10.3.2 AT THE SCENE

10.3.2.1 The Investigation Team

The presence of radiological material at a scene dictates the desire for a number of specialists to be available during the investigation. The skill set required includes health physicists to examine the scene for health and safety hazards, bomb disposal experts to check and disable trigger devices, law enforcement forensic experts to control sample collection and advise on sample handling, storage, and transport, and nuclear forensic specialists to advise on radiological evidence.

The job of the health physicist is to report on the levels of radioactivity that exist within the site and help advise on decisions relating to protective measures (e.g., protective clothing, breathing apparatuses, and dosimetry) that may need to be taken by persons entering the site. The protective measures that need to be taken will depend on factors such as the type of radiation (α, β, γ, and neutron), the activity of the source, whether the radioactive material is sealed or open to the environment, and the chemical and physical properties of the material. The use of nondestructive analysis techniques such as handheld γ spectroscopy or neutron counting should enable identification of the material. This information can then be used to make an assessment on the possible health risks associated with workers entering the site. The protection measures provided should be consistent with national guidelines or, if these are not sufficient, consistent with IAEA guidelines [25,26].

Once these initial actions have been taken, bomb disposal experts may then enter the site to check for and disable any trigger devices that may be present. Techniques such as portable x-ray imaging and ion mobility may be used to identify the composite structure of a sample and analyze for the presence of explosives, respectively. Once the site is deemed safe, the task of evidence identification, documentation, and collection can begin.

10.3.2.2 Sample Collection

The collection of radiological material should be conducted in accordance with standard methods recommended by national bodies and those used by national law enforcement experts. The regimes used may differ from country to country based on forensic doctrine and national law. Therefore, in all cases the collection, documentation, and storage of the materials should be consistent with national chain-of-custody procedures [27].

The procedures for locating and documenting radiological evidence are similar to those used for traditional forensics [2]. The use of a grid system, photographic documentation, and precise drawings or mapping with referenced coordinates (e.g., the global positioning system [GPS]) showing the location of any evidence (radioactive or traditional) is essential. It is advisable that a radiological survey, referenced to a grid system or map is used to determine the extent of the contamination and the establishment of cordon and control areas [14]. The use of radiation detection equipment, as described earlier, is vital for locating and identifying the radioactive isotopes.

The objective of the crime scene expert is to collect evidence for analysis that may provide clues to the origin of the material. Hence the radioactive material and related samples, such as source containers with unique identifiers, are both potential indicators as to the origin of radioactive material. If the radioactive sample is contained within a vessel or lead-shielded container, the job of sample collection is simplified. For this scenario, the material should be collected and secured with care so as not to destroy any potential traditional forensic evidence (e.g., fingerprints, fibers, biological evidence, etc.). In situations where the radioactive material is widely dispersed, the task of collection is more difficult. If possible, it is recommended that radioactive samples be extricated from nonradioactive material (i.e., contaminants). However, this may not always be easily achieved [28]. The handling of traditional evidence from this scenario is also problematic due to the presence of radioactive material. In all cases, the collection of either radioactive or traditional samples should be conducted, if possible, in a manner that will not destroy or modify the other.

International organizations, such as the IAEA and the ITWG's INFL program, are working to provide advice and support to the international community on issues pertaining to the collection of radiological samples. Details can be found in a number of publications [29,30]. Moreover, both the IAEA and INFL are currently fine tuning procedures for the sampling of seized materials, the shipping of samples, and the analysis and evaluation of experimental results.

10.3.2.3 Sample Storage and Transportation

Once the collection of samples is completed, the task of temporary storage and transportation of the items to a suitable laboratory will need to be considered. Temporary storage of samples may be required for two main reasons. First, there may be a requirement to analyze samples in the field to enable the identification of the radionuclides present, to address occupational health and safety issues, and to ensure compliance with national laws and guidelines. Second, it may be necessary to store items temporarily while the required approvals for transporting the samples to alternative locations are sought. In either case, a temporary storage facility must be secure and meet the mandatory safety requirements needed to handle the level of radioactivity present within the samples. Furthermore, the facility must have the required licensing or permits needed to store radioactive materials and must meet the chain-of-custody requirements of national law enforcement agencies.

The transportation of the samples to appropriate laboratories will require the use of suitable packaging procedures to ensure there is no cross contamination of samples and that national requirements regarding the safe and secure transportation of radioactive materials are satisfied [31,32].

10.3.3 THE NUCLEAR FORENSICS LABORATORY

10.3.3.1 Introduction

Prior to performing analyses there is a need for the facilities conducting nuclear forensic analysis to be appropriately licensed to handle radioactive materials, to have appropriate document control and chain-of-custody procedures, to have appropriate quality assurance programs in place, and to have the required infrastructure, expertise, and facilities to undertake the required analyses [19,27,28,33]. Assuming these nontrivial issues have been resolved, the next step is to perform a number of analyses on the samples.

The role of the nuclear forensic scientist is to apply a number of appropriate techniques to elucidate information that may provide clues about the material. As with traditional forensics, there exist no steadfast procedures. The techniques used depend on the physical and chemical properties of the samples. Figure 10.1 details, in flow chart form, the main stages of identification of materials of unknown origin, which is based on procedures outlined in [34].

A number of publications have discussed at length the expertise and facilities a laboratory must possess in order to conduct nuclear forensics [2,19,28]. Of particular importance are mass spectrometry measurements such as inductively coupled plasma mass spectrometry (ICP-MS), secondary ion mass spectrometry (SIMS), accelerator mass spectrometry (AMS), and thermal ionization mass spectrometry (TIMS), because these techniques can provide isotopic information [7,35–37]. Radiometric techniques such as high-resolution γ spectroscopy (HRGS) also play an important role and are invaluable in identifying radioactive materials and the corresponding isotopes.

Ultimately, nondestructive analyses are preferred to those that modify or destroy potential evidence. Moreover, analysis techniques may be precluded from use if the quantity of sample required for the analysis would result in the destruction of a high proportion of a sample. Therefore, law enforcement officers must decide whether the benefits of a technique are worth the loss or partial loss of a

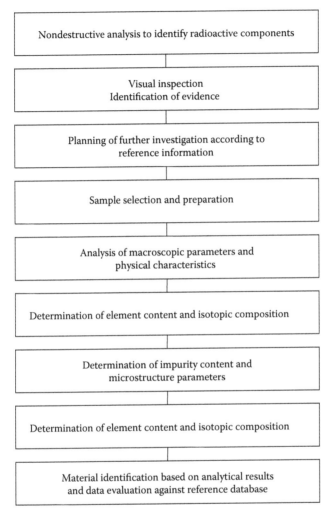

FIGURE 10.1 Flow chart for the analysis of nuclear and radioactive forensic samples adapted from [34].

sample. National laws that govern the use and preservation of evidence will need to be considered prior to any analysis being undertaken.

A number of useful characterization techniques are listed in Table 10.4 and classified with respect to the capability of providing imaging, bulk, and microanalytical data. A comprehensive list of techniques and their capabilities is outlined in Table 10.5. Radiation detection will not be revisited in this section, as most of the relevant issues have already been discussed. Guidance in the selection and use of these techniques does exist in both the general literature and from international workshops [2,7,19,23,28]. Clearly an exhaustive list and description of

TABLE 10.4
A List of Useful Instrumentation Likely to Be Used in a Nuclear Forensic Laboratory

Analysis Type	Measurements	Suitable Techniques
Imaging	Photography	Conventional or digital photography
	Radiography	X-ray imaging
	Microscopy	Optical and electron microscopy
Bulk analysis	Macroscopic characterization*	See note
	Elemental analysis	TIMS, XRF, ICP-MS, PIXE
	Trace elemental analysis (inorganic)	ICP-MS, AMS, NAA, PIXE
	Organic analysis	GC-MS, CHNS analyzer, vibrational spectroscopy, NMR
	Isotopic analysis	HRGS, ICP-MS, SIMS, AMS
	Crystal structure	XRD and ED
	Bulk environmental sampling	AMS, TIMS, ICP-MS, α, β, γ spectrometry
	Particle environmental sampling	SIMS, fission track TIMS, SEM, EDX/WDX
Microanalysis (or particle analysis)	Electron microscopy	SEM, TEM
	Elemental analysis	WDX, EDX, SIMS
	Particle analysis	SIMS, TIMS, fission track, SEM, EDX/WDX

* Macroscopic characterization includes weight, density, radiography, viscosity, surface area, particle size, and surface roughness measurements.

Note: AMS, accelerator mass spectrometry; CHNS, carbon-hydrogen-nitrogen-sulfur; ED, electron diffraction; EDX, energy dispersive x-ray; GC-MS, gas chromatography mass spectrometry; HRGS, high-resolution γ spectroscopy; ICP-MS, inductively coupled plasma mass spectrometry; NAA, neutron activation analysis; NMR, nuclear magnetic resonance; SEM, scanning electron microscopy; SIMS, secondary ion mass spectrometry; TIMS, thermal ionization mass spectrometry; WDX, wavelength dispersive x-ray; XRD, x-ray diffraction; XRF, x-ray fluorescence.

these techniques is beyond the scope of this discussion; however, a number of the most relevant techniques are listed and discussed.

10.3.3.2 Imaging Techniques

The optical characteristics of a sample may provide evidence that identifies a material and its origin. Some containers used for radionuclides have distinctive shapes or structures, such as pigtails used for x-ray imaging. Furthermore, many of these containers have markings that are descriptive of a sample's point of origin. The visual properties of the radioisotope may be indicative of its chemical form or oxidation state. The use of optical microscopy can reveal information about a sample such as homogeneity or the presence of microscopic impurities. It follows that documenting visual characteristics is one method of sample identification and this can be done by the use of photographic equipment.

TABLE 10.5
Common Nuclear Analytical Techniques and the Information Obtained from the Measurements

Type	Technique	Minimum Detection Limits (MDL)/Resolution	Information
Physical	Visual inspection	0.1 mm spatial resolution	Macroscopic properties: texture, size, processing artifacts, tooling marks and shape of solid objects (e.g., nuclear fuel pellet dimensions [pellet diameter, height, inner hole diameter] are unique to a given manufacturer).
	Optical microscopy (OM)	1 μm spatial resolution	
Microstructural	XRD	MDL ~ 5 atom %	Structure of inorganic and organic crystalline materials, particle morphology, inclusions (or occlusions), and size distribution of powder samples. This information can be indicative of the manufacturing process.
	SEM	1.5 nm spatial resolution	
	TEM	0.1 nm spatial resolution	
Chemical	GC-MS	MDL ~ parts per million	Identification of trace organic constituents, structure and association of chemical and molecular species (e.g., uranium oxide can be found in many different forms — UO_2, U_3O_8, or UO_3).
	Infrared (IR) spectroscopy	~5–15 μm spatial resolution	
	NMR	MDL ~ parts per million	
Elemental	Mass spectrometry:		Identification of major, minor and trace elements in radioactive material. For example, minor elements define the function of the nuclear material (e.g., erbium or gadolinium are burnable poisons) and trace elements may be indicative of processing or manufacturing processes (e.g., iron and chromium residues from stainless steel tooling or calcium, magnesium, or chlorine residues from water-based cleaning processes).
	SIMS	MDL 0.1 ppb–10 ppm: 0.2–1 μm spatial resolution	
	TIMS	MDL ~ picogram to nanogram	
	ICP	MDL ~ picogram to nanogram	
	Glow discharge (GD-MS)	MDL ~ 0.1 ppb–10 ppm	
	EDX	MDL 0.1–2 atom %: 1 μm spatial resolution	
	XRF	MDL ~ 10 ppm	

(continued)

TABLE 10.5 (continued)
Common Nuclear Analytical Techniques and the Information Obtained from the Measurements

Type	Technique	Minimum Detection Limits (MDL)/Resolution	Information
Isotopic	HRGS Radioanalytical counting methods	MDL ~ nanogram to microgram MDL ~ femtogram to picogram	Fission or neutron-capture products: indisputable evidence that the material has been in a nuclear reactor (e.g., ^{236}U or ^{129}I are indicative of nuclear processes).
	Mass spectrometry: SIMS	MDL 0.1 ppb–10 ppm: 0.2–1 μm spatial resolution	Decay (daughter) products act as fingerprints for the type and operating conditions of a given reactor and are used to determine the age after enrichment/purification from the "parent" isotopes in the material.
	TIMS	MDL ~ picogram to nanogram	
	ICP	MDL ~ picogram to nanogram	

Note: EDX, energy dispersive x-ray; GC-MS, gas chromatography mass spectrometry; ICP, inductively coupled plasma; NMR, nuclear magnetic resonance; SEM, scanning electron microscopy; SIMS, secondary ion mass spectrometry; TEM, transmission electron microscopy; TIMS, thermal ionization mass spectrometry; XRD, x-ray diffraction; XRF, x-ray fluorescence.

Another useful imaging technique is electron microscopy. Scanning electron microscopy (SEM) can provide visual information at a spatial resolution on the order of 1 nm [38]. The technique is capable of identifying crystal morphologies and therefore the presence of multiple phases [39]. It is also useful for studying the distribution of particle size above the spatial resolution limit and can yield qualitative information on sample porosity [40]. Topographical information is obtained by the use of secondary electrons, while backscattered electrons yield information related to the average atomic number of the area being imaged. The latter is observed as contrast variations within the image.

Transmission electron microscopy (TEM) is capable of higher magnification than SEM and typically has a spatial resolution on the order of 0.1 nm, which allows extremely small structural features to be examined [40,41]. The use of a thin sample cross section enables electrons to be passed through the sample. The resultant images enable the user to observe structural features of the material, such as particle size, porosity, crystal morphology, and the presence of individual grains, stacking faults, twin boundaries, and dislocations. Electron diffraction enables crystal structures to be determined from individual areas of a sample. Information obtained from both imaging and electron diffraction can be used to determine the processing history of materials. This information is highly valuable in providing clues for tracing the source of the material. Excellent examples highlighting the use of the technique to analyze plutonium-bearing samples are detailed in recent review articles [23,42].

10.3.3.3 Bulk Analysis

Bulk analysis techniques are those that probe the macroscopic properties of a sample. Standard techniques such as weight, density, viscosity, surface area, particle size, crystallography, and surface roughness measurements yield valuable information; however, it is likely that more sophisticated methods will need to be employed [34]. These techniques can basically be categorized as either elemental analyses or isotopic analyses.

10.3.3.3.1 Elemental Techniques

The use of elemental analysis techniques such as the inductively coupled plasma (ICP) methods, x-ray fluorescence spectroscopy, particle induced x-ray emission (PIXE), carbon-hydrogen-nitrogen-sulfur (CHNS) analysis, and gas chromatography mass spectrometry (GC-MS) can all be used for bulk sample analysis [28,34,43]. Moreover, each of these techniques can yield complementary information useful for characterizing forensic samples.

The major ICP-based methods are inductively coupled plasma atomic emission spectroscopy (ICP-AES), inductively coupled plasma atomic fluorescence spectrometry (ICP-AFS), and ICP-MS. All these methods involve a sample being converted to an aerosol and transported into a plasma, which results in a unique vaporization, atomization, excitation, and ionization source for atomic emission and mass spectrometry [44]. In ICP-AES, the radiation emitted by the analyte is measured at characteristic wavelengths and this signal is used to identify and quantify the elements present. In ICP-MS, the tail of the plasma is extracted into a low-pressure interface and the ions focused and transmitted to a mass analyzer [45]. For ICP-AFS, a primary excitation source, such as a laser or cathode lamp, is used to excite atomic fluorescence from atomic and ionic analyte species [44].

The success of ICP analysis techniques is primarily due to the low detection limits (ppm to ppb depending on the element), the large number of elements that can be analyzed, the precision of the techniques (relative standard deviation of 0.2% to 3%), and the wide dynamic concentration ranges (4 to 11 orders of magnitude) for many elements [44]. However, ICP-MS is generally considered the most powerful method of the three due to its superior detection limits and the ability of this technique to provide isotopic information.

Inductively coupled plasma methods have benefited from the development of a number of methods used to introduce a sample into the plasma. These methods include separation techniques such as gas chromatography (GC) [46], liquid chromatography (LC), capillary electrophoresis (CE) [47], ion exchange chromatography (IEC) [48], and ablation techniques for the direct analysis of solids, such as laser [49], arc, and spark ablation [48]. The technique has also benefited by the ongoing development of mass spectrometers. The development of multi-collector ICP-MS (MC-ICP-MS) enables isotopes of interest, within the limits set by the mass analyzer, to be analyzed simultaneously rather than sequentially. The use of a time-of-flight analyzer (ICP-TOF-MS) enables all isotopes to be analyzed simultaneously. Both MC-ICP-MS and ICP-TOF-MS are proving to be valuable techniques for situations where a limited amount of sample is available or where shorter analysis times are required.

The power of ICP techniques is the ability to ascertain major, minor, and trace elements within a sample. The techniques have been used in traditional forensics for either matching samples or tracing samples back to a point of manufacture. Such analyses have been performed on a variety of samples such as glass [50], bullets [51,52], and paint [53]. Examples of the techniques used for radiological forensics are more limited and primarily involve the use of ICP-MS to obtain both elemental and isotopic data. Examples include the use of ICP-MS for semiquantitative studies of the trace elements and isotopic ratios within yellow cake samples as unique identifiers [54], the use of ICP-MS for the detection of nuclear activities by analyzing plant matter from the surrounding environment for elements such as cobalt, nickel, lanthanum, cesium, samarium, thorium, and uranium [55] and the use of the technique for elemental fingerprinting of nuclear materials [56,57].

Two other useful elemental analysis techniques are x-ray fluorescence (XRF) and PIXE. In both techniques, the excitation of electrons from inner core levels of individual atoms results in vacancies that are filled by electrons from outer core levels. The result is the emission of characteristic x-rays whose intensities are proportional to the concentration of the atoms responsible for each characteristic emission, provided that there is no thickness-dependent or energy-dependent absorption of x-rays and that a constant fraction of the core level vacancies result in x-ray emission [58]. Therefore materials of known composition that are preferably similar to the sample of interest are generally used as calibration standards, although recent studies have also employed the use of Monte Carlo simulation-based quantification schemes to simulate the spectral response [59].

X-ray fluorescence is an analysis technique that is widely used for the examination of samples containing elements from sodium to plutonium. XRF is generally classified as either energy dispersive x-ray fluorescence (ED-XRF) or wavelength dispersive x-ray fluorescence (WD-XRF). An energy dispersive instrument utilizes an energy analyzing detector upon which all the resultant x-rays are focused. A wavelength dispersive instrument uses a diffraction crystal to focus x-rays of specific wavelength upon a detector. By rotating the crystal, the wavelength range is scanned. While ED-XRF systems are faster and less expensive, WD-XRF is more sensitive and has higher resolution [60].

Commercially available XRF systems typically employ x-ray tubes as the excitation source; however, fixed radioactive sources can also be used, particularly in portable devices. Characteristic x-rays can be measured using a variety of detectors such as NaI, lithium doped silicon detectors, and Peltier-cooled PIN detectors [61]. A PIN detector works in the same way as a p-n junction, but it has an intrinsic layer between the p-n junctions, hence the term PIN. For portable instruments solid-state room temperature detectors such as CdZnTe and mercuric iodide are typically used [60,61]. Recent events such as the development of micro-XRF, which enables small particles or fibers to be examined, have enabled the technique to be expanded to analyzing trace quantities of samples.

X-ray fluorescence is used widely in traditional forensic analysis to analyze samples such as glass from automobile headlights [62], fibers [63], environmental forensics [64], coins [65], and printer toner [66]. It follows that similar applications will apply to the analysis of radioactive samples, however, few reports exist in the literature at the present time.

The PIXE technique is analogous to XRF except high-energy particles are used as a primary source. Sample irradiation is usually achieved by the use of protons with energies between 2 and 4 MeV. An accelerator is typically used to produce such particles. The use of protons means that the technique probes only the top 10 to 60 μm of a sample, depending on the energy of the incident beam and the energy of characteristic x-rays. Hence it is important that the analyzed region is representative of the whole sample [67]. The detection of the resultant x-rays is usually performed using energy dispersive semiconductor detectors such as lithium doped silicon detectors or HPGe detectors. Depending on the element and instrumental factors, species can be measured down to concentrations on the order of 1 to 100 ppm [60]. As with XRF, wavelength dispersive crystal spectrometers do exist, however, the wavelength dispersive technique is not commonly used for PIXE.

From the literature, PIXE is less prominent as an analytical technique than XRF and this is primarily due to the requirement of an accelerator. However, PIXE has been used for several traditional forensic applications, including the analysis of ink [68,69], explosives [70], gunshot residue [71], bone [72], and trace metals on skin [73]. The use of PIXE for forensic analysis of radioactive material has not been identified in the literature to date. However, the technique has considerable potential.

The elemental analysis of organic molecules that may be present in radioactive evidence can be measured by a number of techniques, including GC-MS, CHNS analysis, nuclear magnetic resonance, and vibrational spectroscopy [74,75]. The benefit in both identifying and quantifying such materials is that the presence of organic materials may be indicative of processes used to produce or reprocess radioactive materials. Furthermore, these techniques may prove useful in identifying organic materials associated with traditional forensic evidence that may assist in the identification of the source of the material.

10.3.3.3.2 Isotopic Techniques

Other bulk analysis techniques that have proven to be extremely useful in the study of radioactive materials are isotopic analysis methods. One of the most useful techniques, ICP-MS, has already been described in detail. Another technique used is AMS.

Accelerator mass spectrometry is the technique of choice for the detection of long-lived radionuclides that cannot be analyzed with conventional radiometric and spectrometric methods. AMS utilizes an ion accelerator and a beam transport system as an ultrasensitive mass spectrometer to provide multiple stages of mass and charge analysis and element identification. The determination of radionuclides is typically conducted by cesium ion sputtering a sample of interest. The resultant negative ions produced from the sample are then accelerated in a tandem accelerator to energies in the megaelectron volt (MeV) range. The negative ions then interact with a terminal stripper, which results in the loss of electrons. The positively charged species are then accelerated a second time by the same potential. The benefit of the terminal stripper is that it results in the dissociation of molecular ions and therefore the elimination of isobaric interferences. The ions then undergo multiple stages of mass and charge analysis. This separation process enables individual isotopes to be detected and recorded [76].

Accelerator mass spectrometry has an isotopic abundance sensitivity down to one part in 10^{15} and detection limits as low as 10^4 atoms for ^{14}C and other long-lived ($T_{1/2} = 10^3$ to 10^6 yr) cosmogenic isotopes present in the environment [77]. The technique has also proven useful in the detection of long-lived isotopes such as ^{236}U, ^{239}Pu, ^{240}Pu, ^{99}Tc, and ^{237}Np, which are an enduring legacy from nuclear processes such as atomic bomb testing and nuclear reactor operations [77,78]. In forensic science, AMS is a valuable high-sensitivity technique for the isotopic fingerprinting of uranium and plutonium isotopes.

Accelerator mass spectrometry is not a competitive technique for the measurement of the isotopic ratios of abundant isotopes such as ^{235}U:^{238}U, which can be measured more effectively using ICP-MS. This is primarily due to instrumental factors and the laborious sample preparation methods. However, the technique is useful for analyzing rare isotopes such as ^{236}U (an indicator of uranium irradiation in a nuclear reactor), and ^{233}U (which is an indicator of thorium irradiation).

The virtual absence of ^{236}U in nature enables AMS researchers to determine the presence of nuclear irradiation processes from environmental samples. For example, in nature, the highest concentration of ^{236}U occurs in uranium ores in quantities not exceeding ^{236}U:^{238}U of 1×10^{10}. Anthropogenic ^{236}U is produced principally by thermal neutron capture of ^{235}U. In spent or used nuclear fuel, the ^{236}U:^{238}U ratio builds up to 0.1 to 0.5%. Researchers have demonstrated that ^{236}U can be measured by AMS in microgram samples with an isotopic sensitivity of 10^9 for ^{236}U:^{238}U, with the potential of achieving sensitivities in the range of 10^8 to 10^{14} [79–81]. This enables accurate analyses to be conducted on minute quantities of samples, such as those collected from environmental swipe samples. Hence AMS is a powerful technique and plays a key role in a number of nuclear monitoring programs.

Thermal ionization mass spectrometry (TIMS) is another mass spectrometry technique that has found use in the field of nuclear science. The technique requires only small quantities (nanogram to micrograms) of sample deposited on a filament (usually high-purity rhenium or tantalum) and heated until the material evaporates and ionizes. The low-energy ions are then analyzed via mass spectrometry. Typically single sector field mass spectrometers are used for ion separation and result in an isotope ratio precision better than 0.01%, while detection limits for this technique can be as low as 10^{12} [82]. The use of multiple ion collector systems allows the simultaneous measurement of different isotopes.

Thermal ionization mass spectrometry has been used extensively for the characterization of nuclear materials, with much of the seminal research in the field of nuclear forensics being conducted by researchers at the ITU [37,54,56]. TIMS has been used to obtain isotopic abundance data, enabling both the age of nuclear material and the geographical origin of nuclear materials to be established. More information on ITU research has recently been published in a review by Mayer et al. [23].

10.3.3.4 Particle Analysis

Particle analysis techniques are those that probe microscopic areas of a sample. As with the bulk analysis techniques, both elemental and isotopic analyses are possible. The ability to analyze particulates or small areas of a bulk sample is convenient for a number of reasons. Where destructive techniques are employed and only a small quantity of a sample is available, very little sample need be sacrificed in order to obtain physical and chemical information. Furthermore, the ability to analyze small areas of a bulk sample enables the scientist to identify the presence of heterogeneity within a sample. However, care should be exercised when drawing conclusions from microanalytical data. The presence of external contaminants or unidentified sample heterogeneity are possible scenarios that could lead to erroneous interpretations of experimental results.

Many of the bulk analysis techniques discussed previously have been adapted to provide microscopic analysis capabilities. The incorporation of laser ablation as a sample introduction method for ICP-MS enables small particulates to be analyzed. Techniques such as micro-XRF and micro-PIXE and even micro-AMS are also available. However, there exist some techniques that are primarily microanalytical in nature. Two of these will be discussed: SIMS and energy dispersive x-ray analysis (EDX).

Secondary ion mass spectrometry is an ultra-high-vacuum microanalytical technique capable of analyzing particles of submicron dimensions [82]. The technique utilizes a focused primary ion beam (typically Cs^+ or O^+) to produce secondary ions from a sample which are then analyzed by a mass spectrometer. The fact that secondary ions are being interrogated means that the depth resolution of the technique is in the range of a few nanometers. The detection limits of the technique are element dependent, however, parts per billion concentrations are achievable [82]. The quantification of elemental data from SIMS is difficult due to matrix effects. Hence matrix matched standards are required for accurate analyses.

Although the technique has been underutilized by the traditional forensics community, with a very limited number of studies conducted [83], SIMS has proven to be a unique tool for the analysis of nuclear materials. SIMS has been used for the characterization of uranium and plutonium particles in an effort to determine the age and origin of nuclear materials [84,85] and to identify the point of origin (geolocation) of uranium oxides using $^{18}O/^{16}O$ (^{18}O) isotopic ratio methods [86].

Energy dispersive x-ray analysis is an elemental analysis technique that is typically incorporated within electron microscopes. When electrons interact with a sample, inner core electrons can be excited from individual atoms, resulting in vacancies that are filled by electrons from outer core levels, resulting in the emission of characteristic x-rays. The detection of these x-rays enables individual elements within a sample volume of less than 1 μm^3 to be quantified [87]. The EDX technique enables a microscopic area of a sample to be analyzed by this method. As with PIXE, the quantification of elements can suffer from thickness-dependent or energy-dependent x-ray absorption effects. Therefore standards are required to obtain meaningful results. The EDX technique is widely used in both conventional and radiological forensic applications, enabling individual areas of a microscopic sample to be interrogated. The ease with which a sample can be analyzed enables it to be analyzed quickly and allows EDX to be used as an initial screening tool.

10.4 CONCLUSION

The emergence of illicit trafficking in nuclear and radioactive materials is a serious concern in light of the recent increased threat of terrorism. The need for strategies to detect and locate the source of these materials is vital in limiting the effectiveness of radioactive materials as a terrorist tool. Significant progress has been made in recent times, however, more needs to be done to ensure the safety and security of the international community are achieved.

This chapter highlights current capabilities in the field of nuclear detection and forensics by explaining current methods, procedures, and strategies in a general context. Clearly each country has different requirements dictated by national laws, geographical location, and level of funding for equipment and personnel. However, the fundamental strategies for detection and analysis remain the same.

REFERENCES

1. Ferguson, C.D., *The Four Faces of Nuclear Terrorism*, Center for Nonproliferation Studies, Monterey Institute of International Studies, Monterey, CA, 2004.
2. Drielak, S.C., *Hot Zone Forensics Chemical, Biological, and Radiological Evidence Collection*, Charles C Thomas, Springfield, IL, 2004.
3. IAEA, *Safeguards Glossary*, International Safeguards Verification Series No. 3, IAEA, Vienna, 2002.
4. IAEA, *Categorization of Radioactive Sources, Revision of IAEA-TECDOC-1191*, *Categorization of Radiation Sources*, IAEA-TECDOC-1344, IAEA, Vienna, 2003.
5. Ferguson, C.D., Kazi, T., and Perera, J., *Commercial Radioactive Sources; Surveying the Security Risks*. Occasional Paper 11, Center for Nonproliferation Studies, Monterey Institute of International Studies, Monterey, CA, 2003.
6. IAEA Board of Governors Conference, *Nuclear Security — Measures to Protect Against Nuclear Terrorism*, GOV/2004/50-GC(48)/6, August 11, 2004.
7. Moody, K.J., Hutcheon, I.D., and Grant, P.M., *Nuclear Forensic Analysis*, CRC Press, Boca Raton, FL, 2005.
8. U.S. Department of Defense, *Proliferation: Threat and Response*, Office of the Secretary of Defense, January 2001.
9. Tanaguchi, T. and Nilsson, A., *Hotspots, Weak Links: Strengthening Nuclear Security in a Changing World*, IAEA Bulletin 46/1, IAEA, Vienna, 2004.
10. Ferguson, C.D., *Reducing the Threat of RDDs*, IAEA Bulletin 45/1, IAEA, Vienna, 2003.
11. IAEA, *IAEA Illicit Trafficking Database Fact Sheet 1993–2004*, IAEA, Vienna, 2004, available at http://www.iaea.org/ NewsCenter/Features/RadSources/PDF/ fact_figures2004.pdf.
12. Cameron, G., Potential sources of radionuclides from terrorist activities: new challenges in radioecology, presented at the International Conference on Radioactivity in the Environment, Monaco, September 2002.
13. IAEA, *Detection of Radioactive Materials at Borders*, IAEA-TECDOC-1312, IAEA, Vienna, 2002.
14. IAEA, *Response to Events Involving the Inadvertent Movement or Illicit Trafficking of Radioactive Materials*, IAEA-TECDOC-1313, IAEA, Vienna, 2002.
15. IAEA, *Advances in Destructive and Non-Destructive Analysis for Environmental Monitoring and Nuclear Forensics*, IAEA Proceedings Series, Karlsruhe, Germany, October 21–23, 2002.
16. ICRP, *Recommendations of the International Commission on Radiological Protection*, Publication 60, International Commission on Radiological Protection, Stockholm, 1990.

17. ICRU, *Quantities and Units in Radiation Protection and Dosimetry*, Report no. 51, International Commission on Radiological Units and Measurements, Bethesda, MD, 1993.

18. NCRP, *Limitation of Exposure to Ionizing Radiation*, Report no. 116, National Council on Radiation Protection, Bethesda, MD, 1993.

19. IAEA, *Safeguards, Techniques, and Equipment*, International Nuclear Verification Series no. 1 (revised), IAEA, Vienna, 2003.

20. Rodnyi, P.A., Progress in fast scintillators, *Radiat. Meas.*, 33, 505, 2001.

21. Balcerzyk, M., Moszynski, M., and Kapusta, M., Comparison of LaCl3:Ce and NaI(Tl) scintillators in gamma-ray spectrometry, *Nucl. Instrum. Meth. A*, 537, 50, 2005.

22. Friedlander, G., Kennedy, J.W., and Miller, J.M., *Nuclear and Radiochemistry*, 2nd edition, John Wiley & Sons, New York, 1964.

23. Mayer, K., Wallenius, M., and Ray, I., Nuclear Forensics — a methodology for providing clues on the origin of illicitly trafficked nuclear material, *Analyst*, 130, 433, 2005.

24. Koch, L., *Traces of Evidence: Nuclear Forensics and Illicit Trafficking*, IAEA Bulletin 45/1, IAEA, Vienna, 2003.

25. IAEA, *Preparedness and Response for a Nuclear or Radiological Emergency, Safety Requirements*, IAEA Safety Standards Series no. GS-R-2, IAEA, Vienna, 2002.

26. IAEA, *International Basic Safety Standards for Protection Against Ionizing Radiation and for the Safety of Radiation Sources*, IAEA Safety Series no. 115, IAEA, Vienna, 1996.

27. Metz, H.O.E., *Legal and Scientific Scrutiny of Forensic Sciences and Experts*, International Conference on Advances in Destructive and Non-Destructive Analysis for Environmental Monitoring and Nuclear Forensics, IAEA-CN-98/26, Karlsruhe, Germany, 2002.

28. IAEA, *Nuclear Forensic Support. Reference Document for Responding to Illicit Events Involving Nuclear or Other Radioactive Materials*, IAEA Nuclear Security Series no. 2, IAEA, Vienna, 2004.

29. IAEA, *Destructive Analysis and Evaluation Services for Nuclear Material Accountability Verifications*, IAEA STR-69/Rev.4, IAEA, Vienna, 2003.

30. IAEA, *Sample Collecting Procedure for Swipe Samples*, IAEA Safeguards Manual, Form WP EM1 Rev. 3, IAEA, Vienna, 2002.

31. IAEA, *The Physical Protection of Nuclear Material and Nuclear Facilities*, INFCIRC/225 Rev. 4, IAEA, Vienna, 1999.

32. IAEA, *Regulations for the Safe Transportation of Radioactive Material*, Safety Standards Series no. ST-1, IAEA, Vienna, 1996.

33. ISO, *General Requirements for the Competence of Testing and Calibration Laboratories*, ISO 17025, International Organization for Standardization, Geneva, 1999.

34. IAEA, *Provision of Nuclear Forensic Support to Member States for the Characterisation of Seized Nuclear Material*, IAEA Report of the Consultants Group Meeting February 17–19, 2003, IAEA, Vienna, 2003.

35. Wallenius, M., Peerani, P., and Koch, L., Origin determination of plutonium material in nuclear forensics, *J. Radioanal. Nucl. Chem.*, 236, 317, 2000.

36. Erdmann, N., Betti, M., Stetzer, O., Tamborini, G., Kratz, J.V., Trautmann, N., and van Geel, J., Production of monodispersed uranium oxide particles and their characterisation by scanning electron microscopy and secondary ion mass spectrometry, *Spectrochim. Acta B*, 1565, 55, 2000.

37. Hotchkis, M.A.C, Child, D., Fink, D., Jacobsen, G.E., Lee, P.J., Mino, N., Smith, A.M., and Tuniz, C., Measurement of U-236 in environmental media, *Nucl. Instrum. Meth. B.*, 172, 659, 2000.

38. Zaluzec, N.J., Electron energy loss in advanced materials, in *Transmission Electron Energy Loss Spectrometry in Materials Science*, Disko, M.M., Ahn, C.C., and Fultz, B., eds., Minerals, Metals, and Materials Society, Warrendale, PA, 1992.

39. Ray, I.L.F., Schubert, A., and Wallenius, M., The concept of a "microstructural fingerprint" for the characterization of samples in nuclear forensic science, in *Advances in Destructive and Non-Destructive Analysis for Environmental Monitoring and Nuclear Forensics Book of Extended Synopses*, IAEA-CN-98, IAEA, Vienna, 2002.

40. Williams D.B., *Practical Analytical Electron Microscopy in Materials Science*, Philips Electronics, Murray Hill, NJ, 1983.

41. Ray, I.L.F., Wiss, T., and Thiele, H., Recent developments and case studies in nuclear forensic science, in *Advances in Destructive and Non-Destructive Analysis for Environmental Monitoring and Nuclear Forensics Book of Extended Synopses*, IAEA-CN-98, IAEA, Vienna, 2002.

42. Zocco, T.G. and Schwartz, A.J., A brief history of TEM observations of plutonium and its alloys, *JOM*, 55, 24, 2003.

43. Tölgyessy, J. and Klehr, E.H., *Nuclear Environmental Chemical Analysis*, Ellis Horwood, Chichester, UK, 1987.

44. Montaser, A., McLean, J.A., Liu, H., and Mermet, J.M., An introduction to ICP spectrometries for elemental analysis, in *Inductively Coupled Mass Spectrometry*, Montaser A., ed., Wiley-VCH, New York, 1997.

45. Turner, I.L. and Montaser, A., Plasma generation in ICP-MS, in *Inductively Coupled Mass Spectrometry*, Montaser A., ed., Wiley-VCH, New York, 1997.

46. Chong, N.S. and Houk, R.S., Inductively coupled plasma — mass spectrometry for elemental analysis and isotope ratio determination in individual organic compounds separated by gas chromatography, *Appl. Spectrosc.*, 41, 66, 1987.

47. Kuczewski, B., Marquardt, C.M., Seibert, A., Geckeis, H., Volker Kratz, J., and Trautmann, N., Separation of plutonium and neptunium species by capillary electrophoresis-inductively coupled plasma-mass spectrometry and application to natural groundwater samples, *Anal. Chem.*, 75, 6769, 2003.

48. Taylor, H.E., Huff, R.A., and Montaser, A., Novel applications of ICPMS, in *Inductively Coupled Mass Spectrometry*, Montaser A., ed., Wiley-VCH, New York, 1997.

49. Gray, A.L., Solid sample introduction by laser ablation for inductively coupled plasma source mass spectrometry, *Analyst*, 110, 551, 1985.

50. Buscaglia, J.A., Elemental analysis of small glass fragments in forensic science, *Anal. Chim. Acta*, 288, 17, 1994.

51. Keto, R.O., Analysis and comparison of bullet leads by inductively-coupled plasma mass spectrometry, *J. Forensic Sci.*, 44, 1020, 1999.

52. Dufosse, T. and Touron, P., Comparison of bullet alloys by chemical analysis: use of ICP-MS method, *Forensic Sci. Int.*, 91, 197, 1998.

53. Hobbs, A.L. and Almirall, J.R., Trace elemental analysis of automotive paints by laser ablation-inductively coupled plasma-mass spectrometry (LA-ICP-MS), *Anal. Bioanal. Chem.*, 376, 1265, 2003.

54. Wallenius, M., Mayer, K., Tamborini, G., and Nicholl, A., Investigation of correlations in chemical impurities and isotope ratios for nuclear forensic purposes, in *Advances in Destructive and Non-Destructive Analysis for Environmental Monitoring and Nuclear Forensics Book of Extended Synopses*, IAEA-CN-98, IAEA, Vienna, 2002.

55. Buchmann, J.H., Sarkis, J.E.S., and Rodrigues, C., Environmental monitoring used to identify nuclear signatures, *J. Radioanal. Nucl. Chem.*, 258, 139, 2003.

56. Mayer, K., Rasmussen, G., Hild, M., Zuleger, E., Ottmar, H., Abousahl, S., and Hrnecek, E., Application of isotopic fingerprinting in nuclear forensic investigations: a case study, in *Advances in Destructive and Non-Destructive Analysis for Environmental Monitoring and Nuclear Forensics Book of Extended Synopses*, IAEA-CN-98, IAEA, Vienna, 2002.

57. Momoshima, N., Kakiuchi, H., Maeda, Y., Hirai, E., and Ono, T., Identification of the contamination source of plutonium in environmental samples with isotopic ratios determined by inductively coupled plasma mass spectrometry and alpha-spectrometry, *J. Radioanal. Nucl. Chem.*, 221, 213, 1997.

58. Thomas, J.M. and Thomas, W.J., *Principles and Practice of Heterogeneous Catalysis*, 1st ed., VCH Publishers, Weinheim, 1996.

59. Török, S., Osan, J., Vincze, L., Alfody, B., Kerkapoly, A., Vajda, N., Perez, C.A., and Falkenberg, G., Comparison of nuclear and X-ray techniques for actinide analysis of environmental hot particles, *J. Anal. Atom. Spectrom.*, 18, 1202, 2003.

60. Török, S.B., Labar, J., Injuk, J., and VanGrieken, R.E., X-ray spectrometry, *Anal. Chem.*, 68, 467, 1996.

61. Potts, P.J., Ellis, A.T., Holmas, M., Kregscimer, P., Streli, C., West, M., and Wobrauschek, P.M., X-ray spectrometry, *J. Anal. Atom. Spectrom.*, 15, 1417, 2000.

62. Suzuki, Y., Kasamatsu, M., Sugita R., Ohta, H., Suzuki, S., and Marumo, Y., Forensic discrimination of headlight glass by analysis of trace impurities with synchrotron radiation X-ray fluorescence spectrometry and ICP-MS, *Bunseki Kagaku*, 52, 469, 2003.

63. Koons, R.D., Comparison of individual carpet fibers using energy dispersive X-ray fluorescence, *J. Forensic Sci.*, 41, 199, 1996.

64. Wiarda, W., de Bruijn, R.P., and van der Peijl, G.J.Q., Analytical chemistry for environmental forensics, *Forensic Sci. Int.*, 136, 109(suppl.), 2003.

65. Hida, M., Mitsui, T., and Minami, Y., Forensic investigation of counterfeit coins, *Forensic Sci. Int.*, 89, 21, 1997.

66. Trzinska, B.M., Differentiation among black toners originating from the same model of copiers (printers) or the same type of cartridges, *Forensic Sci. Int.*, 136, 76(suppl. 1), 2003.

67. Grimes, G.W., Analysis of individual environmental particles using microPIXE and nuclear microscopy, *X-ray Spectrom.*, 27, 221, 1998.

68. Vogt, C., Becker, A., and Vogt, J., Investigation of ball point pen inks by capillary electrophoresis (CE) with UV/Vis absorbance and laser induced fluorescence detection and particle induced X-ray emission (PIXE), *J. Forensic Sci.*, 44, 819, 1999.

69. Vogt, C., Vogt, J., Becker, A., and Rohde, E., Separation, comparison and identification of fountain pen inks by capillary electrophoresis with UV-visible and fluorescence detection and by proton-induced X-ray emission, *J. Chromatogr. A*, 781, 391, 1997.

70. Lane, D.W. and Wicks, D.C., PIXE, a new technique for the trace element analysis of high explosives, *Nucl. Instrum. Meth. B*, 161, 792, 2000.
71. Sen, P., Panigrahi, N., Rao, M.S., Varier, K.M., Sens, S., and Mehta, G.N., Application of proton-induced X-ray emission technique to gunshot residue analyses, *J. Forensic Sci.*, 27, 330, 1982.
72. Warren, M.W., Falsetti, A.B., Kravchenko, I.I., Dunnam, F.E., Van Rinsvelt, H.A., and Maples, W.R., Elemental analysis of bone: proton-induced X-ray emission testing in forensic cases, *Forensic Sci. Int.*, 125, 37, 2002.
73. Cullander, C., Grant, P.G., and Bench, G., Development of a low-metal adhesive tape to detect and localize metals in or on the stratum corneum at parts per million levels, *Skin Pharmacol. Appl. Skin Physiol.*, 14(suppl. 1), 46, 2001.
74. Roeges, N.P.G., *A Guide to the Complete Interpretation of Infrared Spectra of Organic Structures*, John Wiley & Sons, New York, 1994.
75. Hendra, P., Jones, C., and Warnes, G., *Fourier Transform Raman Spectroscopy Instrumentation and Chemical Applications*, Ellis Horwood, Chichester, UK, 1991.
76. Tuniz, C., Bird, J.R., Fink, D., and Herzog, G.F., *Accelerator Mass Spectrometry: Ultrasensitive Analysis for Global Science*, CRC Press, Boca Raton, FL, 1998.
77. Hotchkis, M.A.C., Child, D., Fink, D., Jacobsen, G.E., Lee, P.J., Mino, N., Smith, A.M., and Tuniz, C., Measurement of 236U in environmental media, *Nucl. Instrum. Meth. B*, 172, 659, 2000.
78. Jacobsen, G.E., AMS measurement of 129I, 36Cl, and 14C in underground waters from Mururoa and Fangataufa atolls, *Nucl. Instrum. Meth. B*, 172, 666, 2000.
79. Hotchkis, M., Child, D., and Tuniz, C., Application of accelerator mass spectrometry for 236U analysis, *J. Nucl. Sci. Technol.*, 39, 532, 2002.
80. Berkovits, D., Feldstein, H., Ghelberg, S., Hershkowitz, A., Navon, E., and Paul, M., 236U in uranium minerals and standards, *Nucl. Instrum. Meth. B*, 172, 372, 2000.
81. Zhao, X.L., Kilius, L.R., Litherland, A.E., and Beasley, T., AMS measurement of environmental U-236 preliminary results and perspectives, *Nucl. Instrum. Meth. B*, 126, 297, 1997.
82. Becker, J.S., Mass spectrometry of long-lived radionuclides, *Spectrochim. Acta. B*, 58, 1757, 2003.
83. Chen, C.Y., Ling, Y.C., Wang, J.T., and Chen, H.Y., SIMS depth profiling analysis of electrical arc residues in fire investigation, *Appl. Surf. Sci.*, 203, 779, 2003.
84. Tamborini, G. and Betti, M., Characterisation of radioactive particles by SIMS, *Mikrochim. Acta*, 132, 411, 2000.
85. Erdmann, N., Betti, M., Stetzer, O., Tamborini, G., Kratz, J.V., Trautmann, N., and van Geel, J., Production of monodisperse uranium oxide particles and their characterization by scanning electron microscopy and secondary ion mass spectrometry, *Spectrochim. Acta B*, 55, 1565, 2000.
86. Tamborini G., Phinney, D., Bildstein, O., and Betti, M., Oxygen isotopic measurements by secondary ion mass spectrometry in uranium oxide microparticles: a nuclear forensic diagnostic, *Anal. Chem.*, 74, 6098, 2002.
87. Williams, D.B., and Carter, C.B., *Transmission Electron Microscopy: A Textbook for Material Science*, Plenum Press, New York, 1996.

11 Radiation Protection Programs

R. J. Emery and M. A. Charlton

CONTENTS

11.1 INTRODUCTION

Radiation protection programs strive to prevent or minimize the harmful effects of radiation sources for those individuals in laboratories involved with the analysis of radioactivity in food and the environment. Sources of radiation inherent to these analytical processes and procedures include ionizing waveforms, particulate radiation, and frequently nonionizing radiation. Sources of ionizing radiation may be used as encapsulated standards for the calibration of counting equipment or in dispersible forms for radiolabeling or internal standardization procedures. Ionizing radiation may also be encountered in the form of radiation producing devices, such as analytical x-ray machines, electron microscopes, or x-ray diffraction devices. Sources of nonionizing radiation, in particular high-energy lasers, are also increasingly being used in analytical devices. The unknown analytical sample in the lab may also contain radioactivity. Samples of food and environmental media contain myriad radionuclides in variable concentrations stemming from natural sources or from environmental releases. With all of these different types of sources that might be present in any analytical lab, and the various pathways for potential exposure, the development of a vigilant radiation protection program to protect the health of the individuals associated with the lab activities is considered to be a necessity.

Laboratory safety programs may be considered integral to an overall philosophy of quality control and improvement. A robust safety program prevents contamination, promotes laboratory hygiene, and espouses the "do no harm" philosophy. The enhanced quality embedded within these elements prevents laboratory injuries, improves sample analysis, and reduces laboratory overhead costs. Therefore laboratories engaged in quality management programs often dedicate resources to safety enhancements.

A radiation protection program is, in effect, a management system that affords an organization the ability to anticipate, recognize, evaluate, and control sources of radiation that might be present in the workplace. Radiation protection programs represent more than just monitoring for the radiation levels present. Robust radiation protection programs include considerations for facility design and engineering controls, personal protective equipment, administrative controls, records review, professional development, and emergency preparedness. Such comprehensive approaches to safety programs have been recognized as standard industry practice, and are considered so important that they are required by some regulatory agencies. Although variability exists among various regulatory entities, a finite set of recognized prudent radiation protection program elements are identifiable. This chapter discusses these common elements and provides examples of the measures that can be employed to create a successful program that protects the health and safety of individuals in the analytical laboratory work setting. Other hazards within the analytical laboratory may require similar management systems. Many laboratories possess biological agents, chemicals, and physical agents in addition to the radiological sources outlined in this chapter. These hazards should warrant additional management systems beyond the scope of this chapter.

Figure 11.1 outlines a pragmatic schema for describing the overarching principles of anticipation, recognition, evaluation, and control of radiation sources in the laboratory. Within each principle are subprocedures or considerations which the laboratory should consider to complement their radiation protection program.

11.2 ANTICIPATION

The first phase in the development of a comprehensive radiation protection program is anticipating the radiation sources to be encountered. In an effort to anticipate potential workplace hazards, safety must be included in the overall laboratory mission. This tangible management support is critical for new or developing radiation safety programs. Strong executive support transfers into prompt anticipation and remediation of occupational hazards.

The anticipation phase typically consists of a review of the overall mission of the laboratory and then the creation of a simple process flowchart that tracks the radiation sources as they pass through the organization. Figure 11.1 contains a conceptual schema to assist in the development of a laboratory process flowchart. It is important to include in this process diagram both the sources inherent

Process phase	Considerations
Delivery	Notification for deliveries
Receipt	Radionuclide expected
	Physical form
	Amount
	Frequency of receipt
	Methods for receipt monitoring
	Addition to inventory
	Interim storage
	Security of facility during receipt and interim storage
Preparation and use	Transport to worksite
	User training
	Protective equipment
	Engineering controls
	Manipulations
	Chemical reactions
	Mechanical manipulations
	Worksite safety surveys
	Monitoring
	Emergencies
	Quality Assurance / Quality Control
	Consideration of pathways for releases
	Postings, access controls
	Data analyses and interpretation
Disposition	How will waste or unused sources accumulation occur?
	Options for return to supplier?
	Means for assay for verification of content
	Storage means
	Processing
	Disposal recycling
	Security
	Removal from inventory
	Releases in other forms
	Waste
	Water
	Air

FIGURE 11.1 Generic process considerations for the delivery, receipt, preparation, use, and release of radiation sources.

in the samples to be analyzed and any sources inherent in the analytical tools and procedures as well.

A typical process flow diagram begins with the delivery and receipt of the radiation source. Laboratories should be designed so that sources are received in a controlled area that is away from normal operations. Keeping the source receipt area away from normal operations prevents the possibility of facility contamination if a package is found to be leaking and minimizes the impact of background radiation levels that can adversely impact sensitive radioanalytical procedures. Since some sources may arrive in heavy shipping containers, or may be in various forms of environmental media, consideration must be given to material handling aspects, such as the use of carts or lifts. Upon receipt, the radiation source must be characterized and inventoried so that a complete accounting of the radiation sources present at any time can be maintained. During the receipt phase, consideration must be given to the radiological monitoring of the transport package to verify integrity. Provisions for interim storage of any source must be made so that the source is properly secured and maintained in appropriate environmental conditions. For example, some samples may need to be maintained in a frozen state, whereas others may need to be maintained at room temperature conditions at all times. Other samples may hold the possibility of offgassing either potentially hazardous gases or nuisance odors, which may warrant the need for storage with local exhaust ventilation. All of these types of requirements should be anticipated prior to the initiation of activities.

After the source receipt phase, the typical process flow leads to the preparation of the source for use or analysis. In this phase, needs for source handling, contamination control, shielding, and local exhaust ventilation should be anticipated. Accommodations should also be made for upset conditions. For example, if a sample leaks, the pathways for fluid flow should be anticipated. Similarly, if the potential for gases or vapors may be present, the fate of these should be considered as well.

Since it is not uncommon for laboratory analyses to subject samples to elevated temperatures, pressures, or chemical reactions in order to extract or isolate targeted components of interest, such processes should also be anticipated, as they can result in releases and possible exposures.

The last stage of the process analysis considers the release, discharge, or disposal of the source. By anticipating the need for space and equipment to address the accumulation and subsequent disposal of waste materials, the radiation protection program will be developed in a manner that addresses the entire scope of operations.

Once a general process flow has been diagrammed, then certain operating parameters can be circumscribed. Estimates describing the number of sources or samples to be received and the average daily and weekly volumes help establish operating bounds for the organization. Such operating parameters are necessarily limited by aspects such as organizational staffing and facility space. Within these operating bounds, accommodations should be made for possible emergency situations, such as when a massive number of samples might be received due to an unusual event, along with envisioned general increases in volume due to organizational growth. These operating boundaries can then serve to drive facility design or modification needs and will aid in the facility permitting process as well.

Armed with the information gained from the anticipation phase of radiation protection program development, the focus can now be directed toward the recognition phase of the process.

11.3 RECOGNITION

Since humans cannot detect the presence of radiation with any of our sensory pathways, we must rely on other means to recognize its presence. Thus, recognition of possible radiological hazards is typically accomplished through a combination of worker education and administrative access controls and postings.

Worker education should be considered a cornerstone for any radiation protection program. An educated workforce can lead to the installation of a safety culture wherein safety becomes an unquestionable part of every aspect of work. When this type of environment is installed, all of the other programmatic issues fall neatly into place. Although specific regulatory requirements regarding radiation safety training vary (Table 11.1 shows the training elements for radiation workers in Texas), all should enable workers to answer the basic following questions:

- What are the risks inherent to my job, and where are they?
- What steps do I take to perform my job in a safe manner?
- Where can I obtain additional information or assistance?
- What do I do in case of an emergency?

Equally important to providing this basic information, educational programs should also serve as a platform for conveying an organizational commitment to safety and genuine concern for its workers. All too often, excellent educational content is provided via a format that does not effectively convey this message. For example, when a new employee is provided basic radiation safety training via videotape or computer terminal, an unintended message could be that the organization is not truly dedicated to this aspect of operations and is more interested in fulfilling some regulatory requirement. Radiation protection programs should make a concerted effort to avoid this unintended outcome.

TABLE 11.1
Radiation Protection Topics Required by Regulatory Authorities in Texas (25 TAC 289.203(c))

Topic	Regulatory Reference
Storage, transfer, use of workplace radiation sources	289.203(c)(1)(A)
Health protection problems associated with radiation	289.203(c)(1)(B)
Precautions and procedures needed to minimize exposure	289.203(c)(1)(B)
Instructed in applicable radiation protection regulations	289.203(c)(1)(C)
Instructed to report any incident or violation	289.203(c)(1)(D)
Emergency response procedures and warning	289.203(c)(1)(E)
Radiation exposure reports involving the employee	289.203(c)(1)(F)

To verify that the necessary educational content has been understood by workers, some type of educational assessment tool is needed. This may be in the form of a test or a series of signed acknowledgements, but regardless of the format, it is important to ensure in documented form that the student left the training session with the knowledge to perform work safely, and where to turn if questions arise.

An essential part of any radiation safety educational effort includes information on how to recognize where radiation might be present. Workers should be educated about the various warning signs and barriers that may be placed around areas where radiation sources are used. Descriptions of actual source containers are also useful.

11.4 EVALUATION

Once the source term for the work area has been established and the specific locations of use established, then evaluation of the radiation protection program can begin. Typical program evaluations consist of routine surveys to ensure that radiation levels are being maintained as low as reasonably achievable (ALARA) and that contamination is controlled within workspaces and at acceptable levels. Routine surveys should not be limited merely to the detection of radiation, and should include an assessment of programmatic aspects such as the presence of postings, documented worker training, and a review of regular work practices.

11.5 CONTROL

Radiation protection programs focus control efforts in three primary phases: prior to the use of radiation sources, during the use of radiation sources, and at the time of ultimate disposition of the source. Each phase of radiation exposure control employs distinct management techniques. The most effective radiation protection program requires a team-based approach with support from executive management, regulatory authorities, facility planners, radiation safety personnel, the laboratory director, and laboratory staff.

11.5.1 PREEXPOSURE CONTROLS

A guiding principle of radiation protection practice involves minimizing or preventing radiation exposure before laboratory work begins. This could include consideration of the types of research protocols envisioned, facility construction, engineering control in the form of directional airflow, or security controls in the form of locks and identification card readers. In the laboratory setting, two of the most common administrative controls are peer review safety committees and consideration of radiation source substitution.

Many regulatory authorities promulgate standards that mandate health care and research settings convene a properly constituted "Radiation Safety Committee." In general, a facility Radiation Safety Committee possesses the ability to approve new uses of radioactive material, new radionuclides, or even new radioactive material laboratories. The goal of the peer Radiation Safety Committee is to evaluate the hazards of radiation exposure and recommend control measures to the investigator. This peer review methodology for hazard assessment and control has a solid foundation in the laboratory due to the common presence of other institutional review committees (e.g., Institutional Review Board).

Radiation source substitution focuses on the availability of alternative research techniques to minimize or prevent exposure to radioactive materials. For example, if the laboratory requests the use of ^{32}P (E_{max} = 1.7 MeV B$^-$), source substitution philosophy dictates the consideration of ^{33}P (E_{max} = 0.25 MeV B$^-$). In this example, a ^{32}P laboratory nucleotide may be easily substituted with ^{33}P to accomplish the same scientific goals with a lower energy product. The most effective source substitution occurs prior to exposure and before the laboratory generates data. Therefore formally incorporating these goals into the Radiation Safety Committee's charter and operations may be helpful.

11.5.2 Laboratory Exposure Controls

Radiation safety programs employ a tiered approach to managing radiation exposures during routine laboratory operations. This multifaceted approach includes aggressive employee safety training, "dry run" walk-throughs, laboratory director feedback, workplace surveillance, exposure monitoring, and pragmatic radiation protection program review. When taken together as a systematic approach, this exposure minimization plan is circular, with the continual goal of reducing laboratory radiation exposures.

The dynamic nature of the laboratory work setting dictates an aggressive worker safety training program. Most regulatory authorities will prescribe certain radiation safety training topics. Table 11.1 illustrates the common topics required by the radiation control authority in Texas. In reviewing Table 11.1, these topics may be considered rather general and not specific to the laboratory setting. Most laboratory directors will require significantly more detailed treatment of occupational hazards in order to prevent hazardous exposures in the laboratory setting. Radiation protection standards require the level or duration of training be commensurate with the level of hazard presented by the radiation source. Laboratory safety training also commonly uses "dry run" walk-throughs and continual feedback from the laboratory director.

The "dry run" method of training enables a laboratory worker to progress stepwise through a new laboratory protocol without the inclusion of radioactive material. Laboratory workers may then plan out details such as the physical layout of the laboratory bench, placement of portable shielding, critical equipment, and radioactive waste containers. This important training initiative generally results in lower radiation doses for new laboratory workers by minimizing the time around radiation sources and improving process knowledge.

Workplace surveillance programs enable an unbiased observer to review the use, storage, and containment of radiation sources in the laboratory setting. These observations are then presented to the laboratory director in order to reduce radiation exposures in the laboratory. Workplace surveillance programs may be initiated by the laboratory director or the facility radiation safety personnel. A common approach involves the use of a published survey tool, removable contamination surveys, and an ambient radiation level survey. The survey tool or checklist enables a trained observer to evaluate the same laboratory situations in each facility laboratory. A further benefit of the survey tool is that the laboratory director or staff may periodically self-assess the safety of their program. Figure 11.2 provides an example of a common laboratory radiation safety survey tool.

All radiation sources must have caution signs and hazard warnings denoting the presence of ionizing radiation in the workplace. This signage generally takes the form of the universal "trefoil" symbol with yellow background/magenta lettering or yellow background/black lettering. Figure 11.3 is an example of the common radiation trefoil symbol.

11.6 CONCLUSION

Ionizing radiation presents an important risk to the general public and in many workplaces. The preventive measures described in the text outline prudent steps for eliminating or mitigating the hazard posed by these ionizing radiation sources. The comprehensive philosophy of anticipation, recognition, evaluation, and control of ionizing radiation sources yields a framework for the safe and healthful use of these sources.

Further refinements in the risk factors, biological outcomes, uses, and technology surrounding radiation exposure should be anticipated. New international recommendations for radiation protection are routinely revised and reissued. This process lends itself to pragmatic review of all operations with exposure to radiation hazards. Therefore the guidelines suggested throughout the text should be viewed as a current evaluation of the status, but continuous improvement, work practice controls, and engineering controls should be adopted.

The use of potential carcinogens in the workplace places a heavy burden on the radiation protection program administrators because of the potential for serious biological endpoints. A sensible approach to evaluating, mitigating, or eliminating the risk to occupationally exposed individuals is critically important. These steps, taken in conjunction with standard laboratory practices, provide a solid foundation for engaging in the benefits of ionizing radiation while offsetting the negative outcomes.

University of Texas-Houston health science center
Environmental Health and Safety Department
Radiation Safety Division
Laboratory Safety Evaluation Record

Date Performed:_____   Page: 1
Date Printed: _1/13/2006_____

Procedure: Evaluate each of the following items according to the requirements of the *Radiation Safety Manual*,
June 1996. Place a check in the appropriate space for either Y (YES), N (NO), or N/A (Not
Applicable). Enter comments in the provided space.

	Y	N	N/A	Comments?
General Safety				
General housekeeping orderly?	☐	☐	☐	_____
Current emergency contact phone numbers posted?	☐	☐	☐	_____
Hazard communication training attendance?	☐	☐	☐	_____
Linear air flow rate in hood adequate?	☐	☐	☐	_____
Measured linear flow rate:_____lfpm				
Is the hood air flow laminar?	☐	☐	☐	_____
No food or drink observed in laboratory?	☐	☐	☐	_____
Fire Safety				
Fire egress unobstructed?	☐	☐	☐	_____
Fire extinguisher available?	☐	☐	☐	_____
Electrical circuit load appears normal?	☐	☐	☐	_____
Physical Safety				
Absence of trip hazards?	☐	☐	☐	_____
Compressed gas cylinders secured?	☐	☐	☐	_____
Personal protective equipment used?	☐	☐	☐	_____
Guards in place for mechanical hazards	☐	☐	☐	_____
Biological Safety				
Biohazard laboratories properly posted?	☐	☐	☐	_____
Universal precautions utilized?	☐	☐	☐	_____
Biological safety cabinet certified (annual)?	☐	☐	☐	_____
Ultraviolet lamps used properly & posted?	☐	☐	☐	_____
Biohazard waste properly stored?	☐	☐	☐	_____
Chemical Safety				
NFPA rating present?	☐	☐	☐	_____
Chemicals stored properly?	☐	☐	☐	_____
No flammables stored in refrigerator?	☐	☐	☐	_____
Chemical waste properly stored?	☐	☐	☐	_____
Radiation Safety				
Appropriate CRAM signs posted (door, hood, ref, etc.)?	☐	☐	☐	_____
Properly documented lab survey records present?	☐	☐	☐	_____
Wipe test equipment appropriate & functioning?	☐	☐	☐	_____
Current *Radiation Safety Manual* available?	☐	☐	☐	_____
Current NTE & emergency procedures posted?	☐	☐	☐	_____
Radionuclide storage & security adequate?	☐	☐	☐	_____
Personnel monitoring utilized and appropriate?	☐	☐	☐	_____
Survey instrument available, calibrated, & functioning?	☐	☐	☐	_____
Radioactive waste stored properly?	☐	☐	☐	_____
No additional safety concerns?	☐	☐	☐	_____

Any unsatisfactory safety condition or concern must be relayed to the appropriate Environmental Health & Safety Division

Relayed To: Date: Concern(s):

FIGURE 11.2 Radioactive material laboratory safety evaluation survey tool.

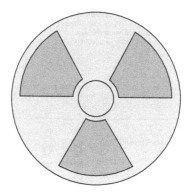

FIGURE 11.3 Common radiation trefoil symbol. The color version has magenta coloring on a yellow background.

11.7 SUPPLEMENTAL READING

Charlton, M.A. and Emery, R.J., An analysis of reported incidents involving radiopharmaceuticals for the development of intervention strategies, *Health Phys.*, 81, 585, 2001.

Emery, R.J., Adding value to your radiation protection program, in *Management and Administration of Radiation Safety Programs*, Roessler, C.E., ed., Medical Physics Publishing, Madison, WI, 1998.

Emery, R.J., Charlton, M.A., and Goodman, G.R., Texas radiation protection program outcomes as indicated by regulatory compliance activities from 1988 to 1997, *Health Phys.* 78, 335, 2000.

Emery, R.J., Charlton, M.A., and Mathis, J.L., Estimating the administrative costs of regulatory noncompliance: a pilot method for quantifying the value of prevention, *Health Phys.*, 78(5 suppl.), S40, 2000.

Emery, R.J., Charlton, M.A., Orders, A.B., and Hernandez, M., Using fault tree analysis to identify causes of non-compliance: enhancing violation outcome data for the purposes of education and prevention. *Health Phys.* 80(suppl. 1), S16, 2001.

Emery, R.J., Pollock, J., and Charlton, M.A., Notices of violation issued to Texas radioactive material licensees inspected in 1995, *Health Phys.*, 73, 706, 1997.

Texas Department of Health, Texas regulations for the control of radiation, Bureau of Radiation Control, Austin, TX, 2002.

U.S. Nuclear Regulatory Commission, Standards for protection against radiation, Title 10 CFR part 20, 1991.

U.S. Nuclear Regulatory Commission, Uses of radioactive material, NUREG/BR-0217, U.S. Nuclear Regulatory Commission, Washington, DC, 1996.

12 Regulations

F. J. Bradley and R. M. Pratt

CONTENTS

12.1 INTRODUCTION

12.1.1 BACKGROUND

Regulations for control of radioactivity in food and the environment are myriad and complex. International and national bodies have formulated maximum permissible contamination limits in response to the 1986 Chernobyl accident and, more recently, in preparation for future radiological emergencies, either accidental or by malevolent intent. Individual countries have promulgated sets of regulatory limits, some based on international standards, some generated internally. To list control values for all countries would be impractical; therefore, this chapter will present a limited selection of regulations and recommendations from international agencies and some individual nations.

Since radioactivity in food, the environment, and drinking water involves public exposure, tables in this chapter present concentration limits based on the concept of dose limitations to the public. For comparison and completeness, occupational dose limits for regulated industries, issued by the International Atomic Energy Agency (IAEA) and the U.S. Nuclear Regulatory Commission (NRC), are presented in Section 12.3.4 and Section 12.4.5, respectively.

Methodologies for derivation of concentration limits in food and water are discussed, with examples provided. An area of concern is radionuclides in soil, especially following decommissioning of formerly licensed or regulated facilities. Generic soil limits are not provided since they are site specific, but a decision-making statistical methodology to demonstrate compliance with limits, the Multiagency Radiation Survey and Site Investigation Manual (MARSSIM), is briefly covered in Section 12.4.5.

While most regulatory limits are based on doses above natural background radiation, some values include background, such as drinking water standards, which are discussed in Section 12.5 and Section 12.6.

All foods have some radioactivity arising from naturally occurring radionuclides, and some people have declared that this is beneficial. Natural radioactivity in matter arises mainly from ^{3}H, ^{14}C, ^{40}K, ^{226}Ra, natural thorium (Th-nat), natural uranium (U-nat), and their decay products. Thoron and radon (^{220}Rn and ^{222}Rn) are ubiquitous noble gases and can cause especially high inhalation doses averaging 1.2 mSv/yr with a range of 0.2 to 10 mSv/yr. The United Nations Scientific Committee on the Effects of Atomic Radiation (UNSCEAR) [1] has provided an estimate of worldwide average public radiation exposures, as presented in Table 12.1. This table provides a perspective for the public exposure limits recommended by various agencies in this chapter and indicates that naturally occurring radionuclides impose an internal ingestion dose of 0.3 mSv/yr or 30 mrem/yr. According to the Department for Environment, Food and Rural Affairs, United Kingdom (DEFRA) [2], approximately 60% of the annual internal ingestion background dose arises from ^{40}K; the remaining 40% is from the other naturally occurring radionuclides. Potassium is regulated by the body so that adults have

TABLE 12.1
Average Radiation Dose from Natural Sources

Source	Worldwide Average Annual Effective Dose (mSv/yr)	Typical Range (mSv/yr)
External exposure		
Cosmic rays	0.4	0.3–1.0
Terrestrial gamma rays[a]	0.5	0.3–0.6
Internal exposure		
Inhalation (mainly radon)	1.2	0.2–10[b]
Ingestion (food and drinking water)	0.3	0.2–0.8
Total	2.4	1–10

[a] Terrestrial exposure is due to radionuclides in the soil and building materials.

[b] Dose from inhalation of radon may exceed 10 mSv/yr in certain residential areas.

Source: UNSCEAR, 2000 [1].
See http://www.who.int/water_sanitation_health/dwq/gdwq3/en.

a fairly constant potassium content. The other naturally occurring radionuclides vary greatly among individuals, depending on their culture, diet, and food sources. Individuals in Kerala, India, and Pocos del Cobdas, Brazil have evolved in a total background average dose level of about 24 mSv/yr (10 times the norm) with apparently no detectable ill effects.

There is a long history of regulating toxic chemicals, such as lead and arsenic, in food and commodities, and in the 1950s the concept of regulating radioactivity in the environment, especially in air and water, was formalized. New York State Industrial Code, Rule 38 [3] listed maximum permissible concentrations (MPC) in units of microCuries per milliliter (μCi/ml) in air and water based on the then-current doses recommended by the National Committee on Radiological Protection (NCRP) [4]. At about the same time, the U.S. Atomic Energy Commission (AEC) — later the regulatory side became the NRC — issued "Part 20, Standards for Protection Against Radiation" (see Section 12.4.5). These recommendations differentiated between occupationally exposed workers and the public, with the public MPC set at about 3% of the worker MPC.

Two events, worldwide fallout from atmospheric testing of nuclear weapons and the Chernobyl nuclear reactor meltdown, galvanized many regulatory agencies to determine what impact such events had on foodstuffs and to issue regulations governing their transnational transport.

12.1.2 OVERVIEW

This chapter presents two classes of regulations. The first class embodies recommendations issued by international organizations that, in most cases, are not legally binding and the second class of regulations represents those issued by national governments that, in most cases, have some legal status. Most guidelines specify limits on radioactivity in food and drinking water. The IAEA has issued a set of recommendations covering the broad topic of contamination of commodities.

The limits presently in force and characterized in this chapter are as follows:

Chernobyl contamination related limits:
  Food and Agriculture Organization (FAO), Section 12.3.2
  European Union (EU), Section 12.3.3
  Australia, Section 12.4.1
  Lithuania, Section 12.4.2
  Ukraine, Section 12.4.3
Other limits that address future radiological contaminating events:
  Codex Alimentarius Commission, Section 12.3.1
  EU, Section 12.3.3
  Lithuania, Section 12.4.2
  U.S. Food and Drug Administration (FDA), Section 12.4.4
  Japan, Section 12.4.6
  Canada, Section 12.4.7
Then there are limits covering on-going licensed or regulated operations
  handling radioactivity:

International Atomic Energy Agency (IAEA), Section 12.3.4

U.S. Nuclear Regulatory Commission (NRC), Section 12.4.5

Finally, agencies that address the sensitive topic of radioactivity in drinking water:

World Health Organization (WHO), Section 12.5.1

U.S. Environmental Protection Agency (EPA), Section 12.6.1

New Zealand Ministry of Health, Section 12.6.2

12.2 DERIVATION OF RADIOACTIVITY CONCENTRATION LIMITS IN FOOD AND DRINKING WATER

The methodology for estimating the MPC of radionuclides in food and drinking water is well established and goes back to the earliest regulations in radiation protection. Mathematically, for the ith radionuclide, the equation is

$$MPC_i = \frac{D}{f_i(FI)(DC)_i} \qquad (12.1)$$

where

MPC = maximum permissible concentration (in Bq/kg for solid or liquid and Bq/l for water),

D = maximum recommended dose per unit time per critical organ (in mSv/yr),

f = fraction of food intake that is contaminated (dimensionless),

FI = food intake per unit time (in kg/yr or l/yr),

DC = dose conversion factor (in mSv/Bq).

Equation 12.1 is used to illustrate the derivation of the various concentration limits throughout the chapter.

Terms used for radioactivity concentration limits by various agencies include MPC, guideline level (GL), action level (AL), maximum acceptable value (MAV), international radionuclide action level for foods (IRALF), intervention level (IL), derived intervention level (DIL), level of concern (LOC), and other similar terms. The annual dose unit is in millisieverts per year (mSv/yr) and usually indicates the committed effective dose equivalent (CEDE). In some cases, the unit represents the committed dose equivalent (CDE), when only the individual tissue or organ is the target. The f factor given in Equation 12.1 may vary from 0.01 to 1.0; the assumed value will be given in the various subsections.

12.3 INTERNATIONAL REGULATIONS FOR RADIOACTIVITY IN FOOD AND COMMODITIES

12.3.1 CODEX ALIMENTARIUS COMMISSION

12.3.1.1 Background

The Codex Alimentarius Commission (CAC) is a joint endeavor of the Food and Agriculture Organization (FAO) and the World Health Organization (WHO) of

TABLE 12.2
Codex Alimentarius Commission, United Nations:
Emergency Food Guideline Levels

Group	Radionuclides	Guideline Level (Bq/kg)
I	^{238}Pu, ^{239}Pu, ^{240}Pu, ^{241}Am	1
II	^{90}Sr, ^{106}Ru, ^{129}I, ^{131}I, ^{235}U	100
III	^{35}S, ^{60}Co, ^{89}Sr, ^{103}Ru, ^{134}Cs, ^{137}Cs, ^{144}Ce, ^{192}Ir	1,000
IV	^{3}H, ^{14}C, ^{99}Tc	10,000

Source: CAC, 2004 [5].
See http://www.criirad.com/criirad/actualites/Dossiers2005/
MenacesRadioactivesAliments/Extrait%20Codex%20Anglais.doc.

the United Nations (UN). The Codex Alimentarius, or Food Code, is the global reference of good practice for consumers, food producers and processors, and national food control agencies in the international food trade. It provides recommendations for GLs for radioactivity in foods to assist UN agencies. The GLs may become the basis for national action levels [5]. They are reproduced in Table 12.2.

The proposed recommendations of the CAC are at step five of the overall acceptance procedure. The GLs are intended to apply to radionuclide contamination in food destined for human consumption and traded internationally. It is suggested that the GLs apply to food after reconstitution (not dried foods) and ready for consumption in the first year after a nuclear accident or malevolent incident. The nuclides in Table 12.2 are those most likely present after such an event. Naturally occurring radionuclides are excluded except for ^{235}U, ^{3}H, and ^{14}C. The nuclides are segregated into four groups with the GLs logarithmically rounded by orders of magnitude (i.e., 1, 10^2, 10^3, and 10^4 Bq/kg).

12.3.1.2 Implementation

Each radionuclide group in Table 12.2 can be treated independently, but for multiple radionuclides within each group, the sum of the concentrations must be less than the GL for that group. If the concentration in food is less than the GL, the food is considered safe for human consumption. When contamination exceeds the GL, the national government must decide whether, and under what circumstances, the food will be distributed. National governments may want to adopt different GLs if the underlying assumptions do not apply.

The GLs are determined using Equation 12.1. The example for the case of ^{90}Sr uses the following assumptions:

D = 1 mSv/yr, committed effective dose,
DC = 2.3 × 10^{-4} mSv/Bq, from the ICRP [6,7],
FI = 550 kg/yr, for adults,
FI = 200 kg/yr, for infants,
  f = 0.1, imported food in the first year following a nuclear accident
    or malevolent incident,
  f = 0.01, minor foods (garlic, truffles, etc.).

$$GL_i = \frac{D}{f_i(FI)(DC)_i}$$

$$GL_{Sr-90} = \frac{1 \text{ mSv/y}}{(0.1)(200 \text{ kg/y})(2.3 \times 10^{-4} \text{ mSv/Bq})}, \text{ for infants}$$

GL_{Sr-90} = 217, rounded to 100 Bq/kg.

In a similar manner, the GLs for other radionuclides can be determined.

12.3.2 FOOD AND AGRICULTURE ORGANIZATION

12.3.2.1 Background

The FAO advises member states on topics of agriculture, production, processing, and storage of food as well as legislation controlling food quality and safety [8]. As a result of the Chernobyl accident in 1986, there was considerable disruption in the worldwide food distribution chain due to a lack of knowledge on radioactive contamination standards for food. The FAO convened a group of technical experts that issued two reports upon which the present recommendations for International Radionuclide Action Levels for Foods (IRALF) are based.

To establish IRALFs, the following underlying principles were followed:

- The IRALF should be simple, uniform and applicable to all food moving in international trade.
- Consumers and food and health authorities can easily understand the IRALF.
- The IRALF should be sufficiently low that no further action is necessary if the food is at or below the limits.

12.3.2.2 Implementation

The IRALFs for three groups of radionuclides were determined by utilizing Equation 12.1. Group I covered ^{90}Sr and ^{131}I; group II, ^{134}Cs and ^{137}Cs; and group III, ^{239}Pu.

The following assumptions were made:

- 100% of the diet is contaminated, $f = 1$.
- For radionuclides with half-lives of less than 70 days, the food intake is for a period of five half-lives. For example, for ^{131}I, FI is the intake over 40 days.
- For radionuclides with half-lives of more than 70 days, the full annual FI is assumed.
- The IRALF from different groups can be applied independently of one another.
- The IRALF for cesium isotopes should be limited by the sum of fractions rule.
- Allowances should be made in applying IRALFs to dried or concentrated food before reconstitution and for food consumed in small quantities, such as herbs and spices (i.e., $f = 0.1$).

Using Equation 12.1 to derive the IRALF for ^{239}Pu in the first year following a radiological incident, make the following substitutions:

$D = 50$ mSv/yr, committed dose equivalent,
$FI = 375$ kg/yr (for a child),
$DC = 1.7 \times 10^{-2}$ mSv/Bq,
$f = 1$.

$$IRALF_{Pu-239} = \frac{50 \text{ mSv/y}}{(1)(375 \text{ kg/y})(1.7 \times 10^{-2} \text{ mSv/Bq})}$$

$GL_{Pu-239} = 8$, rounded to 10 Bq/kg.

The IRALFs become effective in the first and second year following an incident. Table 12.3 gives the derived IRALFs for five radionuclides (^{90}Sr, ^{131}I, ^{134}Cs, ^{137}Cs, and ^{239}Pu), and using the same methodology, IRALFs for other radionuclides can be derived. At the time of the Chernobyl accident, dose coefficients were available for infants and children from Johnson and Dunsford [9] and for adults from ICRP [10] and the lower limit was the recommended IRALF given in the expert report [11]. These values are also given in Table 12.3.

Many countries at the time used a similar methodology to establish limits. The U.S. FDA analyzed 1,035 samples of imported food from a 400 km radius around Chernobyl in the year following April 26, 1986. The findings were that 12 samples exceeded the limits as follows [8]:

- Two cheese samples, ^{131}I.
- Five pasta samples, ^{134}Cs and ^{137}Cs.
- Four spice samples, ^{134}Cs and ^{137}Cs.
- One cheese sample ^{134}Cs and ^{137}Cs.

TABLE 12.3
Food and Agriculture Organization (FAO) International Radionuclide Action Levels in Food (IRALF)

Group	Nuclide	Target Organ	Dose (mSv/yr)	Dose Conversion (mSv/Bq)	Food Intake (kg/yr)	IRALF (Bq/kg)
I	^{90}Sr first year	Bone surface	50	1.9×10^{-3}	375	70
	^{90}Sr following years		10	1.9×10^{-3}		20
	^{131}I first year	Thyroid (infant)	50	2.9×10^{-3}	40	400
II	^{134}Cs first year	Whole body	5	2.0×10^{-5}	750	350
	^{134}Cs following years	(adult)	1	2.0×10^{-5}		50
	^{137}Cs first year	Whole body	5	1.4×10^{-5}	750	500
	^{137}Cs following years	(adult)	1	1.4×10^{-5}		100
III	^{239}Pu first year	Bone surface	50	1.7×10^{-2}	375	10
	^{239}Pu following years	(infant)	10	1.7×10^{-2}		2

Source: FAO [11].
See http://www.criirad.com/criirad/actualites/Dossiers2005/MenacesRadioactivesAliments/
Extrait%20Codex%20Anglais.doc.

The total value of food imports from the region totaled US$5 billion and the impounded imports US$0.2 million, so the economic impact from these findings was insignificant.

12.3.3 EUROPEAN UNION

12.3.3.1 Background

Regulations for radioactivity in food in the European Union (EU) are in a state of flux. Two sets of regulations are in force; the first set applies to food imported into the EU following the Chernobyl accident and the second set addresses future radiological incidents resulting in potential food contamination. Steps are being taken to rationalize and harmonize the standards.

The first set of regulations (designated as Council Regulations European Economic Communities [EEC] No. 737/90) applies to imported food products originating in third-world countries. The regulation has been amended several times and Council Regulations European Communities (EC) No. 616/2000 extended this regulation to March 31, 2010 [12]. Table 12.4 gives the maximum permissible limits for imported foods into the EU following the Chernobyl accident.

TABLE 12.4
European Union: Maximum Permissible Levels for Imported Food Into EU Following the Chernobyl Accident

Radionuclide	Milk, Milk Products, and Foodstuffs* (Bq/kg)	All Other Food Products (Bq/kg)
^{134}Cs + ^{137}Cs	370	600

* Intended for infants 4 to 6 months old.

Source: Official Journal of the European Communities [12].

The second set of regulations was passed by the EC in 1987 [13] for future radioactive food contamination incidents and was amended in 1989. These limits are called interventional levels (ILs) and are reproduced in Table 12.5. They are applicable for 3 months postincident or until amended. They apply to four radionuclide groups and five food groups and follow the recommendations of the ICRP [14]. There have been complaints about the regulations since the ^{137}Cs IL for baby foods is 370 Bq/kg for the Chernobyl contamination and 400 Bq/kg for

TABLE 12.5
European Union: Intervention Levels

Group	Radionuclide	Baby Food[a] (Bq/kg)	Dairy Products[b] (Bq/kg)	Minor Foods[c] (Bq/kg)	Other Foods[d] (Bq/kg)	Liquid Foods[e] (Bq/kg)
I	Isotopes of strontium Mainly ^{90}Sr	75	125	7,500	750	125
	Isotopes of iodine Mainly ^{131}I	150	500	20,000	2,000	500
II	α emitters of plutonium and trans-plutonium elements	1	20	800	80	20
III	All other nuclides with $T_{1/2}$ >10 days, mainly ^{134}Cs, ^{137}Cs	400	1,000	12,500	1,250	1,000

[a] Foodstuffs meant for feeding of infants in the first 4 to 6 months of life.
[b] Milk and cream only.
[c] Foods consumed in very small quantities, including herbs, spices, fats, oils, preserved fruits and nuts, caviar, and truffles.
[d] All foods not listed.
[e] Fruit and vegetable juices, bottled water, beer, wine, spirits, and vinegar.

Source: Official Journal of European Communities [13].
See http://www.es.lancs.ac.uk/casestud/case3.htm.

any future radiological event (see Table 12.4 and Table 12.5). But considering the statistical nature of radioactive decay and background subtraction, there is no significant difference between these values. More significant differences exist between the tables under the heading: Other Foods for ^{137}Cs. The limit is 1250 Bq/kg in Table 12.5 and 600 Bq/kg in Table 12.4.

12.3.3.2 Inspection and Enforcement

Under EEC Regulation No. 737/90 [12] (see Table 12.4), member states are required to monitor for compliance of imported food from third countries outside the EU. Member states are required to provide information regarding noncompliance and, in cases of repeated offenses, the EU may impose a prohibition on the importation of food from those countries. All imported food must be accompanied by a certificate stating that ^{134}Cs plus ^{137}Cs content is within Table 12.4 limits.

12.3.4 INTERNATIONAL ATOMIC ENERGY AGENCY

12.3.4.1 Background

The IAEA is the pivotal agency of the UN for nuclear safety and, since its formation in 1957, has issued the Basic Safety Series (BSS) [15], which are periodically updated. These documents provide member states with guidance and recommendations on the best practices for nuclear safety and radiation protection.

Dose limits from the Basic Safety Series No. 115-1 are

Public Exposure Dose Limits

II-8. The estimated average doses to the relevant critical groups of members of the public that are attributable to practices shall not exceed the following limits:

(a) an effective dose of 1 mSv in a year;
(b) in special circumstances, an effective dose of up to 5 mSv in a single year provided that the average dose over five years does not exceed 1 mSv per year;
(c) an equivalent dose to the lens of the eye of 15 mSv in a year; and
(d) an equivalent dose to the skin of 50 mSv in a year.

Throughout the nuclear complex, including industry, research institutes, universities, and hospitals where persons are working with radioactivity, there has been a cry for exempt limits for radionuclides in commodities. In response, the General Conference of the IAEA passed a resolution in 2000 [16] for the director general to develop "radiological criteria for long-lived radionuclides in commodities (especially foodstuffs and wood)."

12.3.4.2 Implementation

To implement the resolution, the IAEA formed a technical committee and, with assistance from specialized UN agencies and comments from member states, developed the safety guide entitled *Application of the Concepts of Exclusion, Exemption and Clearance* [17]. The guide created a basis for the derivation of radionuclide concentration limits in bulk amounts of materials and provided for the application of limits to commodities in trade (see Table 12.6). It covers both

TABLE 12.6
IAEA: Intervention Levels for Radionuclides in Bulk Amounts of Material

Group	Radionuclides	Intervention Level (Bq/kg)
I	^{129}I	10
II	^{22}Na, ^{46}Sc, ^{54}Mn, ^{56}Co, ^{60}Co, ^{65}Zn, ^{94}Nb, ^{106}Ru, ^{110m}Ag, ^{125}Sb, ^{134}Cs, ^{137}Cs, ^{152}Eu, ^{154}Eu, ^{182}Ta, ^{207}Bi, ^{229}Th, ^{232}U, ^{238}Pu, ^{239}Pu, ^{240}Pu, ^{242}Pu, ^{244}Pu, ^{241}Am, ^{242m}Am, ^{243}Am, ^{245}Cm, ^{246}Cm, ^{247}Cm, ^{248}Cm, ^{249}Cf, ^{251}Cf, ^{254}Es	100
III	^{14}C, ^{24}Na, ^{36}Cl, ^{48}Sc, ^{48}V, ^{52}Mn, ^{59}Fe, ^{57}Co, ^{58}Co, ^{75}Se, ^{82}Br, ^{85}Sr, ^{90}Sr, ^{95}Zr, ^{95}Nb, ^{96}Tc, ^{99}Tc, ^{103}Ru, ^{105}Ag, ^{109}Cd, ^{113}Sn, ^{124}Sb, ^{123m}Te, ^{132}Te, ^{136}Cs, ^{140}Ba, ^{140}La, ^{139}Ce, ^{155}Eu, ^{160}Tb, ^{181}Hf, ^{185}Os, ^{190}Ir, ^{192}Ir, ^{204}Tl, ^{206}Bi, ^{232}Th (includes thorium series), ^{233}U, ^{235}U (includes actinium series), ^{238}U (includes uranium series), ^{237}Np, ^{236}Pu, ^{243}Cm, ^{244}Cm, ^{248}Cf, ^{250}Cf, ^{252}Cf, ^{254}Cf	1,000
IV	^{7}Be, ^{18}F, ^{38}Cl, ^{40}K, ^{43}K, ^{47}Ca, ^{51}Mn, ^{52m}Mn, ^{56}Mn, ^{52}Fe, ^{55}Co, ^{62m}Co, ^{65}Ni, ^{69m}Zn, ^{72}Ga, ^{74}As, ^{76}As, ^{91}Sr, ^{92}Sr, ^{93}Zr, ^{97}Zr, ^{93m}Nb, ^{97}Nb, ^{98}Nb, ^{90}Mo, ^{93}Mo, ^{99}Mo, ^{101}Mo, ^{97}Tc, ^{97}Ru, ^{105}Ru, ^{115}Cd, ^{111}In, ^{114m}In, ^{125}Sn, ^{122}Sb, ^{127m}Te, ^{129m}Te, ^{131m}Te, ^{133}Te, ^{133m}Te, ^{134}Te, ^{126}I, ^{130}I, ^{131}I, ^{132}I, ^{133}I, ^{134}I, ^{135}I, ^{129}Cs, ^{132}Cs, ^{138}Cs, ^{131}Ba, ^{143}Ce, ^{144}Ce, ^{153}Gd, ^{181}W, ^{187}W, ^{191}Pt, ^{198}Au, ^{203}Hg, ^{200}Tl, ^{202}Tl, ^{203}Pb, ^{203}Po, ^{205}Po, ^{207}Po, ^{225}Ra, ^{230}Pa, ^{233}Pa, ^{230}U, ^{236}U, ^{240}Np, ^{241}Pu, ^{242}Cm, ^{254m}Es	10,000
V	^{3}H, ^{35}S, ^{42}K, ^{45}Ca, ^{47}Sc, ^{51}Cr, ^{53}Mn, ^{61}Co, ^{59}Ni, ^{63}Ni, ^{64}Cu, ^{86}Rb, ^{85m}Sr, ^{87m}Sr, ^{91}Y, ^{91m}Y, ^{92}Y, ^{93}Y, ^{97m}Tc, ^{99m}Tc, ^{105}Rh, ^{109}Pd, ^{111}Ag, ^{115m}Cd, ^{113m}In, ^{115m}In, ^{129}Te, ^{131}Te, ^{123}I, ^{125}I, ^{135}Cs, ^{141}Ce, ^{142}Pr, ^{147}Nd, ^{149}Nd, ^{153}Sm, ^{152m}Eu, ^{159}Gd, ^{166}Dy, ^{166}Ho, ^{171}Er, ^{170}Tm, ^{175}Yb, ^{177}Lu, ^{188}Re, ^{191}Os, ^{193}Os, ^{194}Ir, ^{197m}Pt, ^{199}Au, ^{197}Hg, ^{197m}Hg, ^{201}Tl, ^{227}Ra, ^{231}U, ^{237}U, ^{239}U, ^{240}U, ^{239}Np, ^{234}Pu, ^{235}Pu, ^{237}Pu, ^{249}Bk, ^{253}Cf, ^{253}Es, ^{255}Fm	100,000
VI	^{31}Si, ^{32}P, ^{33}P, ^{55}Fe, ^{60m}Co, ^{69}Zn, ^{73}As, ^{77}As, ^{89}Sr, ^{90}Y, ^{96m}Tc, ^{103}Pd, ^{125m}Te, ^{127}Te, ^{131}Cs, ^{134m}Cs, ^{143}Pr, ^{147}Pm, ^{149}Pm, ^{151}Sm, ^{165}Dy, ^{169}Er, ^{171}Tm, ^{185}W, ^{186}Re, ^{191m}Os, ^{193m}Pt, ^{197}Pt, ^{211}Ac, ^{226}Th, ^{243}Pu, ^{242}Am, ^{246}Cf	1,000,000
VII	^{58m}Co, ^{71}Ge, ^{103m}Rh, ^{254}Fm	10,000,000

Source: IAEA, 2004 [17].
See www.iaea.org/About/Policy/GC/GC48/Documents/gc48-8.pdf.

natural and man-made radionuclides. The guide recommends a graded approach for exclusion, exemption, and clearance and recommends that the values be verified in their application. The levels listed in Table 12.6 are used for exclusion (pursuant to BSS, paragraph 1.4); exemption (pursuant to BSS, paragraph 2.17, paragraph 2.18 and Schedule 1), and clearance (pursuant to BSS, paragraph 2.19).

12.4 NATIONAL REGULATIONS FOR RADIOACTIVITY IN FOOD AND COMMODITIES

12.4.1 AUSTRALIA

12.4.1.1 Background and Implementation

Australian Directive Canberra Act 2600 (1987), regulating radioactivity in food, was issued in response to the Chernobyl accident and remains in force [18]. Following the accident, the Minister for Community Services and Health issued an order banning the importation of any contaminated food items. A surveillance program to check for radioactivity levels in food upon arrival in Australia is in force. Only one contamination limit, for ^{137}Cs, is specified in the order. See Table 12.7.

12.4.2 LITHUANIA

12.4.2.1 Background

Lithuania has two sets of limits for edible food applicable in different circumstances and another set of limits for animal feedstuffs. The first set of limits, valid for exported food (see Table 12.8), address contamination resulting from the Chernobyl accident. This is to ensure compliance with the EU ILs for imported food (see Section 12.3.3). Contamination limits for feedstuffs are given in Table 12.9 and apply to Chernobyl contamination. Contamination limits for edible food, which apply for three months following a future radiological incident, are given in Table 12.10.

TABLE 12.7
Australia: Maximum Permissible Concentration of Radioactivity in Food

Radionuclide	Maximum Radioactive Concentration in Foodstuffs (Bq/kg)
^{137}Cs	600

Source: Australian Directive [18].
Email Geoff.Williams@arpansa.gov.au.

TABLE 12.8

Lithuania: Maximum Permissible Concentrations of Radioactive Contamination in Foodstuffs Following the Chernobyl Accident

Foodstuffs	Radionuclides	Maximum Permissible Concentration (Bq/kg)
Milk and milk products, foodstuffs for babies 4 to 6 months old	^{134}Cs and ^{137}Cs	370
Other foodstuffs	^{134}Cs and ^{137}Cs	600

Source: Lithuanian Hygiene Norm [19].
See http://www.aaa.am.lt/files/0.666753001095316895.doc.

TABLE 12.9

Lithuania: Permissible Levels of Contamination in Feedstuffs

Groups of Animals on Feedstuffs	Radionuclides	Permissible Level (Bq/kg)
Pigs	^{134}Cs and ^{137}Cs	1250
Poultry, lambs, and calves	^{134}Cs and ^{137}Cs	2500
Others	^{134}Cs and ^{137}Cs	5000

Source: Lithuanian Hygiene Norm [19].
See http://www.aaa.am.lt/files/0.666753001095316895.doc.

12.4.2.2 Enactment

The Minister of Health, by Order No. 739 (December 11, 1998), promulgated MPCs for radionuclides in food, feedstuffs, and drinking water as listed in the Lithuanian Hygiene Norm HN 84:1998 [19]. Food contamination MPCs from the Chernobyl accident are included in the norm and are tabulated in Table 12.8. The food concentration limits apply to baby food, milk, other foods (except minor foods, which have a higher MPC by a factor of 10 [i.e., $f = 0.1$]), liquid food, and drinking water. The MPCs also apply to raw materials going into food. As an added safeguard to ensure compliance with Table 12.8 limits, Lithuania has imposed limits on animal feedstuffs for cesium isotopes (Table 12.9). They apply to feed for pigs, poultry, lambs, calves, and other animals.

Table 12.10 lists MPCs for four groups of radionuclides and four types of foods in case of future radiological emergencies. The four groups of nuclides are those that might occur after a reactor incident. Group IV does not include the naturally occurring radionuclides of ^{3}H, ^{14}C, and ^{40}K. These MPCs parallel EU limits for future radiological emergencies (see Section 12.3.3).

TABLE 12.10
Lithuania: Maximum Permissible Concentrations of Radionuclides in Foodstuffs and Raw Materials After a Future Nuclear or Radiological Accident

Group	Radionuclides	Foodstuffs for Babies (Bq/kg)	Milk (Bq/kg)	Other Foodstuffs (Except Those Used in Small Amounts) (Bq/kg)	Liquid Foodstuffs (Including Drinking Water) (Bq/kg)
I	Strontium isotopes, especially [90]Sr	75	125	750	125
II	Iodine isotopes, especially [131]I	150	500	2000	500
III	Plutonium and trans-plutonium α-emitting isotopes, especially [239]Pu, [241]Am	1	20	80	20
IV	Other radionuclides with $T_{1/2} > 10$ days, especially [134]Cs, [137]Cs	400	1000	1250	1000

Note: [14]C, ^{3}H, and [40]K are not included in group IV.

Source: Lithuanian Hygiene Norm [19].

Email rsc@rsc.lt.
See http://www.aaa.am.lt/files/0.666753001095316895.doc.

12.4.2.3 Inspection and Enforcement

Under the order, imported and exported food is monitored for radioactivity. The Lithuanian Radiation Protection Services conducts these measurements and completes the laboratory certificates required for the export of mushrooms and forest berries to EU member states.

12.4.3 UKRAINE

12.4.3.1 Background

From April 26 to May 6, 1986, Unit Four of the Chernobyl Nuclear Power Station exploded and the core melted, spewing fission and activation products all over the globe. Estimates of long-lived radionuclides released are [20]

- ^{137}Cs, 8.6×10^{16} Bq (2.3 MCi; 1.5 MCi in 2005).
- ^{90}Sr, 8×10^{15} Bq (0.22 MCi; 0.14 MCi in 2005).
- ^{239}Pu, 3.4×10^{13} Bq (0.92 kCi; no change).
- ^{240}Pu, 5.3×10^{13} Bq (1.4 kCi; no change).

Ukraine was heavily contaminated with the larger particles containing strontium and plutonium isotopes that were deposited close to the reactor site. Smaller particulates of cesium and iodine isotopes were spread all over the Northern Hemisphere. Radioactivity in food has been a major concern in Ukraine and its neighbors in Europe ever since. The most heavily contaminated areas were evacuated, an exclusion zone was set up, and radioactivity limits in food were established.

12.4.3.2 Implementation

Ukrainian regulations governing radioactive contamination were issued initially in 1991 for the most heavily affected regions of Kiev, Volynski, and Zhytomyr. New updated regulations were issued and approved by the Ministry of Health in 1997, effective January 1, 1998, for acceptable levels of ^{137}Cs and ^{90}Sr in food for 16 food groups, including drinking water (AL-97). These are still in force and are reproduced in Table 12.11. The standards are based on a typical Ukrainian diet and should limit public exposure to less than 1 mSv/yr, committed effective dose equivalent, if enforced. These limits were established by the National Commission on Radiation Protection of the Population of Ukraine in cooperation with the Committee for Hygiene Regulations of the Ministry of Health Protection [20].

If an individual consumes a standard diet within the AL-97 limits for ^{137}Cs he will receive 1 mSv/yr or less and a similar amount for ^{90}Sr. But if the food is contaminated with both ^{137}Cs and ^{90}Sr, the limit is determined by the sum of fractions formula for each food item to maintain the individual dose at less than 1 mSv/yr (committed effective dose equivalent).

12.4.3.3 Inspection and Enforcement

Ukraine is in a recovery phase following the acute phase of the Chernobyl accident of 1986 in which 29 persons died of radiation sickness and 130,000 people were evacuated in a 30 km (18.6 mile) radius of the reactor site. Today, monitoring of the environment is done by numerous agencies. Radioactivity in food is spot-checked, and special measurements will be made only after future releases of a large amount of activity. Measurements for the radioactive content of building materials and timber are also required. Ukraine puts the responsibility on the producers and manufacturers of food and commodities for compliance with AL-97 limits, as given in Table 12.11. Besides radioactive decay, natural processes have diluted the Chernobyl contamination in the environment, but one must be cautious since there may be some reconcentration processes at work.

TABLE 12.11
Ukraine: Acceptable Levels for ^{137}Cs and ^{90}Sr in Foodstuffs and Potable Water (1997)

Foodstuffs	AL: ^{137}Cs (Bq/kg)	AL: ^{90}Sr (Bq/kg)
Bread and bread products	20	5
Potatoes	60	20
Vegetables (root and leafy)	40	20
Fruits	70	10
Meat and meat products	200	20
Fish and fish products	150	35
Milk and milk products	100	20
Egg per unit	6	2
Water (per l)	2	2
Milk concentrated	300	60
Milk powdered	500	100
Fresh wild berries and mushrooms	500	50
Dried wild berries and mushrooms	2500	250
Drug plants (herbs)	600	200
Others	600	200
Special infant food	40	5

Source: UNECE 1997 [20].
See www.unece.org/env/epr/studies/ukraine/chapter04.pdf.

12.4.4 U.S. FOOD AND DRUG ADMINISTRATION

12.4.4.1 Background

The FDA Center for Food Safety and Applied Nutrition (CFSAN) issued the Compliance Policy Guide (CPG) for radioactivity in food starting in June 1986 in response to the Chernobyl accident. In the original CPG, the concentration limit term used was levels of concern (LOC). In recent years, ILs have been used since the CAC, FAO, and WHO use the term. The term, in recent CPG revisions, is now derived intervention level (DIL) [21]. In some cases, DILs are higher than the LOCs due to different underlying assumptions in their derivation. The only concern in the original CPG guide was for accidents at reactors and other large sources of radioactivity releases, but the latest CPG addresses radiological accidents and malevolent intent that may contaminate the food supply.

The CPG limits are based on the following public dose limits:

- $D = 5$ mSv/yr (500 mrem/yr), committed effective dose equivalent.
- $D = 50$ mSv/yr (5000 mrem/yr), committed dose equivalent to individual organ or tissue.

These values are as recommended in the ICRP publication, *Protection of the Public in Event of a Major Radiological Accident: Principals for Planning* [14]

12.4.4.2 Promulgation

Derived intervention levels are not absolute upper limits and, due to the many conservative assumptions in their derivation, they leave room for flexibility in their enforcement. CPG is a "should" and not a "shall" regulation. There are other regulations under which enforcement action may be taken. Enforcement actions are based on radioactivity measurements or circumstances surrounding the contamination. Various federal statutes exist under which foodstuffs can be seized or detained at a port of entry.

12.4.4.3 Derived Intervention Levels

Fortunately an explanation of the derivation of DILs is given in a lucid presentation with all the underlying assumptions and dose factors in *Accidental Radioactive Contamination of Human Food and Animal Feeds: Recommendations for State and Local Agencies* [22]. DILs in Table 12.12 are derived for five radionuclide groups from a detailed analysis of total diet for six age groups: 3 months, 1 year, 5 years, 10 years, 15 years, and adult. The diets are based on U.S. Department of Agriculture (USDA) and U.S. Environmental Protection Agency (EPA) studies [23–25].

The *f* factor in Equation 12.1 determines what fraction of the food intake (*FI*) is assumed to be contaminated. In an actual accident scenario, it is assumed that alternate food sources would be available over time, therefore $f = 0.1$, as recommended by the CAC and FAO, but the FDA uses $f = 0.3$ to account for some subgroups that may not have access to alternate food sources. Finally, for infants (3 months and 1 year), $f = 1$ due to the great dependence on narrow food types. With these assumptions, the DILs were obtained.

TABLE 12.12
U.S. FDA Derived Intervention Levels

Group	Radionuclides	Derived Intervention Level Bq/kg	Derived Intervention Level pCi/kg
I	^{90}Sr	160	4,300
II	^{131}I	170	4,600
III	^{134}Cs + ^{137}Cs	1,200	32,000
IV	^{238}Pu + ^{239}Pu + ^{241}Am	2	54
V	^{103}Ru + ^{106}Ru	$\frac{C_3}{6800} + \frac{C_6}{450} < 1$	$\frac{C_3}{180,000} + \frac{C_6}{12,000} < 1$

Source: FDA, July 2004 [21].
See http://www.cfsan.fda.gov/~dms/nucleve2.html.

Example: For ^{90}Sr intake in a 15-year-old child, bone exposure gives the most limiting DIL.

Assume:
   $D = 50$ mSv/yr, committed dose equivalent,
   $f = 0.3$,
   $FI = 869$ kg/yr,
   $DC = 1.2 \times 10^{-3}$ mSv/yr.

$$DIL = \frac{50 \text{ mSv/y}}{(0.3)(869 \text{ kg/y})(1.2 \times 10^{-3} \text{ mSv/Bq})}$$

$$DIL = 160 \text{ Bq/kg.}$$

For the other four groups of nuclides a similar analysis determines the most limiting value. Also, it is assumed that the values can be applied independently for each radionuclide group. In the case of ^{103}Ru and ^{106}Ru the combination DIL is limited by the sum of the fractions rule because of the wide disparity in their individual DILs.

The original selection of radionuclides in Table 12.12 was based on Chernobyl experience. Using the same methodology, DILs were determined for 15 additional radionuclides. These results are given in Table 12.13, but are not formally part of the CPG.

12.4.4.4 Surveillance and Enforcement

While the CPG provides recommended DILs in the food supply, the values are not regulatory upper limits. An ongoing surveillance program of radioactivity in food under CFSAN is in place to detect any deviation from background levels. The program surveys around U.S. nuclear power plants and imported food at the borders. γ-spectrum analysis is done to quickly identify photon-emitting nuclides, and results are available within a few days. ^{90}Sr, a β emitter, analysis is more tedious and takes 1 to 2 weeks for results. As noted, enforcement can be taken or prosecution can occur under various statutes.

12.4.5 U.S. NUCLEAR REGULATORY COMMISSION

12.4.5.1 Background

The NRC regulations for occupational and public exposure to radiation have a long history. The original regulations were promulgated 50 years ago under the authority granted to the U.S. Atomic Energy Commission (AEC), a predecessor agency of the NRC. The authorizing authority was contained in the Atomic Energy Act of 1954, amended many times since that date. The regulations are promulgated in the Code of Federal Regulations (CFR) cited as 10 CFR Part 20 [26]

TABLE 12.13
U.S. FDA DILs for Other Radionuclides

Radionuclide	Derived Intervention Level (Bq/kg)
^{89}Sr	1,400
^{91}Y	1,200
^{95}Zr	4,000
^{95}Nb	12,000
^{132}Te	4,000
^{129}I	56
^{133}I	7,000
^{140}Ba	6,900
^{141}Ce	7,200
^{144}Ce	500
^{237}Np	4
^{239}Np	28,000
^{241}Pu	120
^{242}Cm	19
^{244}Cm	2

Source: FDA [22].
See http://www.fda.gov/cdrh/dmqrp/84.html.

for exposure limits. The regulations cover possession, use, and disposal of three broad classes of radionuclides:

- Source material: natural uranium, natural thorium, and depleted uranium.
- Special nuclear material: plutonium, ^{325}U, ^{233}U.
- By-product material: fission products and activation products.

Since this chapter covers mainly public exposure, the occupational concentration limits in air and water for various nuclides will not be listed, but they are easily accessed at the NRC website at www.nrc.gov, then click on links to Part 20 and specific nuclides of interest.

As specified in 10 CFR Part 20 [26], public dose limits are:

§20.1301 Dose limits for individual members of the public.

(a) Each licensee shall conduct operations so that –

   (1) The total effective dose equivalent to individual members of the public from the licensed operation does not exceed 0.1 rem (1 mSv) in a year, exclusive of the dose contribution from background radiation, from any administration the individual has received from exposure, to individuals administered radioactive material and release under §35.75, from voluntary participation in medical

research programs, and from the licensee's disposal of radioactive material into sanitary sewerage in accordance with §20.2003, and

(2) The dose in any unrestricted area from external sources, exclusive of the dose contribution from patients administered radioactive material and released in accordance with §35.75, does not exceed 0.002 rem (0.02 mSv) in any one hour.

(b) If the licensee permits members of the public to have access to controlled areas, the limits for members of the public continue to apply to those individuals.

(c) Notwithstanding (a)(1) of this section, a licensee may permit visitors to an individual who cannot be released, under §35.75, to receive a radiation dose greater than 0.1 rem (1 mSv) if –

(1) The radiation dose received does not exceed 0.5 rem (5 mSv); and

(2) The authorized user, as defined in 10 CFR Part 35, has determined before the visit that it is appropriate.

(d) A license applicant may apply for prior NRC authorization to operate up to an annual dose limit for an individual member of the public of 0.5 rem (5 mSv). The licensee or license applicant shall include the following information in this application:

(1) Demonstration of the need for and the expected duration of operations in excess of the limit in paragraph (a) of this section;

(2) The licensee's program to assess and control dose within the 0.5 rem (5 mSv) annual limit; and

(3) The procedures to be followed to maintain the dose as low as is reasonably achievable.

(e) In addition to the requirements of this part, a licensee subject to the provisions of EPA's generally applicable environmental radiation standards in 40 CFR Part 190 shall comply with those standards.

(f) The Commission may impose additional restrictions on radiation levels in unrestricted areas and on the total quantity of radionuclides that a licensee may release in effluents in order to restrict the collective dose.

The public concentration limits for selected radionuclides are given in Table 12.14. An example of how they were derived is given as follows:

Example: inhalation exposure to ^{90}Sr for long-term deposition (Y retention class).

Assume:

$D = 0.5$ mSv/yr, committed effective dose equivalent, includes a factor of 0.5 to cover all age groups

FI (air intake) $= 7.2 \times 10^9$ ml/yr,

$f = 1$,

$DC = 3.4 \times 10^{-4}$ mSv/Bq [10].

TABLE 12.14

U.S. NRC Air and Water Concentration Limits in the Environment for Selected Radionuclides

		Effluent Concentrations		Releases to Sewers
Radionuclide	Class	Air (μCi/ml)	Water (μCi/ml)	Monthly Average Concentration (μCi/ml)
^{3}H	Water	1×10^{-7}	1×10^{-3}	1×10^{-2}
^{14}C	Monoxide	2×10^{-6}	—	—
	Dioxide	3×10^{-7}	—	—
	Compounds	3×10^{-9}	3×10^{-5}	3×10^{-4}
^{60}Co	W	2×10^{-10}	3×10^{-6}	3×10^{-5}
	Y	5×10^{-11}	—	—
^{90}Sr	D	3×10^{-11}	5×10^{-7}	5×10^{-6}
	Y	6×10^{-12}	—	—
^{131}I	D, all compounds	2×10^{-10}	1×10^{-6}	1×10^{-5}
^{134}Cs	D, all compounds	2×10^{-10}	9×10^{-7}	9×10^{-6}
^{137}Cs	D, all compounds	2×10^{-10}	1×10^{-6}	1×10^{-5}
^{192}Ir	D	4×10^{-10}	1×10^{-5}	1×10^{-4}
	W	6×10^{-10}	—	—
	Y	3×10^{-10}	—	—
^{226}Ra	W, all compounds	9×10^{-13}	6×10^{-8}	6×10^{-7}
^{232}Th	W	4×10^{-13}	3×10^{-8}	3×10^{-7}
	Y	6×10^{-13}	—	—
^{235}U	D	3×10^{-12}	3×10^{-7}	3×10^{-6}
	W	1×10^{-12}	—	—
	Y	6×10^{-14}	—	—
^{238}U	D	3×10^{-12}	3×10^{-7}	3×10^{-6}
	W	1×10^{-12}	—	—
	Y	6×10^{-14}	—	—
^{238}Pu	W	2×10^{-14}	2×10^{-8}	2×10^{-7}
	Y	2×10^{-14}	—	—
^{239}Pu	W	2×10^{-14}	2×10^{-8}	2×10^{-7}
	Y	2×10^{-14}	—	—
^{241}Am	W	2×10^{-14}	2×10^{-8}	2×10^{-7}
	Y	2×10^{-14}	—	—

Notes: D, W, and Y refer to three classes of radioactive material particles with an activity median aerodynamic diameter (AMAD) of 1 μm with a retention in the pulmonary region of the lung in approximately days (D), weeks (W), or years (Y).

To convert values of μCi/ml to Bq/l, multiply by 3.7×10^7.

Source: NRC [26].

See http://www.nrc.gov/reading-rm/doc-collections/cfr/part020/appb/#A.

$$MPC = \frac{0.5 \ \text{mSv/y}}{(1)(7.2 \times 10^9 \ \text{ml/y})(3.4 \times 10^{-4} \ \text{mSv/Bq})}$$

$MPC = 2 \times 10^{-7}$ Bq/ml (6×10^{-12} μCi/ml).

12.4.5.2 Inspection and Enforcement

Persons possessing radioactive material, as defined in the regulations (Title 10 CFR), must obtain a license to possess and use radioactive material and to dispose of it in an acceptable manner. Inspections are conducted on a priority basis according to application, nuclide, quantity, and hazard. Nuclear power reactors have onsite NRC inspectors. Violations of regulations can result in fines, and in a few cases, due to willful neglect leading to injury, incarceration. Under Section 274 of the Atomic Energy Act of 1954, as amended, some licensing, inspection, and enforcement functions are delegated to individual states where the state governor has signed an agreement with the NRC. These agreement states must promulgate and enforce regulations that are compatible with those of the NRC.

Clean up of radioactively contaminated sites for unrestricted use is a common occurrence in modern industrial societies. What release criteria to use, and whether a site has met the criteria, has been a contentious issue. Normally, release criteria is dose based, depending on the jurisdiction and future use of the site. The dose criteria may be 5, 1, 0.5, 0.25, 0.15, 0.1, or 0.04 mSv/yr. Based on the release dose, one can determine the derived concentration guidance level (DCGL) for various exposure scenarios. The problem is then to determine if the site meets the DCGL. MARSSIM [27] is a statistical tool that aids in demonstrating compliance with site release criteria. Unfortunately this approach can be expensive and probably will only be utilized at major radioactively contaminated sites, and even then the approach sometimes fails when the release criteria are changed.

12.4.6 JAPAN

12.4.6.1 Background

Japan, with a modern industrial economy and a population of about 125 million tightly packed on four islands (Honshu, Kyushu, Shikoku, and Hokaido), utilizes copious amounts of electricity. Due to limited indigenous fossil fuel sources, Japan produces 30% of its electric power from 51 nuclear power plants. There is a strong nuclear support industry, including fuel fabrication installations. Cognizant of the possibility of nuclear accidents, Japan has a Nuclear Safety Commission, which has developed a set of emergency guidelines, entitled "Emergency Preparedness of Nuclear Installations" [28]. The original guide was promulgated in June 1980 and the latest revision is dated June 2001. The Tokaimura accident in September 1999 taxed the response system and now the guidelines include standards for notification, sheltering, evacuation, and limits for contamination of edible foods.

TABLE 12.15
Japan: Emergency Preparedness Guidelines for Limits in Food and Drinking Water

Group	Radionuclides	Drinking Water and Dairy Products (Bq/kg)	Vegetables, Grain, Meat, Eggs, Fish (Bq/kg)
I	^{131}I	300	2000
II	^{134}Cs and ^{137}Cs	200	500
III	Uranium isotopes	20	100
IV	α-emitting nuclides of plutonium and transuranic nuclides (^{238}Pu, ^{239}Pu, ^{240}Pu, ^{242}Pu, ^{241}Am, ^{242}Cm, ^{243}Cm, ^{244}Cm)	1	10

Source: The Emergency Preparedness Guidelines "Emergency Preparedness of Nuclear Installations" (Excerpt), Nuclear Safety Commission, Latest Revision: June, 2001 [28].
See http://www.jnes.go.jp/bonsaipage/english/an-3-12.htm.

12.4.6.2 Implementation

The guide stipulates an emergency planning zone of 8 to 10 km around nuclear power plants and research reactors with a power level greater than 50 MW. Table 12.15 provides concentration limits for radioactive contamination limits for four radionuclide groups in two food groups. While no information is provided on the *f* values, the portion of the food contaminated, or the dose limit, the limits are consistent with the FAO limits, as described in Section 12.3.2.

12.4.7 CANADA

12.4.7.1 Background

Health Canada, under authority of the Food and Drugs Act [29], is responsible for the safety of all domestic and imported food offered for sale within Canada. Under this authority, Health Canada has promulgated guidelines, called action levels, for radioactivity contaminants in commercial food and public drinking water supplies. This agency succinctly states that the object and implementation of the guidelines in a nuclear emergency are to minimize public health risks and to preserve public confidence in the safety of the public food supply. Enforcement of the guidelines for food is the responsibility of the Canadian Food Inspection Agency under existing rules of coordination with provincial authorities and the food industry. Implementation of public drinking water standards is the responsibility of federal, provincial, or municipal authorities depending on existing protocols.

TABLE 12.16
Canada: Recommended Action Levels for Radionuclides of Potential Significance to Dose from the Ingestion of Contaminated Food

Group	Radionuclides	Fresh Liquid Milk (Bq/kg)	Other Commercial Foods and Beverages (Bq/kg)	Public Drinking Water (Bq/l)
I	^{89}Sr	300	1000	300
II	^{90}Sr	30	100	30
III	^{103}Ru	1000	1000	1000
IV	^{106}Ru	100	300	100
V	^{131}I	100	1000	100
VI	^{134}Cs, ^{137}Cs	300	1000	100
VII	^{238}Pu, ^{230}Pu, ^{240}Pu, ^{242}Pu, ^{241}Am	1	10	1

Source: Health Canada [29].
See www.hc-sc.gc.ca/hecs-sesc/rpb/pdf/01hecs254.pdf.

12.4.7.2 Implementation

Action levels were derived for three food groups: fresh liquid milk, other commercial foods and beverages, and public drinking water for six age groups. These action levels, given in Table 12.16, are for seven of the most significant radionuclides based on past experience, such as the Chernobyl accident. Due to conservatism used in deriving the action levels and the likelihood of alternate food availability in an emergency, the action levels can be applied independently for each food group. For multiple radionuclide contaminants in each food group, the standard sum of fractions rule is recommended. As indicated above, these action levels, except public drinking water values, are the responsibility of the Canadian Food Inspection Agency under existing protocols with the individual provinces and territories.

12.4.7.3 Comparison of Standards for Radioactivity in Food

Health Canada guidelines [29] provide an overview of the various recommendations on radioactivity in food in a unique table. The table has been updated and reproduced in Table 12.17 in amended form. It is helpful in gaining an understanding of the various regulations and recommendations now in force and their underlying premises, as well as their complexity. This is also an area in flux. For example, IAEA standards have now been issued covering a broadly defined category called commodities. We have updated the Codex reference with their recent recommendations and dropped Health Canada's reference to the WHO recommendations, since WHO now follows the Codex Alimentarius recommendations.

TABLE 12.17

Comparison of Methodologies Presently in Use by Various Organizations (Adapted from Health Canada Guidelines [29])

Organization	Intervention Level (mSv/yr)	Food Groups	Contamination Factor (f)	Action Level Groups	Implementation
Health Canada	1 (per food group)	3	$f = 1$ for fresh liquid milk; $f = 0.2$ for all other foods	Individual radionuclides	Applied independently between food groups; all radionuclides additive within a single food group
IAEA	Optimized action levels derived from cost-benefit analysis	2	Not applicable	7	Applied independently between food groups; all radionuclides additive within a single food group
Codex Alimentarius	1	Applies to total diet	$f = 0.1$, except minor foods; $f = 0.01$	4	Applied independently to each radionuclide group, but within each group the sum of concentrations must be less than the action level
U.S. FDA	5, CEDE 50, CDE for thyroid and bone	Applies to total diet	$f = 0.3$, except $f = 1$ diet for infants 3 months to 1 year	5	Each radionuclide group action level can be applied independently, but within each group the DILs are summed except for ruthenium isotopes

Source: authors.

12.5 INTERNATIONAL REGULATIONS FOR RADIOACTIVITY IN DRINKING WATER

12.5.1 WORLD HEALTH ORGANIZATION

12.5.1.1 Background

The WHO is charged with advising member states on matters of good health practice. Since 1981 WHO has issued three editions of its publication *Guidelines for Drinking Water Quality, Volume 1, 3rd Edition* [30]. It is well known that the single most important measure that can be taken to enhance worldwide public health is to improve drinking water quality. Fortunately radioactive contaminants in drinking water are not a common water quality problem. But it is of public concern, and public health officials must screen for the presence of radioactivity in drinking water.

Drinking water standards are different from most limits in this chapter because they apply to public drinking water supplies with the assumption that individuals are drinking the water throughout their entire lifespan. The latest WHO standard is based on a public committed effective dose of 0.1 mSv/yr (10 mrem/yr). This dose limit is set at 10% of the ICRP recommended public dose of 1 mSv/yr above the natural background radiation level. It is explicitly stated, in the case of radiological incidents, that temporary elevated radioactive contamination standards in drinking water may be used. This dose standard is premised on the linear no threshold theory, which holds that some radiation, no matter how low, may present some incremental risk of cancer. In many areas around the world, people drink mineral waters with a high radiation content for their health, on a temporary basis.

12.5.1.2 Implementation

There are two standards for maintaining clean drinking water recommended by WHO. One is a screening standard set at a very low level that can be implemented by most drinking water authorities around the world. The WHO screening standard is set at 0.5 Bq/l (gross α activity) and 1 Bq/l (gross β activity). If the screening standard is exceeded, specific analysis must be performed to identify the nuclides present. GLs for selected radionuclides are given in Table 12.18. In case more than one nuclide is present, the sum of fractions limitation should be used to ensure that the dose limit is not exceeded.

Guidance levels exclude ^{40}K activity, which is ubiquitous, and its content in the human body is controlled by homeostasis. ^{40}K activity should be determined separately and subtracted from the gross β activity. Radon (^{222}Rn) and thoron (^{220}Rn) are also ubiquitous and should be determined separately. They are noble gases and are given off by drinking water in the water supply system and should not normally interfere with screening counts. These nuclides should also be evaluated on a separate basis because they may contribute to an inhalation and external dose in homes and working spaces. The WHO *Guidelines on Drinking*

TABLE 12.18
WHO Drinking Water Standards
for Selected Radionuclides

Radionuclides	Dose Conversion (mSv/Bq)	Guidance Level (Bq/l)[a]
^{3}H	1.8×10^{-8}	10,000
^{14}C	5.8×10^{-7}	100
^{60}Co	3.4×10^{-6}	100
^{89}Sr	2.6×10^{-6}	100
^{90}Sr	2.8×10^{-5}	10
^{129}I	1.1×10^{-4}	1000
^{131}I	2.2×10^{-5}	10
^{134}Cs	1.9×10^{-5}	10
^{137}Cs	1.3×10^{-5}	10
^{210}Pb	6.9×10^{-4}	0.1
^{210}Po[b]	1.2×10^{-3}	0.1
^{224}Ra[b]	6.5×10^{-5}	1
^{226}Ra[b]	2.8×10^{-4}	1
^{228}Ra[b]	6.9×10^{-4}	0.1
^{232}Th[b]	2.3×10^{-4}	1
^{238}U[b,c]	4.5×10^{-5}	10
^{234}U[b]	4.9×10^{-5}	10
^{239}Pu	2.5×10^{-4}	1

[a] Guidance levels are rounded by averaging the log scale values (to 10^{n} if the calculated value was less than 3×10^{n} and greater than 3×10^{n1}).
[b] Natural radionuclides.
[c] The provisional guideline value for uranium in drinking water is 15 µg/l based on its chemical toxicity for the kidney.

Source: WHO, 2004 [30].

See http://www.who.int/water_sanitation_health/dwq/gdwq3/en.

Water Quality [30] recommend the pylon technique for determination of radon activity, which uses a water degassing unit and Lucas scintillation chamber. WHO recommends a GL of 100 Bq/l for ^{222}Rn.

Example: to determine drinking water GLs, use Equation 12.1.

Assume for ^{14}C:
$D = 0.1$ mSv/yr, committed effective dose equivalent,
$f = 1$,
$FI = 730$ l/yr,
$DC = 5.8 \times 10^{-7}$ mSv/Bq [7].

$$GL = \frac{0.1 \text{ mSv/y}}{(1)(730 \text{ L/y})(5.8 \times 10^{-7} \text{ mSv/Bq})}$$

$GL = 236$ Bq/kg.

As described in the WHO [30], the value is rounded as follows: If GL is between 3×10^n and $3 \times 10^{n-1}$, then the GL = 10^n. Therefore, in this case, the GL of 236 is between 30 and 300, then GL = 100 Bq/l.

12.5.1.3 Inspection and Enforcement

The WHO recommends that all new public drinking water supplies should be screened for their radionuclide content to comply with the screening standards mentioned above. For good statistical results, it is recommended that samples should be taken quarterly in the first year and subsequently every five years after installation of a water supply system.

In case the screening standard is exceeded, then more sophisticated radio-chemical analysis is necessary. In rare instances where GLs are exceeded, installation of a filtration system or alternate public water supplies may need to be considered, remembering the cost and the significant safety factors that are incorporated in the GLs in Table 12.18.

12.6 NATIONAL REGULATIONS FOR RADIOACTIVITY IN DRINKING WATER

12.6.1 U.S. Environmental Protection Agency Drinking Water Standards

12.6.1.1 Background and Implementation

The EPA is empowered by law [31] to set enforceable standards for public drinking water supplies in the U.S. The drinking water standards assume a water intake (FI) of 2 l/day, 365 days/yr, and a public dose limit of 0.04 mSv/yr (4 mrem/yr). This dose limit is defined as the dose equivalent and is based on the methodology and terms in earlier publications of the NCRP [32]. The regulation has two standards. One standard is defined as the maximum contaminant level goal (MCLG), which is zero, and the second is maximum contaminant level (MCL). Four groups of radionuclides are listed (see Table 12.19): group I, α particles; group II, β particles and photon emitters; group III, ^{226}Ra plus ^{228}Ra; and group IV, uranium.

Using the methodology of the NCRP, one can derive drinking water maximum permissible concentrations for other selected radionuclides, and these concentration limits are listed in Table 12.20 [31]. Obviously, at the low dose limit, the only human detriment arises from cancer risk, and this is based on the linear no-threshold

TABLE 12.19
U.S. EPA Primary Drinking Water Standards

Nuclides	MCLG		MCL	
	pCi/l	Bq/l	pCi/l	Bq/l
α particles (excluding uranium, ^{226}Ra, and ^{228}Ra)	0	0	15 (see Table 12.20)	0.56 (see Table 12.20)
β particles and photon emitters	0	0	Internal dose $\leq$ 0.04 mSv/yr (see Table 12.20)	
^{226}Ra and ^{228}Ra (combined)	0	0	5	0.19
Uranium	0	0	30 µg/l	30 µg/l

Source: EPA [31].
See http://www.epa.gov/safewater/mcl.html.

TABLE 12.20
U.S. EPA Derived Drinking Water Standards

Nuclide	pCi/l	Bq/l	Nuclide	pCi/l	Bq/l	Nuclide	pCi/l	Bq/l
^{227}Ac	—	—	^{153}Gd	600	22	^{125}Sb	300	11
^{108m}Ag	—	—	^{3}H	20,000	740	^{147}Sm	15	0.56
^{110m}Ag	90	3.3	^{129}I	1	0.037	^{151}Sm	1,000	37
^{241}Am	15	0.56	^{40}K	—	—	^{90}Sr	8	0.3
^{243}Am	15	0.56	^{54}Mn	300	11	^{99}Tc	900	33
^{207}Bi	200	7.4	^{22}Na	400	15	^{228}Th	15	0.56
^{14}C	2,000	74	^{94}Nb	—	—	^{229}Th	15	0.56
^{109}Cd	600	22	^{59}Ni	300	11	^{230}Th	15	0.56
^{144}Ce	30	1.1	^{63}Ni	50	1.9	^{232}Th	15	0.56
^{36}Cl	700	26	^{237}Np	15	0.56	^{204}Tl	300	11
^{243}Cm	15	0.56	^{231}Pa	15	0.56	^{232}U	20	0.74
^{244}Cm	15	0.56	^{210}Pb	—	—	^{233}U	20	0.74
^{248}Cm	15	0.56	^{147}Pm	587	22	^{234}U	20	0.74
^{57}Co	1,000	37	^{238}Pu	15	0.56	^{235}U	20	0.74
^{60}Co	100	3.7	^{239}Pu	15	0.56	^{236}U	20	0.74
^{134}Cs	80	3.0	^{240}Pu	15	0.56	^{238}U	20	0.74
^{135}Cs	900	33	^{241}Pu	—	—	^{65}Zn	300	11
^{137}Cs	200	7.4	^{242}Pu	15	0.56			
^{152}Eu	200	7.4	^{244}Pu	15	0.56			
^{154}Eu	60	2.2	^{226}Ra	5	0.19			
^{155}Eu	600	22	^{228}Ra	5	0.19			
^{55}Fe	2,000	74	^{106}Ru	30	1.1			

Note: Values are based on an individual dose equal to 0.04 mSv/yr (4 mrem/yr) to the whole body or an organ combined from all β and photon emitters.

Source: EPA [31].
See http://www.epa.gov/oerrpage/superfund/resources/radiation/att_d-clean.pdf.

theory of radiation damage. This dose limit of 0.04 mSv/yr (4 mrem/yr) is about 1.5% of the average background dose that everyone is exposed to on this planet.

12.6.2 NEW ZEALAND

12.6.2.1 Background and Implementation

In 2000, the New Zealand Ministry of Health published a stringent drinking water standard for radioactive contamination [33]. The standard specifies radon concentrations in drinking water that are close to the recently recommended WHO standard for radon in water. Table 12.21 lists the maximum acceptable values (MAVs) for gross α and β activity exclusive of radon and ^{40}K determinands.

TABLE 12.21
New Zealand: Maximum Acceptable Values for Radiological Determinands

Radioactive Constituents	Maximum Acceptable Values (Bq/l)
Total α activity	0.10, excluding radon
Total β activity	0.50, excluding ^{40}K
Radon	100

Source: Drinking Water Standards for New Zealand, 2000 [33]. See http://www.moh.govt.nz.

REFERENCES

1. United Nations Scientific Committee on Effects of Atomic Radiation, New York, 2000.
2. Department for Environment, Food and Rural Affairs, United Kingdom.
3. New York State, *The Industrial Code, Rule 38, Radiation Protection*, Albany, NY, 1955.
4. National Committee on Radiation Protection, *Report of Subcommittee on Permissible Internal Dose*, Handbook 52, National Bureau of Standards, Washington, DC, 1953.
5. Codex Alimentarius Commission, *Contaminants: Guideline Levels for Radionuclides in Food Following Accidental Nuclear Contamination for Use in International Trade, Supplemental to Codex Alimentarius, Vol. XVII*, 1st ed., Joint FAO/WHO Food Standards Program, Rome, 2004.
6. International Commission on Radiation Protection, Publication 60, Pergamon Press, Oxford, 1991.
7. Eckerman, K.F., in *Effective Dose Coefficients for Selected Radionuclides, Appendix A.4, Public Protection from Nuclear, Chemical and Biological Terrorism*, Brodsky, A., Johnson, R.H., Jr., and Goans, R.E., eds., Medical Physics Publishing, Madison, WI, 2004.

8. Randall, A.W., *Radionuclide Contamination of Foods: FAO Recommended Limits*, Food Quality and Standards Service, FAO, Rome, undated.

9. Johnson, J.R. and Dunsford. D.W., *Dose Conversion Factors for Intakes of Select Radionuclides by Infants and Children*, Chalk River Atomic Energy of Canada, Ltd., Canada, 1983.

10. International Commission on Radiological Protection *Limits for Intake of Radionuclides by Workers*, Publication 30, ICRP, Paris, 1979.

11. Food and Agriculture Organization , *Report of the Expert Consideration on Recommended Limits for Radionuclide Content of Food*, FAO, Rome, 1987.

12. Official Journal, Council Regulation (EC) no. 616/2000 and Council Regulation (EEC) no. 737/90, Brussels, 2000.

13. Official Journal, Council Regulation (EC) no. 3954/87, Brussels, 1987.

14. International Commission on Radiation Protection , *Protection of Public in Event of Major Radiation Accidents: Principles for Planning*, Publication 40, Pergamon Press, Oxford, 1984.

15. International Atomic Energy Agency, *International Basic Safety Standards for Protection Against Ionizing Radiation and for the Safety of Radiation Sources*, Safety Series no. 115-1, IAEA, Vienna, 1994.

16. International Atomic Energy Agency, *Radiological Criteria for Radioactivity in Commodities*, Report by the Director General, IAEA, Vienna, 2004.

17. International Atomic Energy Agency, *Application of Concepts of Exclusion, Exemption and Clearance*, Safety Guide RS-G-1.7, IAEA, Vienna, 2004.

18. Australian Directive Canberra Act 2600, issued by the Minister for Community Services and Health, Canberra, 1987.

19. Lithuanian Hygiene Norm, no. 84-1998, approved by Minister of Hygiene, Order no. 739, December 11, 1998.

20. U.N. Economic and Social Council, *Environmental Performance Review of Ukraine*, United Nations, New York, 1999.

21. U.S. Food and Drug Administration, *Radionuclides in Domestic and Imported Foods*, Compliance Policy Guide 7119.14, Section 560.750, FDA, Washington, DC, 2004.

22. U.S. Food and Drug Administration, "Accidental Radioactive Contamination of Human Food and Animal Feeds, Recommendations for State and Local Agencies," *Federal Register* 63:4342.413403, Rockville, MD, August 13, 1998.

23. U.S. Department of Agriculture, *Food Intakes: Individuals in 49 States, Year 1977–1978*, Report no. T-1, U.S. Department of Agriculture, Washington, DC, August, 1983.

24. U.S. Environmental Protection Agency, *An Estimation of the Daily Food Intake Based on Data from the 1977–1978 USDA Nationwide Food Consumption Survey*, EPA 520/I-84-015, EPA, Washington, DC, 1984.

25. U.S. Environmental Protection Agency, *An Estimation of the Daily Average Food Intake by Age and Sex for Use in Assessing the Radionuclide Intake of Individuals in the General Population*, EPA 520/I-84-021, EPA, Washington, DC, 1984.

26. U.S. Nuclear Regulatory Commission, Title 10 Code of Federal Regulations (CFR), Part 20 (cited as 10 CFR Part 20), Standards for Protection Against Radiation, NRC, Washington, DC.

27. U.S. Nuclear Regulatory Commission, *Multi-Agency Radiation Survey and Site Investigation Manual*, NUREG-1575, NRC, Rockville, MD, 2000.

28. Nuclear Safety Commission, *Decision of Emergency Preparedness of Nuclear Installations, Japan*, latest revision June 2001.

29. Health Canada, *Guidelines for the Restriction of Radioactively Contaminated Food and Water Following a Nuclear Emergency*, Minister of Public Works and Government Services, Ottawa, Canada, 2000.

30. World Health Organization, *Guidelines for Drinking Water*, Volume 1, 3rd ed., WHO, Geneva, 2004.

31. U.S. Environmental Protection Agency, *National Drinking Water Regulations*, EPA 570/9-76-003, EPA, Washington, DC, 1976.

32. National Committee on Radiation Protection, *Maximum Permissible Body Burdens and Maximum Permissible Concentrations of Radionuclides in Air and Water for Occupational Exposure*, National Bureau of Standards Handbook 69, NCRP, Washington, DC, 1963.

33. New Zealand Ministry of Health, *Drinking Water Standards*, Wellington, New Zealand, 2000.

ACRONYMS

AEC	U.S. Atomic Energy Commission
AL	Action Level or Acceptable Level
CAC	Codex Alimentarius Commission
CEDE	Committed Effective Dose Equivalent
CPG	Compliance Policy Guide DC Dose conversion factor in mSv/Bq
DEFRA	Department for Environment, Food and Rural Affairs, United Kingdom
DIL	Derived Interventional Level
EEC	European Economic Community
EPA	U.S. Environmental Protection Agency
EU	European Union
f	fraction of uptake
FAO	Food and Agriculture Organization, United Nations
FDA	U.S. Food and Drug Administration
FI	Food intake
GL	Guideline Levels
IAEA	International Atomic Energy Agency, United Nations
ICRP	International Commission on Radiation Protection
IRALF	International Radionuclide Action Levels in Food
MARSSIM	Multi-Agency Radiation Survey and Site Investigation Manual
MAV	Maximum Acceptable Value
MPC	Maximum Permissible Concentration
NCRP	National Commission on Radiation Protection
NRC	U.S. Nuclear Regulatory Commission
PAG	Protective Action Guides

UNSCEAR   United Nations Scientific Committee on Effects of Atomic Radiation
WHO   World Health Organization, United Nations

GLOSSARY

Absorbed dose Absorbed dose means the energy imparted by ionizing radiation per unit mass of irradiated material. The unit of absorbed dose is the Gray (Gy) and the Rad.

Becquerel (Bq) Unit of radioactivity equal to one disintegration per second (dps).

Committed Effective Dose Equivalent The weighted sum of committed dose equivalent to specified organs and tissues over the specified period following an intake of a radionuclide.

   The sum of the products of the weighting factors applicable to each of the body organs or tissues that are irradiated and the committed dose equivalent to each of these organs or tissues. It is the dose that one would receive from an intake for 30, 50 or 70 years to the target tissue or organ, unit is Sv or mSv.

Committed Dose Equivalent The total dose equivalent (averaged over tissue T) deposited over the 50 year period following the intake of a radionuclide. The committed deposition period is 30, 50 or 70 years depending on the regulation.

Curie Unit of radioactivity equal to 3.7×10^{10} nuclear disintegrations per second. One curie = 3.7×10^{10} Bq.

Derived Concentration Guideline Level A derived radionuclide specific activity concentration within a survey unit corresponding to the release criteria. DCGLs are derived from activity/dose relationships through various exposure pathway scenarios.

Derived Interventional Level Concentration limit derived from the interventional level of dose at which introduction of protective measure should be considered. Unit is Bq/kg.

Dose coefficient Conversion coefficient for committed dose equivalent or committed effective dose equivalent per unit of radioactivity. Unit is mSv/Bq.

Dose Equivalent The product of the absorbed dose, the quality factor, and any other modifying factors.

Protective Action Guide Committed effective dose equivalent or committed dose equivalent to an individual organ or tissue that warrants protective action following a release of radioactivity.

Rem Unit of dose equivalent, originally the Roentgen Equivalent Mammal. One rem = 0.01 Sv.

Sievert (Sv) Unit of dose equivalent.

Total Equivalent Dose Equivalent The sum of the deep dose equivalent for external exposure and the committed effective dose equivalent for internal exposure.

13 Food Irradiation: Microbiological, Nutritional, and Functional Assessment

Paula Pinto, Sandra Cabo Verde,
Maria João Trigo, Antonieta Santana, and
Maria Luísa Botelho

CONTENTS

13.1 INTRODUCTION

During the past two decades, the Food and Agriculture Organization (FAO), the International Atomic Energy Agency (IAEA), and the World Health Organization (WHO) have become closely involved with the issue of food irradiation, since several aspects of this technology fall within their operating mandates. Among the main activities of the IAEA is the encouragement of peaceful uses of nuclear energy. The FAO, on the other hand, must guarantee a global reduction of post-harvest losses as well as the advancement of food quality, safety, and nutrition. The WHO is predominantly concerned with global public health, namely through the reduction of foodborne diseases.

Under the tutelage of these three United Nations (UN) agencies, irradiation has become one of the most extensively investigated and controversial technologies in food processing. Expert committees have regularly evaluated studies on the safety and proprieties of irradiated foods and have concluded that the process and the resulting foods are safe. WHO has recently reviewed a previous report, and on the basis of extensive scientific evidence, concluded that food irradiated to any dose appropriate to achieve the intended technological objective is both safe to consume and nutritionally adequate [1]. The experts further conclude that no upper dose limit needs to be imposed.

The increasing consumer demand for "fresh" and natural food products has lead to the improvement of nonthermal technologies such as irradiation and freezing as food preservation processes [2–6]. The nonthermal technologies, like irradiation, have the ability to inactivate microorganisms at ambient or near-ambient temperatures, thus avoiding the deleterious effects that heat has on flavor, color and nutrient value of food [7,8].

Fumigation with methyl bromide and ethylene oxide are also used as disinfestation and microbiological control methods, but restrictive legislation is being applied [9]. In these procedures, the lethal agent residues prevent reinfestation, but usually are also harmful for human health [10]. One of the advantages of irradiation for disinfestation is the absence of chemical residues in food after processing, although packaging and storage conditions are important for preventing reinfestation.

13.2 PRINCIPLES AND FUNDAMENTALS

Food irradiation employs an energy form called ionizing radiation, which relays in the absorption of energy by the materials. Ionizing radiation with wavelengths less than 10^{-10} m, such as γ-rays, x-rays, and electron beams have a higher energy, causing electron transitions and atom ionization, but the energy imparted in the system is not enough to change the nucleus into a radioactive isotope. The mean energy, $d\bar{\varepsilon}$, imparted by ionizing radiation to an incremental quantity of matter, divided by the mass of that matter, dm, is called the absorbed dose (D), given by Equation 13.1. The definition is given strictly for absorbed dose at a point. In radiation processing, it means the averaged over a finite mass of a given material and is read by a calibrated dosimeter in terms of energy imparted per unit of mass [11]:

$$D = \frac{d\bar{\varepsilon}}{dm}.$$ (13.1)

The unit of absorbed dose is joules per kilogram (J/kg) and is expressed in grays (Gy) or multiples of grays (previously the unit name was rad: 1 Gy = 100 rad). The absorbed dose rate or dose rate (D) is the absorbed dose per time unit and is expressed on a per-gray basis (Equation 13.2):

$$\dot{D} = \frac{dD}{dt} \ . \tag{13.2}$$

The sources of radiation allowed for food processing are γ-rays from ^{60}Co and ^{137}Cs, accelerated electrons with less than 10 MeV and x-rays with less than 5 MeV, so that the energy level is not sufficient to induce radioactivity in food [12]. The one prevailing requirement for an energy source to be employed in food irradiation is that the energy levels must be below those that could possibly cause the food to become radioactive. After that requirement is met, sources are considered on the basis of their practical and economic feasibility. Machine sources must produce radiation with relatively simple technology and isotopes must be sufficiently long lived and emit penetrating radiation.

The effect of γ-rays, x-rays, and electron beams are equally effective for equal quantities of energy absorbed. Since x-ray use in food preservation has low efficiency and high production costs, most research has concentrated on the use of γ photons and electron beams. γ-rays are continuously emitted in all directions from radioactive sources and are penetrating. These sources (^{60}Co or ^{137}Cs) must be constantly replenished due to their decay and require more shielding to protect workers [13]. Electron beams are directional and less penetrating, can be turned off for repair or maintenance work, and present no hazard of radioactive materials after a fire, explosion, or other catastrophe.

There is not an industry or group of companies designing facilities exclusively for food irradiation [14]. The design and build up of food irradiation facilities must comply with the good manufacturing practices (GMPs) that are mandatory for all aspects of food trade and has to be licensed for processing food. The design of the facilities must take into account all the regulations about workers' safety and health, as well as radiation monitoring and control. Dosimetry is an important issue in food processing; absorbed dose must be calibrated, monitored, and recorded [15]. The planned dose to be applied to a product is usually a result of previous studies and depends on the purpose of the process (e.g., delay ripening/physiological growth, disinfestations, shelf-life extension, microbial control, etc.) and on the maximum doses that the physical, chemical, and functional properties the product sustains without harmful alterations. The layout of the facility must also foresee the output of the irradiated product, which depends on several factors such as radiation source, dwell time, transportation speed of the product and the bulk density of the material to be irradiated [16]. Before the irradiation process, the dose uniformity ratio (which is defined as the maximum dose divided by the minimum dose absorbed on the product) and product geometry vs. density must be optimized and dose distribution studies must be done.

13.3 DOSIMETRY AND DOSIMETERS

Before radiation processing of any foodstuff is implemented, dosimetry measurements should be made in order to demonstrate the accomplishment with the regulatory requirements [16,17]. Dosimetry commissioning measurements must be done for each new irradiation process, including new products and modifications of sources, strength of activity, and geometry of products. Records of the measurements should be used to support evidence that the process is according the regulatory requirements. Routine dosimetry must relay the commission results and must also be recorded.

The "dosimetry system" includes the radiation sensor and the analytical methods that relate its reproducibility response to ionizing radiation at a location in a given product. Although new dosimetry systems are in development, the most used as reference are the calorimeters to the accelerator electron beam and ferrous sulfate (Fricke) dosimetry for γ rays. A Fricke dose meter is essentially a water-equivalent system that is adequate for food irradiation since it determines the absorbed dose from a reproducible chemical effect based on radiolysis.

Routine dosimeters must be easily handled and must not be expensive, as they are generally used in great quantities, and the choice of dosimeter depends on the dose range applied [11,18].

13.4 BIOLOGICAL ASSESSMENT

The goal of food irradiation is the destruction of certain microorganisms, specifically those causing food spoilage and human diseases. Fundamental research in radiation biology and applied research beyond the enhancement of hygiene and the reduction of food losses have contributed to the present knowledge.

A variety of hypotheses concerning the radiation effects on cells have been proposed and examined. Today it is generally accepted that deoxyribonucleic acid (DNA) represents the most critical target of ionizing radiation.

When ionizing radiation is absorbed by biological material, there is a possibility that it will act on the critical targets in the cell. The biomolecules may be ionized or excited by energy deposition, inducing a chain of events that leads to biological change and cell death. This phenomenon is called the direct effect of radiation, which is the dominant process when dry spores of spore-forming microorganisms are irradiated. Radiation can also interact with other atoms or molecules in the cell, particularly water, originating in free radicals including hydrogen atoms ($H^{\bullet}$), hydroxyl radicals ($OH^{\bullet}$), and solvated electrons (e_s^-), which can diffuse through the cell (Figure 13.1). These reactive intermediates then interact with biomolecules. When such systems are irradiated in the presence of oxygen the radicals formed in the biomolecules are converted into the corresponding peroxyl [19]. This effect is called the indirect effect of radiation and has major importance in vegetative cells, since 80% of the cell is water.

The cumulative amount of absorbed radiation energy required to inactivate microorganisms in a food product depends on several factors. Thus the dose required for each individual application should be established by risk analysis, taking into consideration the contamination level, the hazard involved, irradiation temperatures, oxygen presence, the efficiency of the radiation treatment, and the fate of critical organisms during manufacturing and storage [20].

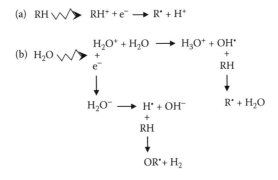

FIGURE 13.1 Genesis of free radicals during: (a) The direct effect of radiation, which involves the simple interaction between the ionizing radiation and critical biological molecules (RH); and (b) the indirect effect of radiation, which involves aqueous free radicals as intermediates in the transfer of radiation energy to biological molecules (RH).

Radiation resistances, even under comparable conditions, vary widely among different microorganisms. The resistance can differ from species to species and between strains of the same species [21]. These radiation sensitivity differences among similar groups of microorganisms are correlated to their inherent diversity with respect to the chemical and physical structure as well their capacity to recover from radiation injuries.

In most cases, radiation survival follows exponential kinetics. In order to characterize organisms by their radiation sensitivity, the D_{10} value is used, which is defined as the dose required to inactivate 90% of a population or the dose of irradiation needed to produce a 10-fold reduction in the population. If N_0 is the initial number of organisms present, N is the number of organisms surviving the radiation dose D, and D_{10} is the decimal reduction dose, the exponential survival plot can be represented mathematically by Equation 13.3 [22]:

$$\log N = -\frac{1}{D_{10}} D + \log N_0. \tag{13.3}$$

The value of D_{10} can be determined by calculating the inverse of the slope of the regression line obtained (Figure 13.2). Inactivation curves may also show curvilinear survival plots and can present an initial shoulder (sigmoidal curves) or an ending tail. In sigmoidal curves, a shoulder is observed at low doses and an exponential phase at higher doses. The shoulder may be explained by multiple targets or certain repair processes being effective at low doses and becoming inoperative at higher doses [23]. The ending tail curves can be interpreted as being caused by a microbial population that is nonhomogeneous with regard to resistivity. A higher portion of the less resistant cells are inactivated first, leaving the more resistant cells to tail out [24].

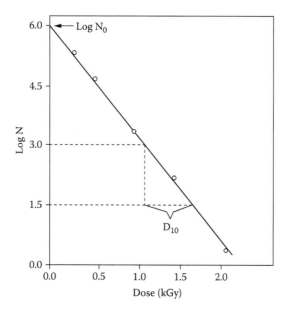

FIGURE 13.2 Typical exponential inactivation curve, where N_0 is the initial number of organisms present, N the number after irradiation with a dose D. The slope of the regression line is $-1/D_{10}$. The value of D_{10} can also be determined graphically as indicated (adapted from Reference 17).

The effectiveness of a given dose depends on intrinsic factors, as reported previously, but also on extracellular environment parameters, such as temperature, gaseous environment, water activity, pH, and the chemical components of the food (Table 13.1), as well as dose rate and postirradiation storage condition.

Elevated temperature treatments synergistically enhance the bactericidal effects of ionizing radiation on vegetative cells, possibly due to the repair systems, which normally operate at or slightly above ambient temperatures and become damaged at higher temperatures [25]. Vegetative microorganisms are considerably more resistant to irradiation at subfreezing temperatures than at ambient temperatures [26]. The decrease in water activity and the restriction of the diffusion of radicals in the frozen state are possible explanations. Otherwise, bacterial spores are less affected by subfreezing temperatures [27], since their core has a low moisture content and appreciable effect on the already restricted diffusion of radicals would not be probable.

The presence of oxygen increases the lethal effects of ionizing radiation on microbial cells. In anaerobic and wet conditions, the resistance levels of vegetative bacteria may be expected to increase by factors ranging from 2 to about 5 compared to those in aerated systems [28]. However, this oxygen effect is not always so evidently observed because irradiation itself causes more or less anoxic conditions in a sample, especially when electron radiation is used. Since part of the effect of ionizing radiation on a microorganism is due to indirect action

TABLE 13.1
Effects on Radioresistivity of Microorganisms of Some Extracellular Environmental Parameters

	Extracellular Environmental Parameters	Effects on Radioresistivity
Gaseous environment	Oxygen	↓
Temperature	High temperatures	↓
	Freezing temperatures	↑
Chemical components	Alcohols	↑
of the food	Carbohydrates	↑
	Proteins	↑
	Sulphydryl-containing compounds	↑
	Quinones	↓
	Nitrites and nitrates	↓
Water content	High	↑

The lower arrow (↓) represents a decrease in the radioresistance; the upper arrow (↑) represents an increase in the radioresistance. (Adapted from Silverman [29].)

mediated through radicals, the nature of the medium in which the microorganisms are suspended obviously plays an important role in determining the dose required for a given microbiocidal effect. The more complex the medium, the greater the competition by its components for the radicals formed by irradiation within the cell, thus "sparing" or "protecting" the microorganisms.

The dose rate of the irradiation process is another parameter that can influence the radiation response of microorganisms. The effect on resistivity usually decreases at high rates [29,30], probably due to the inability of the repair system to respond quickly to the constant induced damage.

Sublethal damage to microorganisms taking place during irradiation can increase their sensitivity to environmental stress factors and other injurious agents (temperature, pH, nutrients, inhibitors, etc.) and synergistic effects of irradiation and certain processes applied in food technology can be encountered [31]. Therefore it is possible in principle to enhance the microbiological effectiveness of irradiation and reduce the dose required for food preservation, thereby improving product quality, by combining the irradiation treatment with other additives and conditions stressful to microorganisms.

Even those foods that are not perishable or are kept from spoiling by methods like freezing can carry pathogenic microorganisms. Mass tourism, worldwide trade in foodstuffs and feedstuffs, mass production of food animals and slaughtering, catering, and ready-to-eat foods have contributed to the worldwide rise of foodborne outbreaks [32]. Mossel [33] lists four epidemiological groups of disease-causing foodborne organisms:

- The "big four": *Salmonella* species, *Campylobacter* species, *Staphylococcus aureus*, and *Bacillus cereus*.
- The "minor culprits": *Shigella*, *Yersinia enterolitica*, *Vibrio parahaemolyticus*, various enterophathogenic and enterotoxinogenic types of *Escherichia coli*, *Clostridium perfringens*, and *Aeromonas hydrophila*.
- The very aggressive, but fortunately less frequently involved organism *Clostridium botulinum*.
- Organisms whose etiological role in food-transmitted disease has only recently or not definitely been established, such as *Cryptosporium parvum* or *Vibrio vulnificus*.

Fortunately the most common and most troublesome bacteria are sensitive to radiation and can be reliably eliminated by doses less than 10 kGy. For example, it has been shown that a relatively low irradiation dose of 1.5 kGy is sufficient to give a 10,000-fold reduction in the number of *E. coli* O157:H7 at 5°C [34]. This irradiation dose is also sufficient to eliminate *Salmonella* and *Campylobacter* from whole-shell eggs without significant adverse effects on the egg quality [35]. *Yersinia* and *Vibrio* spp. also have low resistance to ionizing radiation [36,37]. A dose of 2.5 kGy reduced the number of survivors of four *Shigella* serotypes by more than 6 log-cycles in frozen precooked shrimp in inoculated pack studies [38]. The D_{10} values of *Aeromonas hydrophila* were found to be less than 0.5 kGy in ground fish [39]. Bacterial spores belonging to the genera *Clostridium* and *Bacillus* are of major concern in the microbiology of high-dose irradiated, high-moisture, low-acid foods because several spore-forming species pose serious health hazards, while many others are associated with food spoilage. In general, spores are highly resistant to radiation, heat, and chemicals. Early studies suggest that certain combination treatments have advantages for inactivation of bacterial spores, the most promising being the combination of radiation with heat and food additives [40].

The determination of cell number from mass hyphae-producing molds is sometimes difficult. Their radiation sensitivity is usually not expressed in the form of a D_{10} value. The samples are tested for the presence or absence of survivors after irradiation. The lowest dose giving no survival is regarded as the inactivation dose for the number of spore initially present. The radiation resistances of *Aspergillus* spp. and *Penicillium* spp. are similar to those of less radiation-tolerant vegetative bacteria [41]. In a γ-ray irradiation study, 3 kGy was required to completely inactivate *Aspergillus*, *Rhizopus*, and *Absidia*, whereas a dose of 10 kGy was required for complete inactivation of *Alternaria* and *Fusarium* [42]. If a higher burden of some fungi such as *Alternaria*, *Cladosporium*, or *Culvularia* are present in food, small numbers of them might survive irradiation to dose levels greater than 10 kGy [43]. However, proper primary processing and preirradiation storage of dry commodities should prevent the development of such high-level contamination and should exclude an increase in moisture to levels that would allow any fungal growth.

Viruses are more radiation resistant than bacteria; however, their resistance may vary by as much as 10-fold depending on a number of factors, particularly the concentration of organic material in the suspending medium, the temperature during irradiation, and the degree of dehydration [44]. It has been estimated that carcasses of animals infected with foot-and-mouth virus can be rid of infective viruses with a dose of 20 kGy [45]. Irradiated foods up to 10 kGy must therefore be expected to contain infectious viruses, the same as unheated, dried, salted, or frozen foods. Since conventional heat processing will easily inactivate viruses, the combination of irradiation with a mild heat treatment (such as required for enzyme inactivation) can produce the absence of viable viruses [46].

Radiation effects on parasitic protozoa and helminths are associated with the loss of infectivity, loss of pathogenicity, interruption or prevention of life cycle completion, and death of the parasite. Relatively high doses (4 to 6 kGy) are required to inactivate foodborne parasites. Objectionable sensory changes are induced at these dose levels in raw foods that carry the parasites [47]. However, much lower doses (0.1 to 2 kGy) are adequate to prevent reproduction and maturation, resulting in loss of infectivity [48]. It is safely assumed that controlling microbial pathogens in nonfrozen flesh food with minimum doses of at least 1 kGy should also control infectious parasites that might be present [20].

Irradiation as a disinfestation treatment provides an effective means of disinfesting commodities for quarantine and phytosanitary purposes. The use of irradiation as a quarantine treatment has been argued for several years, but just recently has being developed into a widely adopted method for safeguarding agricultural and natural resources. The objective of any quarantine treatment is to prevent the establishment of quarantine pests possibly present on trade commodities, in areas where such pests are not established or are in limited distribution and are under control. Criteria for effectiveness of a treatment to prevent establishment of a pest species in a new location may be sexual sterilization or physical disablement of adults, inhibition of development to the adult or to an intermediate immature stage, or rarely, immediate mortality. Insects can be present and still alive after irradiation. Radiation technology as a quarantine treatment may be used to inactivate not only insects, but also mites, spider mites, thrips, nematodes, snails, and slugs contaminating grains, fruits, vegetables, cut flowers, fresh herbs, timbers, seedlings, and seeds.

Pest mortality is not always necessary, particularly with insects; the prevention of reproduction should be the goal, which can be accomplished at lower doses than 100% mortality. For example, the sweet potato weevil (*Cylas formicarius elegantulus* [Summers]) treated with 1000 Gy will survive 10 days posttreatment, but only 200 Gy are necessary to sterilize female weevils [49]. Arthropods are more radioresistant than human and other vertebrates, but less resistant than viruses, protozoa, and bacteria [50]. Sensitivity to radiation among families and in particular orders varies sometimes over two orders of magnitude. In general, most insect, mite, and tick families required a sterilization dose of less than 200 Gy. A database compiling radiation doses for arthropod sterilization and disinfestation was developed to support researchers and regulatory agencies dealing with phytosanitary treatments and pest control program operators [51]. This International Database on Insect Disinfestation and Sterilization (IDIDAS) is available at http://www-ididas.iaea.org/ididas/.

The irradiation dose needed for quarantine security is defined at "sufficient to prevent adult emergence" with a maximum allowable limit of 1000 Gy as established by the U.S. Food and Drug Administration (FDA). The efficacy required for a disinfestation treatment (mostly immature stages) varies from country to country and according to whether the treatment is for quarantine or phytosanity purposes. In 1986 a Task Force of the International Consultative Group on Food Irradiation (ICGFI) determined a generic dose of 300 Gy as the minimum needed to achieve quarantine security (99.9968% efficacy at the 95% confidence level) against any stage of any insect species [52]. The advantages and disadvantages of irradiation over other disinfestation treatments are listed in Table 13.2.

When the irradiation is used to delay ripening and senescence of fruits, the food itself is the target. The effects of radiation to induce the delay of ripening are complex. The success with this use of irradiation requires an understanding of the postharvest physiological processes of fruits and treatment that is applied

TABLE 13.2
Advantages and Disadvantages of Irradiation Over Other Disinfestation Treatments

Advantages	Disadvantages
Radiation can be applied in few minutes, while other treatments require hours to days.	It is required a large initial expense for commercial facilities.
Irradiation facilities can be used for a variety of other proposes (inactivation of microorganisms in food, preventing sprouting of roots and tubers, sterilization of medical devices, enhancing gemstone quality, strengthening construction material, wastewater treatment, etc.). Placing commercial irradiators near ports would be reasonable in order to take advantage of their multipurpose uses.	The large maximum:minimum dose ratio (up to 3:1) when applied on a commercial scale to pallet loads means that most of the food products will receive much greater than the minimum effective dose, thus increasing the risk of food damage.
It can be applied to commodities even after they are packed, whereas only cold treatment can be applied to packed commodities.	Although the dose radiation used for disinfestation treatment stops insect development, it does not provide much acute mortality, so live insects may be found by inspectors.
A wide variety of food products tolerate doses required for quarantine security.	Due to safety concerns and facility costs, irradiation will probably not be applied at local packinghouses, but in centralized location, creating an additional transport burden.
Unlike fumigation, there is no residue.	

only at particular stages of fruit development. The delay of senescence often involves retention of fruit firmness longer than is obtained without irradiation. This effect of irradiation appears to be associated with the interference in the normal process of conversion of carbohydrate polymers to smaller molecules, which are the basis of fruit firmness.

Irradiation treatment with very low doses inhibits the sprouting of vegetables such as potatoes, onions, and garlic, effectively replacing the chemicals currently used for this purpose. Irradiation doses ranging from 0.05 to 0.15 kGy inhibit bulb sprouting and are more effective when applied during the dormancy period; specifically within 4 to 6 weeks after harvesting [53]. Ionized bulbs can be stored for several months without heavy spoilage, although ionization and storage can affect changes in the carbohydrate content of onion tissue.

Irradiation can also increase the shelf life of food. Exposure to low-dose irradiation can slow down the ripening and maturation of fruits and vegetables. Ripening of bananas, mangos, and papayas can be delayed by irradiation at up to 1 kGy. Irradiation of mushrooms at 2 to 3 kGy inhibits cap opening and lengthening of the stem [54]. Medium doses (2 to 3 kGy) can be used to control mold growth on strawberries, raspberries, and blueberries, thereby extending their shelf life [55]. Proper dosimetry is a critical control point that ensures an accurate and consistent dose is delivered to each lot processed through the facility, thus the American Society for Testing and Materials (ASTM) standard for dosimetry must be followed [56]. An inaccurate dosimetry system may result in undertreatment of the commodity or overtreatment that can be detrimental to the commodity or surpass the maximum dose allowed.

Safeguarding after treatment is the other critical control point to ensure the integrity of the system. The objective is to address those risks that are not addressed by the actual irradiation procedure. This includes segregating the commodity after treatment to ensure that untreated commodity is not labeled as treated and commingled with treated product. In addition, the commodity must be packaged, held, and shipped in such a manner as to minimize the risks after treatment.

13.5 NUTRITIONAL AND FUNCTIONAL ASSESSMENT

Foods are complex mixtures of chemical compounds whose primary role is to provide sufficient nutrients to meet the nutritional requirements of the human body. The major nutritional components of foods are the macronutrients: proteins, which provide the organism with essential amino acids, and energy; fats and carbohydrates, which are the main sources of energy. Besides sugars and starches (essentially energy providers), carbohydrates also include fibers, which regulate bowel function. Different groups of foods also have different contents of vitamins and minerals, which are required by the human body in various amounts and have several essential functions provided for growth, maintenance, and reproduction [57]. The nutritional quality of a food depends on the bioavailability of the nutrients, which can be affected in a positive or negative way by various processing and preserving technologies.

The free radicals formed during irradiation can react with nutrients and other components of the food, mainly inducing oxidation of metals and ions, oxidation and reduction of carbonyls, elimination of double bonds, decrease of aromaticity, hydroxylation of aromatic rings, and formation of hydroperoxides [58]. These reactions also occur during cooking, roasting, steaming, pasteurization, and other forms of food processing [58]. Total yield of radiolytic products depends on the absorbed radiation dose, water content, and chemical composition of food, temperature, and gaseous environment during irradiation [59].

Meat, fish, milk, and eggs are foods with proteins of high biological value and are generally the main sources of protein in the human diet. Today, the consumption of legumes, especially soybeans, as a protein source is increasing. The biological value of food proteins depend largely on the content and proportion of essential amino acids. Several studies have shown that irradiation of whole foods with doses up to 50 kGy has no effect on the biological value of proteins either from animal or plant origin [17,58,60]. A recent study with a formulated food designed for babies has shown that irradiation with 10 kGy induced losses between zero and 5% for most essential amino acids and only two of the essential amino acids had losses of about 10%. Sulfur-containing and aromatic amino acids are the most sensitive to irradiation and can have a reduction of 13% to 20% with irradiation doses greater than 10 kGy and up to 50 kGy [61]. As recommended by WHO [62], the limit of 10 kGy for elimination of pathogens and extended shelf life can be used for food preservation without significant losses of the nutritional quality of proteins.

The digestibility of plant proteins is generally lower than animal proteins, thus lowering their biological value. However, studies with raw soybeans suggest that irradiation may increase protein digestibility, even with irradiation doses less than 10 kGy [63].

The digestibility of starch may also be changed by irradiation. It has been shown that irradiation of maize and bean flours with doses of 2.5 kGy increased the digestibility of the starch, although higher doses induced a slight reduction in digestibility due to formation of resistant starch (starch with (1-3) bonds) [64]. These results open the possibility of using irradiation processing to reduce the glycemic index of some foods for diabetics and other low sugar diets.

Foods rich in sugars like glucose, fructose, and sucrose can undergo nonenzymatic browning due to Maillard reactions or caramelization, resulting in color and taste changes. Processing these foods with high temperatures or irradiation may lead to an increase in nonenzymatic browning, but only at alkaline pH [65]. However, some studies have shown that irradiating food may cause a decrease in the pH [66,67], thus protecting the food against nonenzymatic browning.

Lipid changes may occur after irradiation due to autoxidative and nonoxidative reactions, leading mostly to formation of hydrocarbons, aldehydes, and ketones [1,68], some of which are responsible for off-flavor or odor generation [69]. Lipid oxidation in foods is generally assessed by means of the thiobarbituric acid reactive substances (TBA-RS) content. In studies with fish and meat, it was shown that TBA-RS values were low (less than about 4 mg MA/kg) for both nonirradiated and irradiated samples with doses less than 5 kGy, after an acceptable storage time (accessed by means of sensorial and microbiological evaluation) [70–72].

Although the intake of fats should be controlled, some fats provide essential fatty acids, linoleic acid, and α-linolenic acid, as well as long-chain polyunsaturated fatty acids (PUFAs) like omega-3 fatty acids, which have been linked to a reduction in coronary heart disease risk [73]. Thus there is an increased concern that irradiation may cause destruction of PUFAs. Based on several studies, the European Scientific Committee on Food [59] concluded that high irradiation doses (50 to 100 kGy) had only marginal effects on essential fatty acids. Furthermore, Geibler et al. [74] only found significant amounts of *cis-trans* isomerization of PUFAs for irradiation doses of 50 kGy or more.

Effects of ionizing radiation on vitamins are well documented. Vitamins D, K, and niacin are highly radiation resistant, and losses due to irradiation have not been observed in several foods, even at high irradiation doses [17]. The other vitamins are more or less sensitive to ionizing radiation depending on the conditions of the irradiation process and on the composition of the food itself. It is well known that irradiation of foods in the presence of oxygen and at room temperature may cause major losses in vitamin E and thiamine (vitamin B_1), which are the most radiation sensitive vitamins. However, if the irradiation process is undertaken at freezing temperatures or with exclusion of air, these losses are substantially reduced and may be even lower than those caused by heat sterilization [1,75].

The most important sources of vitamin C in the human diet are fresh fruits, mainly citrus fruits, and vegetables. Since this vitamin is both heat and radiation sensitive, care should be taken in fruit and vegetable processing technologies. Ionizing radiation in low doses may be used to control insect pests and to extend the shelf life of fresh and minimally processed products.

In strawberries, it has been shown that irradiation doses of 2 kGy did not induce a significant reduction in total vitamin C content during storage up to 10 days for most of the tested varieties [76]. The vitamin C of citrus fruits also does not seem to be affected by low irradiation doses, unlike other treatments used to extend shelf life [77]. In fresh-cut vegetables, radiation doses of 0.5, 1, and 2 kGy had no consistent effect on vitamin C content. The decrease observed mainly during the first week of storage, in all the samples, including nonirradiated samples, indicates that vitamin C loss during storage of fresh-cut vegetables is not affected by ionizing radiation [78].

Potatoes are also important sources of vitamin C in the diet, and depending on the cooking process, losses in the vitamin content are quite different. For example, boiling can reduce the vitamin C content in about 15% and baking can induce a decrease of 40%, as well as storage up to 5 months [76]. The authors have shown that irradiation of potatoes with very low doses (0.15 kGy) sufficient to control sprouting during storage, induce a decrease of about 8% in total vitamin C content initially, but the contents of vitamin C in irradiated and nonirradiated potatoes are the same 5 months after storage.

Besides the well-defined nutrients, foods (especially plant foods) contain several other compounds, some of which have antinutrient and allergenic properties (digestive enzyme inhibitors, lectins), while others like phytosterols, flavonoids, terpenoids, and soluble fibers are known to have biological activities with health benefits [73].

Irradiation of foods with doses up to 10 kGy seems to be effective in inactivating some antinutrients without altering the nutritional quality of the food [58]. On the other hand, it is important that some bioactive components maintain its biological activity after irradiation. Patil and Vanamala [79] observed a small decrease (10 to 15%) in the flavanone content of fruits irradiated with 0.7 kGy. There was no reduction in total carotenoid content with this irradiation dose, although some variations (increases or decreases) were observed for individual carotenoids like β-carotene and lycopene. A recent study with fresh-cut vegetables showed that irradiation with a dose of 1 kGy induces an increase of 14% in the antioxidant capacity of the vegetables [80]. Table 13.3 shows the most important positive and negative effects of irradiation on nutritional quality in various food groups.

Besides nutritional quality, it is also essential that natural and processed foods maintain their color and firmness after irradiation, since these quality factors are of extreme importance for the consumer. A combination of irradiation doses up to 1 kGy (sufficient to reduce the microbial burden), warm water treatment, and packaging in modified atmosphere bags can slow surface browning of fresh-cut lettuce without loss in firmness, thus extending shelf life [78]. Trigo et al. [81] also observed that irradiation of turnips with doses of 0.5 and 1 kGy extended the shelf life without altering surface color and firmness. In other food products, like surimi seafood, neither color nor texture were deteriorated when samples were irradiated with an electron beam up to 4 kGy, at temperatures between 5 and 23°C. On the contrary, if surimi seafood food samples were treated with heat, softening of texture and browning was observed [82].

TABLE 13.3
Effects of Irradiation with Doses up to 10 kGy on Nutritional Quality of Some Foods

Food Groups	General Positive/Negative Effect of Irradiation
Meat	No significant effect on proteins; may induce vitamin B_1 loss
Fish	depending on the irradiation conditions and slight lipid oxidation.
Eggs	
Fruits	May increase antioxidant content; may cause some vitamin C loss.
Vegetables	
Legumes	May increase digestibility of proteins and starch.
Cereals	

Macronutrients are the most important factors in the functional properties of foods, such as viscosity, foaming, emulsification, and gelling capacities. Eggs and egg products (liquid whites, liquid yolks, egg powder) are some of the most used ingredients in food products due to their several functional properties. A decrease in the viscosity of egg whites was observed both in shell eggs and liquid whites irradiated with doses between 0.5 and 5 kGy [83]. This decrease was dependent on the irradiation dose, and for a sanitation irradiation dose of 2 kGy, the reduction was similar to the observed in liquid whites submitted to thermal pasteurization. Although this reduction in viscosity may not affect the foaming capacity of egg whites, it can reduce foam stability [84]. The effect of irradiation on the viscosity of egg yolk and emulsifying capacity is not significant and is also comparable to thermal pasteurization [83,84].

Irradiation of starch also results in a decrease in viscosity which may affect technological properties. For example, irradiation of wheat at doses sufficient to control insect infestation (1 kGy) significantly reduces the stickiness, firmness, and bulkiness of spaghetti [85]. On the other hand, irradiation can produce desirable physical changes in some foods. For instance, bread made from irradiated wheat has greater loaf volume when certain dough formulations are used [86].

13.6 LEGISLATION AND GOVERNMENT REGULATION OF IRRADIATED FOODS

The legislation governing irradiated foods depends of socioeconomic factors and political decisions. Government regulations allow the food industry to utilize this technology and commercialize irradiated foods, such as dried aromatic herbs, spices, and vegetable seasonings imported from other countries, thus preventing cross contamination (microbes and insects), with obvious benefits for consumers. Table 13.4 reviews the foods authorized for treatment with ionizing radiation in countries all over the world (an exhaustive list of foods authorized for irradiation, as well as the dates of approval and permitted absorbed doses can be found on the IAEA website, www.iaea.org).

Although it is a safe technology, irradiation is not yet fully accepted due to a lack of information. In the U.S., more than 40 food products have clearance, but only a few companies are irradiating products for market [14]. Irradiated food must be labeled with a green logo (Figure 13.3) and with the statement "treated with radiation" or "treated by radiation."

In Canada, food irradiation is more restrictive and only seven food products can be irradiated and commercialized [17].

In Latin America, there are several countries with facilities that can irradiate food on a commercial scale [87–89]. In Brazil, there are more than 100 food items approved for irradiation, and in Mexico there are more than 50. Other countries such as Argentina, Chile, Costa Rica, and Cuba have clearance for fewer food items.

TABLE 13.4
Government Regulation of Irradiated Foods

Country	Product
Argentina	Dried fruits and dried vegetables (1.00)[A]; Asparagus, mushrooms (2.00–3.00)[B]; Garlic, onions, potatoes (0.15)[C]; Spices (up to 30)[D]; Strawberry (2.50)[E]
Australia	Herbs, herbal infusions, spices (6.00)[A,C]; Herbs, herbal infusions, spices (30.00)[D]; Fresh fruits (1.00)[F]
Bangladesh	Beans, condiments, dried fish, fruits, legumes, pulses, rice, spices, wheat, wheat products (1.00)[A]; Mango, papaya (1.00)[B]; Onions, potato (0.15)[C]; Fish (2.20), shrimp (5.00), chicken, frog legs (7.00), condiments, spices (10.00)[D]
*Belgium	Garlic, onions, potato, shallots (0.15)[C]; Chicken meat (mechanically recovered), frog legs (frozen), shrimp (frozen) (5.00), egg white (3.00), herbs (dried), spices, vegetables seasonings (dried) (10.00)[D]
Brazil	Any food (**)[A,B,C,D,E,F,G,H]
Canada	Wheat, wheat flour (0.75)[A]; Onions, potato (0.15)[C]; Herbs, spices, dried vegetable seasonings (10.00)[D]
Chile	Beans, cocoa beans, dried fish, fruits, legumes, pulses, rice, wheat, and wheat products (1.00)[A]; Dates (1.00)[B]; Onions, potato (0.15)[C]; Fish, fish products (2.20), cocoa beans (5.00), chicken (7.00), condiments, spices (10.00)[D]; Strawberry (3.00)[E]
China	Condiments, spices (0.5), onions, potato (0.4), apricot, dried fruits, cereal grains (1.00)[A]; Fish, fish products (1.00)[B]; Cocoa beans(0.10–0.20)[C]; Chicken (6.00), cocoa beans, fruits, legumes, dried fish pulses, rice, wheat, wheat products (8.00), apple (10.00)[D]; Dates (0.10), apple (0.40), tomato (4.00)[E]
Costa Rica	Beans, cocoa beans, condiments, fish products, green beans, papaya, pulses, rice, wheat, wheat products (1.00)[A]; Mango (1.00), strawberry (3.00)[A,E]; Onions, potato (0.15)[C]; Fish, fish products (2.20), chicken (7.00), cocoa beans (5.00), condiments (10.00)[D]
Croatia	Cereal grains, cereal muesli, dried fruits and vegetables (1.00)[A]; Fruits, vegetables (3.00)[B,D]; Garlic, ginger, onions, potato, roots, tubers (0.50)[C]; Egg, frozen egg products, egg powder (3.00), chicken, meat, poultry (3.00–7.00), fish, sausages, seafood, shrimp (5.00), frog legs (8.00), dried fruit and vegetables, cereal muesli, enzyme preparations, gum arabic, tea (10.00)[D]; Frozen fruit juices (4.00)[E]; Pork (1.00)[G]; Sterile meals (45.00)[H]
Cuba	Cocoa beans (0.50), dried fish (1.00), dehydrated cocoa, sesame seed (2.00)[A]; Avocado (0.25), mango (0.75)[B]; Onions (0.06), garlic (0.08), potato (0.1)[C]; Bacon and meat products (4.00), meat (5.00), spices (10.00)[D]; Seafood (3.00)[E]
Egypt	Bulbs, garlic, ginger, potatoes, onions, roots, shallots, tubers, and yams (0.20)[C]; Dried garlic, onion, herbs, spices (10.00)[D]
European Union	Herbs (dried), spices, vegetable seasonings (dried) (10.00)[D]
*France	Fruits (dried), vegetables (dried) (1.00)[A]; Garlic, onions, shallots (0.075)[C]; Dehydrated blood, plasma, coagulates, herbs (dried), herbs (frozen), cereal flakes, cereal germ for milk products (10.00), casein, caseinates (6.00), frog legs (frozen), mechanically recovered poultry meat, poultry, shrimp, offal of poultry (5.00), rice flour (4.00), egg white, gum arabic (3.00)[D]

TABLE 13.4 (continued)
Government Regulation of Irradiated Foods

Country	Product
Ghana	Animal feed, pulses, breakfast cereals, cereal grains, cereal products, food animal origin (dried), fruits (dried), vegetables, dry vegetables (1.00)[A,B,F]; Bulbs, garlic, ginger, onions, potato, roots, tubers, shallots (0.2)[C]; Fruits (dried), pulses, breakfast cereals, cereal grains, cereal products, fish, dry fish, nuts, oil seeds, shrimp (5.00), meat, meat products, chicken, chicken products (7.00), herbs, tea, honey, space foods, dried vegetables (10.00)[D]; Fruits, vegetables, dry vegetables (2.50), meat, meat products, poultry, poultry products, frankfurters, fish, fish (dried), shrimp (3.00)[E]; Meat, meat products, poultry, poultry products, seafood, dried fish (2.00)[G]
*Hungary	Pear (1.00), mushrooms (3.00)[B]; Potato (0.10), onions (0.20)[C]; Chicken (4.00), mixed dry ingredients (5.00), spices (6.00)[D]; Cherries, currants, grapes, strawberry (2.50)[E]
India	Dates, figs (dried), raisins (0.75), fish (dried), legumes, pulses, wheat flour, wheat products, shrimp (dried), seafood (dried), rice (1.00)[A]; Mango (0.75)[B]; onions (0.09), garlic, ginger, potato (0.15)[C]; Fish (frozen), seafood (frozen), shellfish (frozen), shrimp (frozen) (6.00), spices (14.00)[D]; Seafood, shellfish, shrimp, chicken products, pork (3.00), chicken, meat, meat products (4.00)[D,E]
Indonesia	Cereal grains, rice, wheat (1.00)[A]; Bulbs, garlic, onions, potato, roots, tubers shallots, ginger (0.15)[C]; Beans, green beans, legumes, pulses (5.00), frog legs, shrimp (frozen) (7.00), spices (10.00)[D]; Fish (dried) (5.00)[E]
Iran	Spices (10.00)[D]
Israel	Fresh and dried fruits and vegetables, beans, cereals (1.00)[A]; Chicken, poultry (7.00), spices, dried vegetables (10.00), animal feed (15.00)[D]; Mushrooms, strawberry (3.00)[E]
*Italy	Garlic, onions and potato (0.15)[C]; Herbs (dried), spices, vegetable seasonings (dried) (10.00)[D]
Japan	Potato (0.15)[C]
Korea, Rep. Of	Chestnuts (0.25), mushrooms (1.00)[A]; Garlic, onions, potato (0.15)[C]; Starch (5.00), enzyme preparations, red pepper paste powder, shellfish powder, soy sauce powder, soybean paste powder, yeast powder, meat (dried), vegetables (dried), (7.00), spices, vegetable seasonings (dried) (10.00)[D]; Sterile meals (10.00)[H]
Libya	Dates (1.00)[A]; Garlic (0.04), onions (0.08), potato (0.1)[C]; Spices (15.00)[D]; Poultry (4.00)[D,E]
Mexico	Bulbs, shallots, garlic, onions (0.20), dried fruits, cereal products, cereal grains, corn products, herbs, rice, rice products, soybean, soybean products, wheat, wheat products (1.00)[A]; Fruits, vegetables (1.00)[B,F]; Ginger, potato, roots, tubers (0.2)[C]; Cocoa (dehydrated), egg (dehydrated), fish, frog legs (fresh or frozen), milk (dehydrated) (5.00), chicken, chicken products (7.00), apricot (dried), beef (dehydrated), condiments (dried), herbs, jujube (dried), soup stock (dehydrated), tea, herbal, fruits (dried), food colors (natural, dehydrated), raisins (10.00)[D]; Fruits, vegetables (2.50), chicken products, fish, frog legs (fresh or frozen) (3.00), chicken (dehydrated/dried) (10.00)[E]; Pork (1.00), fish (2.00)[G]

(continued)

TABLE 13.4 (continued)
Government Regulation of Irradiated Foods

Country	Product
*The Netherlands	Pulses, dried vegetables and fruits, flakes from cereals (1.00)[A]; Gum arabic, egg white, shrimp (3.00), frozen frog legs (5.00), chicken meat (7.00)[D]
New Zealand	Herbs, herbal infusions, spices (6.00)[A,C]; Herbal infusions (10.00), herbs, spices (30.00)[D]; Breadfruit, carambola, custrad apple, longan, litchi, mango, mangosteen, papaya (paw paw), rambutan (1.00)[F]
Pakistan	Beans, breakfast cereals, cereal grains, cereal products, chicken (dehydrated/dried), condiments, corn products, fish (dried), fruits (dried), herbs, jujube (dried), legumes, meat (dried), nuts, poultry (dried), pulses, raisins, rice, spices, vegetables (dried) (1.00)[A]; Fruit, vegetables, vegetables (dried) (1.00)[A,B,F]; Bulbs, garlic, ginger, onions, potato, roots, shallots, tubers, wheat, wheat products (0.2)[C]; Chicken, chicken products, fish, fish products, meat, meat products, poultry, poultry products, seafood (fresh and frozen), shrimp (5.00), condiments, herbs, spices (10.00)[D]; Chicken, chicken products, fish, fish products, meat, meat products, poultry, poultry products, seafood (fresh and frozen), shrimp (3.00), tomato, vegetables (fresh and dried) (2.00)[E]
Philippines	Garlic, onions (0.1)[C]; Spices (6.00)[D]
*Poland	Garlic (0.15), onions (0.06)[C]; Mushrooms, vegetables (dried), spices (10.00)[D]
Russian Federation	Cereals (0.30), rice, dried food concentrates (0.7) dried fruit (1.00) [A]; Onions (0.06), potato (0.3)[C]; Beef, pork and meat products (8.00)[D]; Rabbit (8.00), chicken, poultry (6.00); Fruits (4.00)[E]
South Africa	Avocado (0.1), mango (4.00), garlic (dried), garlic paste, honey, meat, meat products (10.00)[A]; Potato (10.00)[C]; Beef bone extract, beef soup stock (20.00), meat, meat products, fish, baby food, eggs, egg products, fruit jams, cereals, cereal products, dried fruits, soya products, starch, sugar solutions, dietary supplements, sweets, potato chips, dried vegetables (10.00), fruit pulp (5.00), chicken (4.00)[D]; Fruit juices and concentrates, tomato (3.00), sorghum malt beer (1.00)[E]; Sterile meats (50.00)[G]
Syria	Beans, dates, fish (dried), green beans, legumes, mango, papaya, pulses, rice, wheat, wheat products (1.00)[A]; Onions, potato (0.15)[C]; Fish, fish products (2.20), cocoa beans (5.00), chicken (7.00), condiments, spices (10.00)[D]; Strawberry (3.00)[E]
Thailand	Beans, cocoa beans, fish (dried), green beans, jujube (dried), rice, spices, wheat, wheat products (1.00)[A]; Mango, papaya (1.00)[A,B]; Garlic, onions, potato (0.15)[C]; Fish, fish products (2.00), cocoa beans, sausages, shrimp (5.00), chicken (7.00), condiments, spices (10.00)[D]; Nham (raw, fermented pork sausage) (4.00), moo yor (cooked sausage) (5.00)[D,G]
Turkey	Fruits (dried), beef (dehydrated), cereal grains and cereal products, chicken (dehydrated/dried), fish (dried), poultry (dried) (1.00)[A], spices, dried vegetables (10.00)[A,D]; Fruits, vegetables (1.00)[B,F]; Garlic, ginger, onions, shallots, potato (0.20)[C]; Fruits (dried), cereal grains, cereal products, frog legs (frozen), shrimp (5.00)[D,E]; Fish (5.00), bacon, chicken (spiced), meat products, poultry, poultry products (7.00)[D]; Fruit, vegetables (2.50)[E]; Bacon, beef (dehydrated), chicken (spiced), fish (fresh and dried), frog legs (frozen), meat products, poultry (fresh and dried), poultry products, shrimp (3.00)[E,G]; Fish, frog legs (frozen), shrimp (2.00)[G]

TABLE 13.4 (continued)
Government Regulation of Irradiated Foods

Country	Product
Ukraine	Cereal grains (0.30), buckwheat mush (dried), food concentrates (dried), gruel (dried), pudding (dried), rice (0.70), fruits (dried) (1.00)[A]; Onions (0.06), potato (0.3)[C]; Beef, pork and rabbit (raw, semi-prepared) (8.00)[D]; Fruits, vegetables (fresh and dried) (4.00), chicken and poultry (6.00)[E]
*U.K.	Vegetables, pulses, cereals (1.00)[A]; Potatoes, yams, onions, garlic, shallots (0.2)[C]; Poultry (domestic fowls, geese, ducks, guinea fowls, pigeons, quails, turkeys) (7.00)[D]
U.S.	Fruits (fresh and dried), vegetables (fresh and dried) wheat, wheat flour (1.00)[A,B]; Potato, white potatoes (0.15)[C]; Chicken meat (mechanically separated), poultry, poultry products, eggs (whole, fresh) (3.00), meat (4,5–7.00), seeds for sprouting (8.00), enzymes (dehydrated) (10.00), animal feed and pet food (25.00), herbs, spices, vegetable seasonings (30.00)[D]; Pork (1.00)[G]
Uruguay	Potato (0.15)[C]
Vietnam	Corn, fish (dried), green beans, maize, paprika powder (1.00)[A]; Garlic, onions, potato (0.10)[C]
Yugoslavia	Fruits and vegetables (dried), cereal grains, mushrooms (dried), legumes, pulses (10.00)[A]; Garlic, onions, potato (10.00)[C]; Chicken, egg powder, poultry, spices, tea extract, tea, herbal (10.00)[D]

Note: In front of each food or group of foods is the authorized irradiation dose between brackets; superscript letter refers to the purpose of the irradiation: A, disinfestation; B, delay ripening/physiological growth; C, sprouting inhibition; D, microbial control; E, shelf-life extension; F, quarantine treatment; G, Trichina/parasite control; H, sterilization.

* European Union country with positive list of irradiated food.

** The minimum absorbed dose must be sufficient to achieve the intended objective, the maximum absorbed dose must be less than that which would compromise the functional properties or the organoleptic attributes of the food.

Adapted from www.iaea.org.

FIGURE 13.3 International recognized symbol of irradiated food.

Of the 41 countries that have clearance for irradiation, 10 are Asian Pacific countries. However, only three are commercializing irradiated products: China with garlic, Japan with potatoes, and Thailand with "nham" [90].

In Africa, the Republic of South Africa has developed a special interest in food irradiation, being the first country with permission to apply a sterilizing dose to produce and to sell a shelf-stable meat product treated with a combination of heat and irradiation. Other African countries (Egypt, Ghana, Libya, and Syria) have legislation in this field and clearance of several food items.

The European Community began to legislate irradiated foods in 1999. Dried aromatic herbs, spices, and vegetable seasonings were authorized to be irradiated with a maximum overall absorbed dose of 10 kGy [91,92]. In 2002, members states (Belgium, France, Italy, The Netherlands, and the U.K.) published a list of foods and food ingredients authorized for treatment with ionizing radiation [93,94]. In addition, a list of approved food irradiation facilities in the member states and another list for third-world countries was published [95,96]. In the last report from the Commission on Food Irradiation [97], the approximate amount of food irradiated in the EU in 2002 was 20,000 t, and part of this amount was irradiated for export.

Only Canada, India, the U.K., and the U.S. have specific regulations concerning irradiation of food packaging materials [89].

The divergence between the list of foods cleared for irradiation by the governments of almost 40 countries and the short list of facilities actually producing and marketing is remarkable.

13.7 CONSUMER ACCEPTANCE

As mentioned before, irradiation does not influence food nutrients any more than the other conventional technologies. The negative association of irradiated products with nuclear accidents and nuclear weapons causes misconceptions about food irradiation technology. This has led to a nonacceptance of irradiated foods by consumers.

Three ways to help the public understand irradiation technology are consumer surveys with questionnaires interviews, limited test marketing, and actual retail selling. Results of surveys [98–102] show three main behaviors from potential consumer groups: 5% to 10% rejected irradiated food, 55% to 65% were undecided, and 25% to 30% accepted it and believe it is advantageous. The reasons behind rejection are mainly antinuclear convictions and defense of natural food. The behavior of the undecided group may change with improvements in technology.

Limited test marketing of irradiated potatoes, onions, and fruits (papaya, strawberry, and mango) in several countries around the world has shown acceptance by consumers [17,103–107].

In the U.S., market trials showed that irradiated chicken was accepted by the consumers, being bought even when the price was equal to nonirradiated chicken [108]. This limited test marketing suggests that consumers openly accept and buy irradiated foods when they are properly informed. However, information must be clear and concise. In spite of the success of these results, food irradiation in the U.S. and other countries is under development, and major supermarket chains have not yet decided to sell irradiated foodstuffs.

13.8 SAFE FOOD AND CONSUMER SAFETY

Since the first use of irradiation as a method of decontamination in 1951, the scientific community and governmental organizations concerns about the safety of irradiated food and human health. In 1951, the first study with animals fed with irradiated food was performed. Seven years later the U.S. Congress decided that all foods treated by irradiation or with added chemicals should be tested [17]. Since then, hundreds of studies have been performed involving tests with several different animal species (mice, rats, pigs, monkeys, and dogs) fed with irradiated food with dose ranges from 0.1 to 100 kGy [17].

A WHO report [62] stated that 441 studies with animals fed with irradiated food have been performed. More than 250 of them were classified as accepted or accepted with reservation (category A or B, respectively). About 20 were not classified because they were not original studies, while 150 were classified as rejected (R). In this category, the number of animals was not reported or had an insufficient number (less than five), the radiation doses applied were not reported or were less then 0.1 kGy or more than 100 kGy, and other deficiencies. In a report from the Scientific Committee on Food (SCF) [109], no evidence was shown for chronic or carcinogenicity activity and no adverse effects were found on reproductive, growth, or mortality parameters. Another WHO report concluded "that no adverse effects were detected and recommended a dose range of up to 10 kGy." In 1999 the FAO/IAEA/WHO encouraged the use of irradiated food with a maximum dose of 10 kGy [1].

Parallel studies were made to verify if irradiated food is radioactive. A 1986 SCF report concluded that the radioactivity produced was below the detection threshold and was much lower (about 10^5) than that found naturally in fresh food [109].

Also, as mentioned before, numerous studies have been performed to elucidate the effects of irradiation in foodstuffs, namely the identification of radiolytic products and the radiation effects on biomolecules [109]. So far no evidence has been found, even in the toxicological activity of 2-ACBs (these compounds result from the break of the acyl-oxygen bond in triacylglycerols and are not detected in unirradiated foods), as the tests were made with pure 2-ACBs and with concentrations higher than those usually found in irradiated food containing fat [110,111]. Other studies have shown that irradiation reduces the levels of nitro compounds such as nitrosamines in cured meat products [112–115], as well as the levels of biogenic amines [116].

13.9 DETECTION OF IRRADIATED FOOD

Today, several analytical methods are used to detect irradiated foods, not only to verify if all the irradiated foods are correctly labeled, but also to elucidate the toxicological activity of radiolytic products. Despite more than 40 years of research, those analytical methods are sophisticated, expensive, restrictive, and not easy to use and usually it is necessary to use different methods for different kinds of foods.

These methods in the EU must be validated or standardized by the European Committee of Standardization (CEN) [117]. Some of the methods, including those authorized in the EU are

- Electron spin resonance spectroscopy (ESR) [118–120],
- Thermoluminescence (TL) [121],
- Gas chromatography mass spectrometry (GC-MS) or flame ionization detection (GC-FID) [122,123],
- DNA comet assay [124],
- Photostimulated luminescence (PSL) [125],
- Direct epifluorescent filter technique/aerobic plate count (DEFT/APC) [126].

13.10 CONCLUSION

The effectiveness in controlling common foodborne pathogens by irradiation and in treating packaged food (minimizing the possibility of cross contamination prior to consumer use) lead this technology to be mentioned as an effective critical control point in a hazard analysis and critical control points (HACCP) system [127]. However, irradiation it is not a stand-alone process that can guarantee safe food. It must be integrated as part of an overall good manufacturing practice program. Radiation treatment is an emerging technology in an increasing number of countries and more clearances for radiation decontaminated foods will be issued in the near future [19].

REFERENCES

1. *High-Dose Irradiation: Wholesomeness of Food Irradiated with Doses Above 10 KGy*, World Health Organization Technical Report Series 890, WHO, Geneva, 1999.
2. Hite, B.H., The effect of pressure in the preservation of milk, *Agric. Exp. Stn. Bull.*, 58, 15, 1899.
3. Schwartz, B., Effect of X-rays on trichinae, *J. Agric. Res.*, 20, 845, 1921.
4. Jacobs, S.E. and Thornley, M.J., The lethal action of ultrasonic waves on bacteria suspended in milk and other liquids, *J. Appl. Bacteriol.*, 17, 38, 1954.
5. Sale, A.J.H. and Hamilton, W.A., Effects of high electric fields on micro-organisms: III. Lysis of erythrocytes and protoplasts, *Biochim. Biophys. Acta*, 163, 37, 1968.
6. Jeyamkondan, S., Jayas, D.S., and Holley, R.A., Pulsed electric field processing of foods: a review, *J. Food Prot.*, 62, 1088, 1999.
7. Estrada-Girón, Y., Swanson, B.J., and Barbosa-Cánovas, G.V., Advances in the use of high hydrostatic pressure for processing cereal grains and legumes, *Trends Food Sci. Technol.*, 16, 194, 2005.
8. Ross, A.I., Griffiths, M.W., Mittal, G.S., and Deeth, H.C., Combining nonthermal technologies to control foodborne microorganisms, *Int. J. Food Microbiol.*, 89, 125, 2003.

9. Marcotte, M., Irradiation as a disinfestation method-update on methyl bromide phase out, regulatory action and emerging opportunities, *Radiat. Phys. Chem.*, 52, 85, 1998.
10. Farkas, J., Chemical methods of decontamination and their limitations, in *Irradiation of Dry Food Ingredients*, Farkas, J., ed., CRC Press, Boca Raton, FL, 1988.
11. McLaughlin, W.L., Boyd, A.W., Chadwick, K.H., McDonald, J.C., Miller, A., Radiation interactions and dose, in *Dosimetry for Radiation Processing*, McLaughlin, W.L., Boyd, A.W., Chadwick, K.H., McDonald, J.C., Miller, A., eds., Taylor & Francis, London, 1989.
12. Directive 99/2/EC, *Approximation of the Laws of the Member States Concerning Foods and Food Ingredients Treated with Ionizing Radiation*, European Parliament and Council, OJ L 66, 13.3.1999, 16.
13. Jones, J.M., *Food Irradiation in Food Safety*, Eagan Press, St. Paul, MN, 1992.
14. Durante, R.W., Food processors requirements met by radiation processing, *Radiat. Phys. Chem.*, 63, 289, 2002.
15. IAEA, *Natural and Induced Radioactivity in Food*, TECDOC-1287, International Atomic Energy Agency, Vienna, 2002.
16. Codex Alimentarius Commission, *Codex General Standard for Irradiated Food and Recommended International Code of Practice for the Operation of Irradiation Facilities Used for the Treatment of Food*, vol. 15, Codex Alimentarius Commission, Rome, 1984.
17. Diehl, J.F., *Safety of Irradiated Foods*, 2nd ed., Marcel Dekker, New York, 1995.
18. IAEA, *Manual of Food Irradiation Dosimetry*, STI/DOC/10/178, International Atomic Energy Agency, Vienna, 1977.
19. Von Sonntag, C., The chemistry of free-radical-mediated DNA damage, *Basic Life Sci.*, 58, 287, 1991.
20. Farkas, J., Irradiation as a method for decontaminating food — a review, *Int. J. Food Microbiol.*, 44, 189, 1998.
21. Nogueira, F., Botelho, M.L., and Tenreiro, R., Radioresistance studies in *Methylobacterium* spp., *Radiat. Phys. Chem.*, 52, 15, 1998.
22. Lea, D.E., *Actions of Radiations on Living Cells*, 2nd ed., Cambridge University Press, New York, 1955.
23. Davies, R., Sinskey, A.J., and Botstein, D., Deoxyribonucleic acid repair in a highly resistant strain of *Salmonella typhimurium*, *J. Bacteriol.*, 114, 357, 1973.
24. Cerf, O., Tailing of survival curves of bacterial spores, *J. Appl. Bacteriol.*, 42, 1, 1977.
25. Licciardello, J.J., Effect of temperature on radiosensitivity of *Salmonella typhimurium*, *J. Food Sci.*, 29, 469, 1964.
26. Matsuyama, A.T., Thornley, M.J, and Ingram, M., The effect of freezing on the radiation sensitivity of vegetative bacteria, *J. Appl. Bacteriol.*, 27, 110, 1964.
27. Ma, K. and Maxcy, R.B., Factors influencing radiation resistance of vegetative bacteria and spores associated with radappertization of meat, *J. Food Sci.*, 46, 612, 1981.
28. Thornley, M.J., Radiation resistance among bacteria, *J. Appl. Bacteriol.*, 26, 334, 1963.
29. Silverman, G.J., Sterilization by ionizing radiation, in *Disinfection, Sterilization and Preservation*, 3rd ed., Block, S.S., ed., Lea & Febiger, Philadelphia, 1963.
30. Dion, P., Charbonneau, R., and Thibault, C., Effect of ionizing dose rate on the radioresistance of some food pathogenic bacteria, *Can. J. Microbiol.*, 40, 369, 1994.

31. Chowdhury, M.S., Rowley, D.B., Anellis, A., and Levinson, H.S., Influence of post-irradiation incubation temperature on recovery of radiation-injured *C. botulinum* 62A spores, *Appl. Environ. Microbiol.* 32, 172, 1976.

32. Tauxe, R.V., Emerging foodborne diseases: an evolving public health challenge, *Emerg. Infect. Dis.*, 3, 425, 1997.

33. Mossel, D.A.A., Irradiation: an effective mode of processing food for safety, in *Food Irradiation Processing*, STIP/PUB/695, International Atomic Energy Agency, Vienna, 1985.

34. Satin, M., Use of irradiation for microbial decontamination of meat: situation and perspectives, *Meat Sci.*, 62, 277, 2002.

35. Cabo Verde, S., Tenreiro, R., and Botelho, M.L., Sanitation of chicken eggs by ionizing radiation: HACCP and inactivation studies, *Radiat. Phys. Chem.*, 71, 27, 2004.

36. EL-Zawahry, Y.A. and Grecz, N., Inactivation and injury of *Yersinia enterocolitica* by radiation and freezing, *Appl. Environ. Microbiol.*, 42, 464, 1981.

37. de Moraes, I.R., Del Mastro, N.L., Jakabi, M., and Gelli, D.S., Radiosensitivity of *Vibrio cholerae* O1 incorporated in oysters, to (60) Co, *Rev. Saude Publica*, 34, 29, 2000.

38. Cui, S., JIang, T., Li, Y., and Lou, X., Effect of irradiation on the shelf-life of aquatic products, *Wei Sheng Yan Jiu.*, 29, 120, 2000.

39. Palumbo, S.A., Jenkins, R.K., Buchanan, R.L., and Thayer, D.W., Determination of irradiation d-values for *Aeromonas hydrophila*, *J. Food Prot.*, 49, 1003, 1986.

40. Kim, J.H., Stegeman, H., and Farkas, J., Preliminary studies on radiation resistance of thermophilic anarobic spores and the effect of gamma radiation on their heat resistance, *Int. J. Food Microbiol.*, 5, 129, 1987.

41. Blank, G. and Corrigan, D., Comparison of resistance of fungal spores to gamma and electron beam radiation, *Int. J. Food Microbiol.*, 26, 269, 1995.

42. Mohyuddin, M. and Skoropad, W.P., Effects of ^{60}Co gamma irradiation on the survival of some fungi in single samples of each of three different grades of wheat, *Can. J. Bot.*, 48, 217, 1970.

43. Saleh, Y.G., Mayo, M.S., and Ahearn, D.C., Resistance of some common fungi to gamma irradiation, *Appl. Environ. Microbiol.*, 54, 2134, 1988.

44. Grecz, N., Rowley, D.B., and Matsuyama, A., The action of radiation on bacteria and viruses, in *Preservation of Food by Ionizing Radiation*, Josephson, E.S. and Peterson M.S., eds., vol. II., CRC Press, Boca Raton, FL, 1983.

45. Rowley, D.B., Sullivan, R., and Josephson, E.S., Indicators of viruses in foods preserved by ionizing radiation, in *Indicators of Viruses in Water and Food*, Berg, G., ed., Ann Arbor Science Publishers, Ann Arbor, MI, 1978.

46. Adams, W.R. and Pollard, E., Combined thermal and primary ionization effects on bacterial virus, *Arch. Biochem. Biophys.*, 36, 311, 1952.

47. Urbain, W.M., Food irradiation, in *Advances in Food Research*, vol. 24, Chichester, C.O., Mrak, E.M., and Stewart, G.F., eds., Academic Press, New York, 1978.

48. Wilkinson, V.M. and Gould, G.W., *Food Irradiation, A Reference Guide*, Butterworth-Heinemann, Oxford, 1996.

49. Dawes, M.A., Saimi, R.S., Mullen, M.A., Brower, J.H., Loretan, P.A., Sensitivity of sweetpotato weevil (Coleoptera:Curculionidae) to gamma irradiation, *J. Econ. Entomol.*, 80, 142, 1987.

50. Casarett, A.P., *Radiation Biology*, Prentice-Hall, Englewood Cliffs, NJ, 1968.

51. Bakri, A., Heather, N., Hendrichs, J., and Ferris, I., Fifty years of radiation biology in entomology: lessons learned from IDIDAS, *Ann. Entomol. Soc. Am.*, 98, 1, 2005.

52. *Irradiation as a Quarantine Treatment*, International Consultative Group on Food Irradiation, Report of the Task Force Meeting, Chiang Mai, Thailand, 1986.

53. Salunkhe, D.K. and Wu, M.T., Development in technology of storage and handling of fresh fruits and vegetables. *Crit. Rev. Food Technol.*, 4, 15, 1974.

54. Beaulieu, M., D'Aprano, M.B., and Lacroix, M.J., Dose rate effect of gamma irradiation on phenolic compounds, polyphenol oxidase, and browning of mushrooms (*Agaricus bisporus*), *Agric. Food Chem.*, 47, 2537, 1999.

55. Zegota, H., Suitability of Dukat strawberries for studying effects on shelf life of irradiation combined with cold storage, *Z Lebensm Unters Forsch.*, 187, 111, 1988.

56. *Several ASTM Standards*, Vol. 12.02, Annual Book of Standards, American Society for Testing and Materials, Philadelphia, 1997.

57. Berdanier, C., *Handbook of Nutrition and Food*, 1st ed., CRC Press, Boca Raton, FL, 2002.

58. Siddhuraju, P., Makkar, H.P.S., and Becker, K., The effect of ionising radiation on antinutritional factors and nutritional value of plant materials with reference to human and animal food, *Food Chem.*, 78, 187, 2002.

59. *Revision of the Opinion of the Scientific Committee on Food on the Irradiation of Food*, European Commission — Scientific Committee on Food Document SCF/CS/NF/IRR/24 Final, 2003.

60. Wu, D., Ye, Q., Wang, Z., Xia, Y., Effect of gamma irradiation on nutritional components and *Cry1Ab* protein in the transgenic rice with a synthetic *cry1 Ab* gene from *Bacillus thuringiensis, Radiat. Phys. Chem.*, 69, 79, 2004.

61. Matloubi, H., Aflaki, F., and Hadjiezadegan, M., Effect of γ-irradiation on amino acids content of baby foods proteins, *J Food Compost. Anal.*, 17, 133, 2004.

62. World Health Organization, *Safety and Nutritional Adequacy of Irradiated Food*, WHO, Geneva, 1994.

63. Farag, M.D.E.H., The nutritive value for chicks of full-fat soybeans irradiated up to 60 kGy, *Anim. Feed Sci. Technol.*, 73, 319, 1998.

64. Rombo, G., Taylor, J., and Minnaar, A., Irradiation of maize and bean flours: effects on starch physicochemical properties, *J. Sci. Food Agric.*, 84, 350, 2004.

65. Oh, S.H., Effect of pH on non-enzymatic browning reaction during γ-irradiation processing of sugar-glycine solutions., *Food Chem.*, in press.

66. Baraldi, D., Effect of gamma radiation on D-glucose present in apple juice, *J. Food Sci.*, 38, 108, 1973.

67. Lee, Y.S., Oh, S.H., Lee, J.W., Kim, J.H., Rhee, C.O., Lee, H.K., Byun, M.W., Effects of gamma irradiation on quality of cooked rice, *J. Korean Soc. Food Sci. Nutr.*, 33, 582, 2004.

68. Chemical changes in food components caused by irradiation, in *Training Manual on Operation of Food Irradiation Facilities*, International Consultative Group on Food Irradiation, 1st ed., 1992.

69. Ajuyah, A.O., Fenton, T.W., Hardin, R.T., Sim, J.S., Measuring lipid oxidation volatiles in meats, *J. Food Sci.*, 58, 270, 1993.

70. Chouliara, I., Sawaidis, I.N. Panagiotakis, N., and Kontominas, M.G., Preservation of salted, vacuum-packaged, refrigerated sea bream (*Sparus aurata*) fillets by irradiation: microbiological, chemical and sensory attributes, *Food Microbiol.*, 21, 351, 2004.

71. Gomes, H., Silva, E.N., Bolini Cardello, H., and Cippoli, K., Effect of gamma radiation on refrigerated mechanically deboned chicken meat quality, *Meat Sci.*, 65, 919, 2003.

72. Carrasco, A., Tarrega, R., Ramirez, R., Mingoarranz, M.R., and Cara, R., Colour and lipid oxidation changes in dry-cured loins from free-range and intensively reared pigs as affected by ionizing radiation dose level, *Meat Sci.*, 69, 609, 2005.

73. Position of the American Dietetic Association: functional foods, *J. Am. Diet Assoc.*, 104, 814, 2004.

74. Geibler, C., Brede, O., and Reinhardt, J., *cis-trans*-Isomerization of unsaturated fatty acids during γ-irradiation of barley grains, *Radiat. Phys. Chem.*, 67, 105, 2003.

75. Graham, W., Stevenson, M.H., and Stewart, E., Effect of irradiation dose and irradiation temperature on the thiamin content of raw and cooked chicken breast meat, *J. Sci. Food Agric.*, 78, 559, 1998.

76. Graham, W. and Stevenson, M.H., Effect of irradiation on vitamin C content of strawberries and potatoes in combination with storage and with further cooking in potatoes, *J. Sci. Food Agric.*, 75, 371, 1997.

77. Mahrouz, M., Lacroix M., D'Aprano, G., Oufedjikh, H., Boubekri, C., and Gagnon, M., Effect of γ-irradiation combined with washing and waxing treatment on physicochemical properties, vitamin C and organoleptic quality of *Citrus clementina* Hort. Ex. Tanaka, *J. Agric. Food Chem.*, 50, 7271, 2002.

78. Fan, X., Toivonen, P.M., Rajkowski, K.T., and Sokorai, K.J., Warm water treatment in combination with modified atmosphere packing reduces undesirable effects of irradiation on the quality of fresh-cut iceberg lettuce, *J. Sci. Food Chem.*, 51, 1231, 2003.

79. Patil, B.S. and Vanamala, J., Irradiation and storage influence on bioactive components and quality of early and late season 'Rio Red' grapefruit (*Citrus paradisi* Macf), *Postharvest Biol. Technol.*, 34, 53, 2004.

80. Fan, X., Antioxidant capacity of fresh-cut vegetables exposed to ionizing radiation, *J. Sci. Food Agric.*, 85, 995, 2005.

81. Trigo, M.J., et al., Effect of γ radiation on minimally processed lettuce, in *Proc. of Qualidade e Segurança Alimentar*, Instituto Superior de Agronomia, Lisbon, Portugal, 2002, 143.

82. Jaczynski, J. and Park, J.W., Physicochemical properties of surimi seafood as affected by electron beam and heat, *J. Food Sci.*, 68, 626, 2003.

83. Pinto, P., Ribeiro, R., Sousa, L., Verde, S.C., Lima, M.G., Dinis, M., Santana, A., and Botelho, M.L., Sanitation of chicken eggs by ionizing radiation: functional and nutritional assessment, *Radiat. Phys. Chem.*, 71, 35, 2004.

84. Wong, P. and Kitts, D., Physicochemical and functional properties of shell eggs following electron beam irradiation, *J. Sci. Food Agric.*, 83, 44, 2003.

85. Köksel, H., Celik, S., and Tuncer, T., Effects of gamma irradiation on durum wheats and spaghetti quality, *Cereal Chem.*, 73, 507, 1996.

86. Zaied, S.E., Abdel-Hamid, A.A., and Attia, E.A., Technological and chemical characters of bread prepared from irradiated wheat flour, *Nahrung.*, 40, 28, 1996.

87. Del Mastro, N.L., Development of food irradiated in Brazil, *Prog. Nucl. Energy*, 35, 229, 1999.

88. Oliveira, L.C., Present situation of food irradiation in South America and the regulatory perspective for Brasil, *Radiat. Phys. Chem.*, 57, 249, 2000.

89. *ICGFI Database*, International Consultative Group on Food Irradiation (ICGFI), available at http://www.iaea.org/icgfi/introduc.htm.

90. Roberts, P.B., Regulatory aspects of irradiation in the Asia-Pacific region, *Radiat. Phys. Chem.*, 57, 219, 2000.

91. Directive 99/2/EC of the European Parliament and of the Council on the approximation of the laws of the member states concerning foods and food ingredients treated with ionising radiation. OJ L 66, 13.3.1999, 16.

92. Directive 99/3/EC of the European Parliament and of the Council on the establishment of a community list of foods and ingredients treated with ionizing radiation, OJ L 66, 13.3.1999, 24.

93. List of Member States' authorisation of food and food ingredients which may be treated with ionising radiation, OJ C 174, 20.7.2002, 3.

94. List of Member States' authorisation of food and food ingredients which may be treated with ionising radiation, OJ C 56, 11.3.2003, 5.

95. List of approved facilities for the treatment of foods and food ingredients with ionising radiation in the Member States. OJ C 166, 17.7.2003, 2.

96. Commission Decision of 7 October 2004 amending Decision 2002/840/EC adopting the list of approved facilities in third countries for the irradiation of food. OJ L 314, 13.10.2004, 14.

97. Report from the Commission on Food Irradiation for the year 2002, COM (2004) 69 final, Brussels, 25.2.2004.

98. Bruhn, C.M., Sommer, R., and Schutz, H.G., Effect of an educational pamphlet and posters on attitude towards food irradiation, *J. Indust. Irradiat. Technol.*, 4, 1, 1986.

99. The Packer, Fresh Trends, in *A Profile of Fresh Produce Consumer*, Lincolnshire, IL. 1993.

100. Pohlman, A.J., Wood, O.B., and Mason, A.C., Influence of audiovisuals and food samples on consumer acceptance of food irradiation, *Food Technol.*, 48,12, 46, 1994.

101. Resurreccion, A.V.A., Galvez, F.C.F., Fletcher, S.M., and Misra, S.K., Consumer attitudes towards irradiated food: results of a new study, *J. Food Prot.*, 58, 193, 1995.

102. Frenzen, P.D., DeBess, E.E., Hechemy, K.E., Kassenborg, H., Kennedy, M., McCombs, K., and McNees, A., Foodnet Working Group, Consumer acceptance of irradiated meat and poultry meat in the United States, *J. Food Prot.*, 64, 2020, 2001.

103. Uriost, A.M., Croci, C.A., and Curzio, O.A., Consumer acceptance of irradiated onions in Argentina, *Food Technol.*, 44, 137, 1990.

104. *Consumer Attitudes and Market Response to Irradiated Food*, International Consultative Group on Food Irradiation (ICGFI), IAEA, Vienna, Austria, 1999.

105. Laizier, J., Test market of irradiated strawberries in France, *Food Irradiat. Newslett.*, IAEA, Vienna, 11, 45, 1987.

106. Baraldi, D., Technological test at the pre-industrial level on irradiated potatoes: food preservation by irradiation, in *Consumer Acceptance of Irradiated Foods*, Marcotte, M., ed., Nordion International, Kanata, Ontario, Canada, 1977.

107. Bruhn, C.M. and Mason, A., *Science and Society: A Public Information Program on Food Innovations*, Final Report, USDA FY 1994 Special Projects, Project no. 94-EFSQ-1-4141, U.S. Department of Agriculture, Washington, DC, 1996.

108. Fox, J.A. and Olson, D.G., Market trials of irradiated chicken, *Radiat. Phys. Chem.*, 52, 63, 1998.

109. Scientific Committee on Food-SCF, Revision of the opinion of the Scientific Committee on Food on the irradiation of food, Brussels, 2003.

110. Marchioni, E., Raul, F., Burnouf, D., Miesch, M., Delincee, H., Hartwig, A., and Werner, D., Toxicological study of 2-alkylcyclobutanones — results of a collaborative study, *Radiat. Phys. Chem.*, 71, 145, 2004.

111. Sommers, C.H., 2-dodecylcyclobutanone does not induce mutations in the *Salmonella* mutagenecity test or intrachromosomal recombination in *Saccharomyces cerevisae, J. Food Prot.*, 67, 1293, 2004.

112. Jo, C., Ahn, H.J., Son, J.H., Lee, J.W., and Byun, M.W., Packaging and irradiation effect on lipid oxidation, color, residual nitrite content, and nitrosamine formation in cooked pork sausage, *Food Control*, 14,7, 2003.

113. Ahn, H.J., Kim, J.H., Jo, C., Yook, H., and Byun, M.W., Radiolytic characteristics of nitrite by gamma irradiation, *Food Chem.*, 82, 465, 2003.

114. Ahn, H.J., Kim, J.H., Hong-Sun, C.J., Lee, Y.H., and Byun, M.W., N-nitrosamine reduction in salted and fermented anchovy sauce by ionizing irradiation, *Food Control*, 14, 553, 2003.

115. Byun, M.-W., Ahn, H.-J., Kim, J.-H., Lee, J.-W., Yook, H.-S., and Han, S.-B, Determination of volatile N-nitrosamines in irradiated fermented sausage by gas chromatography coupled to a thermal energy analyser, *J Chromatogr. A*, 1054, 403, 2004.

116. Kim, J.H., Ahn, H., Lee, J.W., Park, H., Ryu, G., Kang, I., and Byun, M.W., Effects of gamma irradiation on the biogenic amines in pepperoni with different packaging conditions, *Food Chem.*, 89, 199, 2005.

117. Communication from the commission on food and food ingredients authorised for treatment with ionising radiation in the community, OJ C 241, 29.8.2001, 6.

118. EN 1786, *Foodstuffs — Detection of Irradiated Food Containing Bone — Method by ESR Spectroscopy*, European Committee for Standardization, Brussels, 1996.

119. EN 1787, *Foodstuffs — Detection of Irradiated Food Containing Cellulose — Method by ESR Spectroscopy*, European Committee for Standardization, Brussels, 2000.

120. EN 13708, *Foodstuffs — Detection of Irradiated Food Containing Crystalline Sugar by ESR Spectroscopy*, European Committee for Standardization, Brussels, 2001.

121. EN 1788, *Foodstuffs — Thermoluminescence Detection of Irradiated Food from Which Silicate Minerals can be Isolated*, European Committee for Standardization, Brussels, 2001.

122. EN 1785, *Foodstuffs — Detection of Irradiated Food Containing Fat — GC Analysis of 2-acylcyclobutanones*, European Committee for Standardization, Brussels, 2003.

123. EN 1784, *Foodstuffs — Detection of Irradiated Food Containing Fat — Gas Chromatographic Analysis of Hydrocarbons*, European Committee for Standardization, Brussels, 2003.

124. EN 13784, *Foodstuffs — DNA Comet Assay for the Detection of Irradiated Foodstuffs — Screening Method*, European Committee for Standardization, Brussels, 2001.

125. EN 13751, *Foodstuffs — Detection of Irradiated Food Using Photostimulated Luminescence*, European Committee for Standardization, Brussels, 2002.

126. EN 13783, *Foodstuffs — Detection of Irradiated Food Using Direct Epifluorescent Filter Technique/Aerobic Plate Count (DEFT/APC) — Screening Method*, European Committee for Standardization, Brussels, 2001.

127. U.S. Department of Agriculture, Comments of the American Dietetic Association, Irradiation of meat and meat products: proposed rule, *Federal Register*, 64, 1999, 9089.

Index

A

439

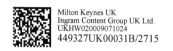

9 780367 453497